Family Medicine: Principles and Practice

Family Medicine:
Principles and Practice

Editor: Clara Wallace

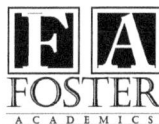

FOSTER
ACADEMICS

www.fosteracademics.com

www.fosteracademics.com

FA
FOSTER
ACADEMICS

Cataloging-in-Publication Data

Family medicine : principles and practice / edited by Clara Wallace.
      p. cm.
Includes bibliographical references and index.
ISBN 978-1-63242-844-8
   1. Family medicine. 2. Families--Health and hygiene. 3. Medicine 4. Medical care. I. Wallace, Clara.
RA418.5.F3 F36 2019
613--dc23

© Foster Academics, 2019

Foster Academics,
118-35 Queens Blvd., Suite 400,
Forest Hills, NY 11375, USA

ISBN 978-1-63242-844-8 (Hardback)

Contents

Preface

This book was inspired by the evolution of our times; to answer the curiosity of inquisitive minds. Many developments have occurred across the globe in the recent past which has transformed the progress in the field.

Family medicine is a branch of primary care concerned with the comprehensive health care of individuals and their families. It focuses on providing continuing care to patients of all genders and ages irrespective of the disease. The primary goals of this field are disease prevention and the promotion of health. A diverse range of acute, chronic and preventive medical care services are delivered by family physicians. This may include routine checkups, counseling for maintaining a healthy lifestyle, health-risk assessments, etc. This book strives to provide a fair idea about this discipline and to help develop a better understanding of the latest advances within this field. It includes some of the vital pieces of work being conducted across the world, on various topics related to family medicine. For all readers who are interested in this medical specialty, the case studies included in this book will serve as an excellent guide to develop a comprehensive understanding.

This book was developed from a mere concept to drafts to chapters and finally compiled together as a complete text to benefit the readers across all nations. To ensure the quality of the content we instilled two significant steps in our procedure. The first was to appoint an editorial team that would verify the data and statistics provided in the book and also select the most appropriate and valuable contributions from the plentiful contributions we received from authors worldwide. The next step was to appoint an expert of the topic as the Editor-in-Chief, who would head the project and finally make the necessary amendments and modifications to make the text reader-friendly. I was then commissioned to examine all the material to present the topics in the most comprehensible and productive format.

I would like to take this opportunity to thank all the contributing authors who were supportive enough to contribute their time and knowledge to this project. I also wish to convey my regards to my family who have been extremely supportive during the entire project.

Editor

Prevalence of pain and its associated factors among the oldest-olds in different care settings

Tina Mallon[1]* , Annette Ernst[1], Christian Brettschneider[2], Hans-Helmut König[2], Tobias Luck[3], Susanne Röhr[3], Siegfried Weyerer[4], Jochen Werle[4], Edelgard Mösch[5], Dagmar Weeg[5], Angela Fuchs[6], Michael Pentzek[6], Luca Kleineidam[7], Kathrin Heser[7], Steffi Riedel-Heller[3], Wolfgang Maier[7,9], Birgitt Wiese[8†], Martin Scherer[1†] for the AgeCoDe & AgeQualiDe study group

Abstract

Background: The prevalence of pain is very common in the oldest age group. Managing pain successfully is a key topic in primary care, especially within the ageing population. Different care settings might have an impact on the prevalence of pain and everyday life.

Methods: Participants from the German longitudinal cohort study on Needs, Health Service Use, Costs and Health-related Quality of Life in a large Sample of Oldest-old Primary Care Patients (85+) (AgeQualiDe) were asked to rate their severity of pain as well as the impairment with daily activities. Besides gender, age, education, BMI and use of analgesics we focused on the current housing situation and on cognitive state. Associations of the dependent measures were tested using four ordinal logistic regression models. Model 1 and 4 consisted of the overall sample, model 2 and 3 were divided according to no cognitive impairment (NCI) and mild cognitive impairment (MCI).

Results: Results show a decline in pain at very old age but nonetheless a high prevalence among the 85+ year olds. Sixty-three per cent of the participants report mild to severe pain and 69% of the participants mild to extreme impairment due to pain with daily activities. Use of analgesics, depression and living at home with care support are significantly associated with higher and male gender with lower pain ratings.

Conclusions: Sufficient pain management among the oldest age group is inevitable. Outpatient care settings are at risk of overlooking pain. Therefore focus should be set on pain management in these settings.

Keywords: Prevalence of pain, Impairment in daily activities, Care setting, Primary care

Background

Due to physical or mental illness or disability 42% of women and 29.6% of men aged 85–89 years receive care in Germany (care is termed according to the German law SGB XI). This number increases again for the 90+ year-olds (67.9% women, 51.8% men) [1]. These numbers show that with the aging population more attention has to

be paid to prevalence and management of pain which goes beyond the treatment with analgesics only and includes alternative options such a relaxation techniques or biofeedback in the oldest age group (85+ years). The presence of daily pain leads to a decline on activities of daily living, especially for cognitive impaired individuals [2–5]. Lower levels of education, female gender and a high Body Mass Index (BMI) seem to entail acute and/or chronic pain [2, 6–8]. Individuals reporting more severe pain were found to score significantly lower in memory tests, for executive function and showed an impaired attentional capacity [2] which has an impact on quality of life and

* Correspondence: t.mallon@uke.de

†Birgitt Wiese and Martin Scherer contributed equally to this work.
[1]Department of Primary Medical Care, Center for Psychosocial Medicine, University Medical Center Hamburg-Eppendorf, Hamburg, Germany
Full list of author information is available at the end of the article

one's independence. Along with other special needs developed with growing age such as geriatric syndromes, frailty, comorbidities, falls and functional decline [9–12] the use of a care service or moving to a care facility is an inevitable consequence in many cases.

The German health care system supplies care at home either with the help of a relative or through a mobile care service. Otherwise moving to a care home or to a facility with "assisted living" (Betreutes Wohnen) which aims at maintaining one's independence by providing helpful services e.g. barrier-free apartment, emergency call, meals and a quick access to care support are other options if care is needed [1].

Acute pain is experienced regularly by up to 49–83% of elderly individuals above the age of 60 living in care homes and 40% of elderly individuals living in the community [13, 14]. Each care setting has its own challenges in dealing with pain and pain management such as shortness of time, lack of staff or lack of knowledge [15] but the effects on pain and the apparent housing situation have not been studied in depth yet. However, studies revealed that patients above the age of 85 were found to be less likely to receive adequate analgesic treatment or even none at all [16] and inadequate pain assessment [6, 17, 18]. Very few studies include the group of over 85 year-olds in their research. Therefore we aimed at uncovering underlying differences in pain prevalence and management and hence our research questions focused on the prevalence of pain in the oldest age group with emphasis on the housing situation, on associated factors with pain and the impact of pain on activities of daily living.

Methods
Study design and sampling
The data were derived from the German longitudinal cohort study on Needs, Health Service Use, Costs and Health-related Quality of Life in a large Sample of Oldest-old Primary Care Patients (85+) (AgeQualiDe) which is considered a follow-on study (follow-up 7 to 9) on Ageing, Cognition and Dementia in Primary Care Patients (AgeCoDe) (75+). In our analysis, we provide cross-sectional results from the baseline of AgeQualiDe that is the 7th follow-up of AgeCoDe. For the initial study 3327 patients had been recruited from over 138 general practitioners (GP) in six German cities (Bonn, Düsseldorf, Hamburg, Leipzig, Mannheim, Munich) in 2003. All GP patients who participated in the study provided written informed consent prior to their participation. Both studies – AgeCoDe and AgeQualiDe – have been approved by the ethics committees of all participating study centres and comply with the ethical standards of the Declaration of Helsinki. Criteria for inclusion in the original study in 2003 were aged 75 and over, the absence

of dementia and a minimum of one contact with the GP per year. Patients had been excluded if one of the following aspects applied: GP consultations only by home visits, lack of the German language, a severe illness with an anticipated fatal outcome within three months, blindness, deafness, inability of consent, residence in a nursing home and not being a patient of the participating GP. The study design of AgeCoDe has been described in detail elsewhere [19]. Within the AgeCoDe study six follow-up waves have been carried out in 1.5 year intervals. With the beginning of follow-up wave 7/ AgeQualiDe baseline 868 individuals are still remaining in the sample. The missing individuals had died before this study wave, refused participation, dropped-out or were otherwise unable to participate. From the baseline sample 757 individuals scored 19 or above in the Mini-Mental-Examination and from them 738 completed the PRS. Mean age of the participants was 88.8 years (SD 2995).

Measures
Pain
The pain assessments were part of a structured clinical interview by trained physicians and psychologists during visits to the participants' homes. Participants were presented with two questions based on the validated version of the German Brief Pain Inventory [20]. First participants had to rate today's severity of pain on a one-dimensional numeric pain rating scale (PRS) ranging from 0 to 100 (no pain to worst pain imaginable). Participants were then grouped and assigned to four categories: "no pain" for participants scoring 0 in the PRS, "mild pain" when scoring between 1 and 30, "moderate pain" when scoring 31–60 and "severe pain" when scoring 61 and above in the PRS. Secondly, participants were asked to rate the impairment with daily activities caused by pain in the last 24 h on a five point Likert-scale, ranging from 1 (no impairment) to 5 (extreme impairment). Furthermore, the use of analgesics was assessed by recording the name and number of all prescribed and over-the-counter drugs the participant used in the last 3 months. All drugs belonging to the Anatomical Therapeutic Chemical–Code subgroup N02 were included in the analgesic use evaluation in our analysis.

Demography and housing
Items on sex, age, Body Mass Index (BMI), level of education and the current housing situation were assessed. Participants were grouped into two age brackets: up until 89 years old and 90+ years old. For BMI participants were grouped into underweight = < 18.5, normal weight = 18.5–24.9, overweight = 25–29.9 and obesity = BMI of 30 or higher. The level of participant's education has been categorized into primary, secondary and tertiary according to the CASMIN criteria [21]. The

housing situation was assessed during the interview by the question "Do you live alone or together with another person in a common-household?" Participants were grouped into "living at home without care support", "living at home with care support", "living in a care-home" and "assisted living".

Cognitive function and clinical variables

Cognitive function was assessed using the Mini-Mental State Examination (MMSE) [22] to detect cognitive impairment. MMSE score below 25 was used as cut-off point for mild cognitive impairment (MCI). Depressive symptoms were measured using the Geriatric Depression Scale [23] consisting of 15 items. A score ranging from 0 to 15 was calculated for each individual (for more details, Weyerer et al. 2008 [19]). Furthermore, the impairments of activities of daily living (IADL) e.g. eating, walking stairs, wash/shower were assessed using the Barthel-Index [24]. A score ranging from 100 (independent from care support) to 0 (dependent on care support) was calculated for each participant.

Statistical analysis

Analyses were carried out for participants who scored 19 and above in the Mini-Mental State Examination (MMSE) ($n = 757$) and from whom we assessed the PRS ($n = 738$).

Demographic and clinical characteristics were assessed. Our dependent variables prevalence of pain and impairment with daily living were divided into the groups mentioned above. Associations were tested using Pearson's $\square^2$ test for categorical variables, one-way ANOVA for continuous variables and Kruskal-Wallis-test for variables that violated assumptions of normality.

Associations of the dependent measures "prevalence of pain" and "impairment with activities of daily living" were then tested with ordinal logistic regression models adjusting for sex, age, education, housing situation, analgesics, BMI, IADL and Depression. Three models were created for prevalence of pain (1–3) and one model for impairment in daily living (4). All models include all factors and categories apart from MMSE. In model 1 MMSE is included for the overall sample. In model 2 we included participants with MMSE above 25 (non-cognitively impaired group – NCI) and in model 3 for participants with MMSE up to 25 (mild cognitively impaired group – MCI). Model 4 has been calculated for the overall sample for impairment in daily living. It was also repeated for the two MMSE groups but no significant differences appeared. Additionally, interaction effects have been calculated for age and living in a care home but showed no statistical significance. Data for MMSE and interaction effects is given upon request.

SAS 9.3 software was used for logistic regression analysis and SPSS Statistics 23 for the remaining statistical analysis. Statistical significance level was set to alpha 0.05.

Results

Demography and prevalence of pain

General and demographic characteristics of our sample are displayed in Table 1. Results are shown for the total sample and stratified by the four categories of pain. Female gender was predominant in the sample (67.5%). Sixty-three per cent of the participants reported mild to severe pain of which 57.5% are male and 65.7% female. Thirty-seven per cent of the participants reported no pain (M: 26.15, SD: 26.68). Assessing the housing situation participants using assisted living show the lowest prevalence of pain (54.2%) followed by care home residents (60%) and participants living at home without care support (61.7%). The highest prevalence of pain was reported by participants living at home with care support (75.2%). Furthermore the latter group reported the highest average pain scores. In this group 39% of the sample reported moderate and 19% severe pain. In contrast, participants living at home without care support and afflicted with pain scored highest in the mild pain category (29.4%).

Of those participants experiencing pain 67.8% did not take any analgesics at the time. Focusing on the cognitive status 51.9% of participants with MCI and 64.3% of participants with NCI reported pain. This difference reached statistical significance ($\square^2$ [3] = 4.45, $p = .035$). In total 229 (31%) participants reported no impairment and 509 (69%) participants mild to extreme impairment due to pain with daily activities.

The bivariate analysis were carried out for the measures age, sex, cognitive impairment (MMSE), analgesics, housing situation, Barthel-Index, BMI and education (see Table 1). Significant differences were appeared between the two age groups ($\square^2$ [3] = 9.18, $p = .027$), for men and women ($\square^2$ [3] = 19.47, $p = <.001$), for the education groups ($\square^2$ [6] = 27.17, $p = <.001$), between use and no use of analgesics ($\square^2$ [3] = 55.01, $p = <.001$) and for the four different housing situations ($\square^2$ [9] = 31.89, $p = <.001$). No significant result was found for the BMI groups nor for Barthel-Index scores. These variables were then put into the multivariate analysis (model 1 – model 4). Results are presented in Table 2.

Model 1 – Overall pain ratings

In model 1 we tested the association of demographic and clinical characteristics on the overall sample. Male sex was statistically significantly associated with lower PRS (OR 0.61, 95% CI 0.45–0.84) while contrary associations were found for age. Individuals between 90 to 94 years of age scored significantly lower in the PRS (OR 0.65, 95% CI 0.48–0.88) than the younger age

Table 1 Sample of Descriptives and Demography

	All N (%)	No Pain N (%)	Mild Pain N (%)	Moderate Pain N(%)	Severe Pain N(%)	Pearson χ^2
Participants (N)	738	273 (37.0)	195 (26.4)	191 (25.9)	79 (10.7)	
Gender						χ^2 [3]= 19.47 p = <.001
Male	240 (32.5)	102 (37.4)	77 (39.5)	42 (22.0)	19 (24.1)	
Female	498 (67.5)	171 (62.6)	118 (60.5)	149 (78.0)	60 (75.9)	
Age (y), M (SD)	88.8 (3.0)					χ^2 [3] = 9.18 p = .027
≤ 89	476 (64.5)	163 (59.7)	134 (68.7)	119 (62.3)	60 (75.9)	
≥ 90	262 (35.5)	110 (40.3)	61 (31.3)	72 (37.7)	19 (24.1)	
Education						χ^2 [6] =27.17 p = <.001
Primary	408 (55.3)	151 (55.3)	90 (46.2)	117 (61.3)	50 (63.3)	
Secondary	226 (30.6)	91 (3.3)	59 (30.2)	59 (30.9)	17 (21.5)	
Tertiary	104 (14.1)	31 (11.4)	46 (23.6)	15 (7.8)	12 (15.2)	
Housing						χ^2 [9] = 1.89 p = <.001
At home[a]	520 (70.5)	199 (72.9)	153 (78.5)	118 (61.8)	50 (63.3)	
At home[b]	105 (14.2)	26 (9.5)	18 (9.2)	41 (21.5)	20 (25.3)	
Assisted living	65 (8.8)	22 (8.1)	11 (5.6)	10 (5.2)	5 (6.3)	
Care home	48 (6.5)	26 (9.5)	13 (6.7)	22 (11.5)	4 (5.1)	
Analgesics*						χ^2 [3] = 5.01 p = <.001
Yes	181 (24.5)	33 (12.1)	42 (21.5)	73 (38.2)	33 (41.8)	
No	546 (74.0)	234 (89.0)	151 (77.4)	115 (60.2)	46 (58.2)	
BMI, M (SD)*	25.2 (3.8)					χ^2 [9] = 8.96 p = .441
Normal weight	340 (49.1)	129 (47.3)	95 (48.7)	83 (43.5)	33 (41.7)	
Underweight	17 (2.5)	9 (3.3)	3 (1.5)	2 (1.0)	3 (3.8)	
Overweight	265 (38.3)	88 (32.2)	69 (35.4)	79 (41.4)	29 (36.7)	
Obese	70 (10.1)	23 (8.4)	18 (9.2)	18 (9.4)	11 (13.9)	
MMSE						χ^2 [3] = 8.30 p = .040
< 25	79 (10.7)	38 (13.9)	16 (8.2)	22 (11.5)	3 (3.8)	
≥ 25	659 (89.3)	235 (86.1)	179 (91.8)	169 (88.5)	76 (96.2)	
Impairment in daily activities*						χ^2 [15] = 521.90 p = <.001
None	229 (31.0)	181 (66.3)	42 (21.5)	6 (3.1)	0 (0.0)	
Mild	215 (29.1)	65 (23.8)	91 (46.6)	47 (24.6)	12 (15.2)	
Medium	158 (21.4)	24 (8.8)	50 (25.6)	73 (38.2)	11 (13.9)	
Moderate	113 (15.3)	3 (1.1)	10 (5.1)	62 (32.5)	38 (48.1)	
Extreme	21 (2.8)	0 (0.0)	1 (0.5)	3 (1.6)	17 (21.5)	

Notes:
M mean
SD standard deviation
Data are presented as number (%)
Alpha was set to 0.05
*Due to missing values not all sums add up to 100%.
[a]Participants without care support.
[b]Participants with care support

bracket. Considering the housing situation higher PRS was significantly associated with participants living at home with care support. There is a 1.6 higher possibility of experiencing pain for this group than living at home without care support (OR 1.60, 95% CI 1.01–2.53). There was also a significant association for analgesics. Participants receiving analgesics experience twice as much pain (OR 2.17, 95% CI 1.48–3.16). Furthermore higher PRS was significantly associated with depression (OR 1.15, 95% CI 1.08–1.22). No significant evidence showed for differences in education, BMI or Barthel-Index.

Table 2 Associations of prevalence of pain for all participants, for participants with MMSE > 25, for participants ≤25 and impairment in daily living for all participants

Variable	Model 1			Model 2			Model 3			Model 4		
	OR	95% CI	p	OR	95% CI	p	OR	95% CI	p	OR	95% CI	p
Gender												
Female	-	-	-	-	-	-	-	-	-	-	-	-
Male	0.61	0.45–0.84	<.01	0.61	0.44–0.84	<.01	0.21	0.05–0.93	0.04	0.59	0.43–0.81	<.01
Age												
<=89	-	-	-	-	-	-	-	-	-	-	-	-
>=90	0.65	0.48–0.88	<.01	0.61	0.44–0.84	<.01	2.17	0.50–9.36	0.30	0.88	0.65–1.19	0.41
Education												
Primary	-	-	-	-	-	-	-	-	-	-	-	-
Secondary	0.75	0.54–1.02	0.07	0.73	0.52–1.01	0.06	4.83	0.71–32.94	0.11	0.76	0.56–1.05	0.09
Tertiary	1.12	0.73–1.71	0.60	1.18	0.76–1.83	0.47	1.31	0.17–10.40	0.79	0.97	0.63–1.48	0.88
Housing												
Living at home[a]	-	-	-	-	-	-	-	-	-	-	-	-
Living at home[b]	1.60	1.01–2.53	0.04	1.70	1.04–2.78	0.04	1.44	0.30–6.90	0.65	1.72	1.08–2.74	0.02
Assisted living	0.71	0.38–1.31	0.27	0.90	0.47–1.71	0.75	<.01	<.001	0.96	0.61	0.33–1.13	0.12
Care home	0.68	0.37–1.24	0.21	0.78	0.39–1.57	0.48	0.08	0.01–0.48	<.01	0.51	0.28–0.93	0.03
Use of Analgesics[c]	2.17	1.48–3.16	<.01	2.13	1.42–3.18	<.01	2.62	0.49–13.98	2.62	2.75	1.88–4.03	<.01
BMI												
Adiposity	1.14	0.71–1.84	0.60	1.17	0.71–1.92	0.53	0.24	0.02–2.81	0.25	1.48	0.92–2.39	0.11
Overweight	1.21	0.89–1.65	0.22	1.19	0.86–1.63	0.30	3.14	0.71–13.99	0.13	1.37	1.01–1.86	0.05
Normal weight	-	-	-	-	-	-	-	-	-	-	-	-
Underweight	0.74	0.29–1.91	0.53	0.55	0.20–1.53	0.25	2.88	0.07–114.06	0.57	1.36	0.05–3.48	0.52
Barthel Index[d]	0.99	0.98–1.01	0.19	0.99	0.98–1.01	0.30	1.01	0.96–1.07	0.64	0.99	0.98–1.01	0.27
Depressive symptoms[e]	1.15	1.08–1.22	<.01	1.14	1.07–1.22	<.01	1.42	1.01–1.99	0.04	1.14	1.07–1.21	<.01
MMSE[f]	0.60	0.35–1.03	0.06	-	-	-	-	-	-	0.69	0.41–1.17	0.17

Notes: *OR* Odds Ratio, Alpha was set to 0.05
[a]Participants without care support
[b]Participants with care support
[c]use of analgesics: dichotomized
[d]Barthel Index: score 0–100
[e]GDS score 0–15
[f]MMSE: score 0–30, cut-off ≤25 for mild cognitive impairment, > 25 no cognitive impairment

Model 2 and 3 - MMSE status

In model two and three we divided the sample in NCI and MCI participants and found significant associations for both groups: Again male sex was significantly associated with lower pain ratings for both groups (NCI: OR 0.61, 95% CI 0.44–0.85 and MCI: OR 0.21, 95% CI 0.05–0.93). Significant associations for age appeared according to model 1 for NCI aged 90 to 94 years old. The older age group scored significantly lower in the PRS (OR 0.61, 95% CI 0.44–0.84). No association with age was found for the group the MCI-participants. Concerning the housing situation living at home with care support was significantly associated with higher ratings on the PRS for NCI (OR 1.70, 95% CI 1.04–2.78) and significantly associated with lower ratings on the PRS for MCI-participants living in a care-home (OR 0.08, 95% CI 0.01–0.48). Also

for both groups higher PRS was significantly associated with depression (NCI: OR 1.14, 95% CI 1.07–1.22 and MCI: OR 1.42, 95% CI 1.01–1.99). Significant associations for analgesics were found for NCI. Those taking analgesics reported twice as much pain (OR 2.12, 95% CI 1.42–3.18). No significant figures appeared for education, BMI or Barthel-Index.

Model 4 - impairment in daily activities

In model 4 we analyzed the impairment in daily activities for the overall sample. Again we found a significant association for lower impairment in daily activities with male sex (OR 0.59, 95% CI 0.43–0.80), analgesics (OR 2.75, 95% CI 1.88–4.03) and depression (OR 1.14, 95% CI 1.07–1.21). The housing situation showed significant less impairment in daily activities for participants living in a care home (OR

0.51, 95% CI 0.28–0.93) and more impairment for participants living at home with care support (OR 1.72, 95% CI 1.08–2.74). For BMI stronger impairment in daily activities was significantly associated with overweight participants (OR 1.37, 95% CI 1.01–1.86). Education and Barthel-Index did not reach statistical significance.

Discussion

This was one of a few existing studies focusing on the prevalence of pain and associated factors such as age, gender, use of analgesics, cognitive state, medication and depression among the population of 85+ year olds.

Age

The study demonstrated a high prevalence of pain (63%) among the age group of 85+ and strong experience impairments with everyday life due to pain (69%). Additionally, our findings suggest that older adults report less pain. These findings are supported by Zyczkowska (2007) [25] who reported decreasing pain scores with growing age for both men and women. The researchers name a changing, more accepting attitude towards pain with increasing age, a "survival bias" meaning only the healthiest managed to reach very old age as possible grounds for these results. In depth research could provide more distinct answers into what leads to these changes in old age and may help overcome fears of ageing.

Gender

Regardless of the cognitive state, men seem to experience less pain and impairment in everyday life due to pain. According to these findings, female gender could increase the risk of experiencing pain. Similar finding have been reported in literature across all age groups [6, 25, 26]. Reasons can be differences in individual pain perception, personal coping strategies or social settings [27, 28]. Gaining a better understanding of the different kinds of pain may also play an important role and may allow deeper insight of coping strategies and physiological factors in men and women [29, 30].

Housing situation

Regarding the housing situation, our data show differences for the housing arrangements chosen in late life. In our sample, 47.8% of women and 34.5% of men aged 90+ years are living in care homes where activities of daily living are reduced and support through care staff is given in many areas [1] which may reduce possible pain hazards. Furthermore, it can be speculated that the availability and home visits of general practitioners are at a higher frequency than in any other housing setting which could have positive effects on pain management. It may also explain why on the other hand participants living at home receiving care experience significantly

more pain and more impairment in activities of daily living. Health care services providing care in the community are generally under immense time pressure and restriction of duties applied by the indication of care level or previous health care assessments e.g. supplying medication, changing bandaging, wash the person. It is also unclear whether pain assessment is part of health care services in the community by default nor if caring relatives focus on the issue. Hence the differences in pain prevalence point to a gap in pain management in outpatient care settings.

Analgesics and cognitive state

Besides reducing pain hazards the use of analgesics plays an important role in pain management. Our results show individuals taking analgesics experience more pain and more impairment in everyday life. This connection may be even stronger due to strong side effects caused by analgesics which further reduce quality of life. Regarding the use of analgesics we found that a large group of participants with pain do not receive analgesics at all which could be explained by missing access to direct medical care, embellishment of pain, refusal to take analgesics, acceptance of pain as one part of growing older or changes in cognitive state. Bauer et al. [31] divided their sample similarly into cognitive unimpaired (CUS) and cognitively impaired participants (CI) with the subgroups of verbal ability (CI-V) and inability (CI-NV) to communicate pain. Though cut-off scores for cognitive impairment varied, the findings point into a similar direction. CUS participants were more likely to receive analgesics while CI participant's risk of not receiving analgesics despite pain indication was significantly increased by up to 2.6 (CI-V) and 3.4 (CI-NV) times. In our sample NCI patients reported twice as much pain despite receiving analgesics. One would have assumed that individuals who are verbally able to express their pain and receive the accurate medication should no longer suffer from pain. This instance may have occurred due to chronic or worsened pain conditions, wrong usage of medication or inadequate medication. In order to minimize the number of adverse side effects patients may also choose to take a lower dosage in order to manage both their level of pain and the adverse side effects. However, giving patients the possibility to address their pain on a regular basis might help to uncover such conflicting circumstances. Maxwell et al. [32] focused on prevalence of pain among nursing home residents and reported one-fifth of the residents with daily pain did not receive analgesics. Also residents aged 75+ years with cognitive impairment or the requirement of an interpreter were significantly less likely to receive an opioid alone or in combination with a non-opioid. This highlights the important fact that changes in cognitive state may hinder the detection of pain and alternative ways to assess the level of pain are needed for patients with cognitive impairment.

In relation to the cognitive state of the participants our results are partly contrary compared to existing literature. Bauer et al. [31] reported higher pain prevalence and less pain related medication for MCI. A pilot study by Monroe et al. [33] indicated greater pain intensity while our data showed significantly lower prevalence of pain for care home settings for MCI participants.

Depression

As for depression our results demonstrated consistent associations with pain and depression as found by a number of previous studies with younger participants [8, 34, 35]. Throughout the data pain and impairments due to pain and depression were highly correlated for very old people. As de Wall [35] showed perceived control plays a crucial role as mediator between pain and the presence of depressive disorders. With growing age perceived control will very likely decline and support will be needed in physical, psychological, medical and social areas of life. Therefore the group of the very old could be considered to be under greater risk of depression and preventive measure should be put in place.

Strength and limitations

The strength of our study lies in the large number of participants aged 85+ who gave extensive insight in their medical, social and psychological aspects of life. The large sample size allowed us to look closer at the connection between cognitive state and the housing arrangement which is becoming more important due to the growing number of individuals using care services.

However, we cannot exclude bias. We focused on pain at the point of time while the interview was performed but did not distinguish between chronic and acute pain in our assessments. The pain assessment was carried out using a simple question. It can be speculated whether the test was suitable for this MCI participants though all participants were verbally able to respond. Also we assessed the medication taken regularly and on demand but analgesics taken in the morning or analgesics not used despite being prescribed could have changed the evaluation. A question whether the medication has been taken in the morning was not included in the assessment. We also did not look at specific pain sites because the interview was already quite extensive.

In order to group the participants into the forms of housing we used the level of care giving through a medical assessment carried out by authorities as an indication which excluded participants receiving support through family members only.

Implications for clinicians and research

The results of the study show that pain scores decrease with age yet the reasons for the results have not been uncovered and can only be speculated upon. In order to explain the differences regarding the housing situation further investigation on the assessment of pain in ambulatory care settings is needed. The integration of routine pain assessments in both ambulatory and care home settings could help to overcome the differences in care settings and lower the number of patients suffering from pain despite taking analgesics. It remains unclear to what extend pain assessments are carried out in the ambulatory care setting in Germany. A general evaluation on this topic may help to identify key aspects in this area. In order to support caring relatives a form of special training or an advisory board may help to sensitize on the topic. For patients with MCI pain assessments should be adapted in order to ensure an accurate treatment and successful aging.

Conclusions

In conclusion, our results give new insight into prevalence of pain and impairment of activities of daily living for the oldest age groups of our society. Even though pain ratings decrease with age pain is still highly prevalent and successful management of pain is indispensable. Especially women and individuals with comorbidities such as depression are more likely to experience pain in very old age. The appropriate utilization of analgesics remains a problematic issue for individuals affected by pain. Also, the form of housing arrangement chosen in late life seems to be associated with the prevalence of pain. Individuals receiving outpatient care experience significantly more pain. These differences point to a gap in pain management especially in outpatient care settings. This could be due to a lack of interaction between care staff and general practitioners or missing standards on pain evaluation. Considering the growing number of individuals aged 85+ the group of the oldest-old shows an increasing demand of care support including management and treatment of pain.

Abbreviations
AgeCode: German Study on Ageing, Cognition and Dementia in Primary Care Patients; AgeQualiDe: Study on needs, health service use, costs and health-related quality of life in a large sample of oldest-old primary care patients; BMI: Body Mass Index; CI: Confidence interval; MCI: Mild Cognitive Impairment; NCI: No Cognitive Impairment; OR: Odds ration; PRS: Pain Rating Scale

Acknowledgements
We want to thank both all participating patients and their general practitioners for their good collaboration.
Members of the AgeCoDe Study Group: Wolfgang Maier (Principal Investigator), Martin Scherer (Principal Investigator), Hendrik van den Bussche (Principal Investigators: 2002–2011), Heinz-Harald Abholz, Christian Brettschneider, Cadja Bachmann, Horst Bickel, Wolfgang Blank, Sandra Eifflaender-Gorfer, Marion Eisele, Annette Ernst, Angela Fuchs, André Hajek, Kathrin Heser, Frank Jessen, Hanna Kaduszkiewicz, Teresa Kaufeler, Mirjam Köhler, Hans-Helmut König, Alexander Koppara, Diana Lubisch, Tobias Luck, Dagmar Lühmann, Melanie Luppa, Tina

Mallon, Manfred Mayer, Edelgard Mösch, Michael Pentzek, Jana Prokein, Steffi G. Riedel-Heller, Susanne Röhr, Anna Schumacher, Janine Stein, Susanne Steinmann, Franziska Tebarth, Carolin van der Leeden, Michael Wagner, Klaus Weckbecker, Dagmar Weeg, Jochen Werle, Siegfried Weyerer, Birgitt Wiese, Steffen Wolfsgruber, Thomas Zimmermann.

Funding

This publication is part of the German Research Network on Dementia (KND), the German Research Network on Degenerative Dementia (KNDD; German Study on Ageing, Cognition and Dementia in Primary Care Patients; AgeCoDe), and the Health Service Research Initiative (Study on Needs, health service use, costs and health-related quality of life in a large sample of oldest-old primary care patients (85+; AgeQualiDe)) and was funded by the German Federal Ministry of Education and Research (grants KND: 01GI0102, 01GI0420, 01GI0422, 01GI0423, 01GI0429, 01GI0431, 01GI0433, 01GI0434; grants KNDD: 01GI0710, 01GI0711, 01GI0712, 01GI0713, 01GI0714, 01GI0715, 01GI0716; grants Health Service Research Initiative: 01GY1322A, 01GY1322B, 01GY1322C, 01GY1322D, 01GY1322E, 01GY1322F, 01GY1322G). Dr. Francisca S. Then has been supported in working on the manuscript by LIFE – Leipzig Research Center for Civilization Diseases, Universität Leipzig. Her collaboration within LIFE was funded by means of the European Social Fund and the Free State of Saxony. We acknowledge support from the German Research Foundation (DFG) and Universität Leipzig within the program of Open Access Publishing. The funders were not involved in the design of the study, in collection, analysis, and interpretation of data, or in writing the manuscript.

Authors' contributions

Analyzed and interpreted the data and drafted the manuscript: TM, BW. Supported in analysis and interpretation of the data and drafting of the manuscript: TL, DL, BW. Acquired the data: TL, CVDL, KH, AF, SM, TM, DW, CB, JW. Conceived and designed the study: BW, HB, HHK, SW, MW, MS, WM, SGRH. Revised the manuscript critically for important intellectual content: AE, CB, HHK, TL, SR, SW, JW, EM, DW, AF, MP, LK, KH, SRH, WM, BW, MS. All authors read and approved the final version of the manuscript.

Ethics approval and consent to participate

Data were derived from the AgeQualiDe study. All GP patients who participated in the study provided written informed consent prior to their participation. The study been approved by the ethics committees of all participating study centers and comply with the ethical standards of the Declaration of Helsinki.

- Ethics Commission of the Medical Association Hamburg (reference number: MC-390/13)
- Ethics Committee of the Medical Faculty of the Rheinische Friedrich-Wilhelms-University of Bonn (reference number: 369/13)
- Medical Ethics Commission II of the Medical Faculty Mannheim/ Heidelberg University (reference number: 2013-662 N-MA)
- Ethics Committee of the Faculty of Medicine of the University of Leipzig (reference number: 309/2007; 333–13-18,112,013)
- Ethical Committee of the Medical Faculty of the Heinrich-Heine-University Düsseldorf (reference number: 2999)
- Ethics Committee of the Faculty of Medicine of the Technical University of Munich (reference number: 713/02 E)

Competing interests

The authors declare that they have no competing interests.

Author details

[1]Department of Primary Medical Care, Center for Psychosocial Medicine, University Medical Center Hamburg-Eppendorf, Hamburg, Germany. [2]Department of Health Economics and Health Services Research, Hamburg Center for Health Economics, University Medical Center Hamburg-Eppendorf, Hamburg, Germany. [3]Institute of Social Medicine, Occupational Health and Public Health (ISAP), University of Leipzig, Leipzig, Germany. [4]Central Institute of Mental Health, Medical Faculty Mannheim, Heidelberg University, Mannheim, Germany. [5]Department of Psychiatry, Klinikum rechts der Isar, Technical University of Munich, Munich, Germany. [6]Institute of General Practice, Medical Faculty, Heinrich-Heine-University Düsseldorf, Düsseldorf, Germany. [7]Department of Psychiatry, University of Bonn, Bonn, Germany. [8]Work Group Medical Statistics and IT-Infrastructure, Institute for General Practice, Hannover Medical School, Hannover, Germany. [9]DZNE, German Center for Neurodegenerative Diseases, Bonn, Germany.

References

1. Ältere Menschen in Deutschland und der Europäischen Union (EU) – Broschüre – Ausgabe 2016 https://www.destatis.de/DE/Publikationen/Thematisch/Bevoelkerung/Bevoelkerungsstand/BroschuereAeltereMenschen0010020169004.html;jsessionid=4409AD30FC9F44669DFC0E4EE918EA28.cae3 12.07.2016 last accessed on 12th August 2016, 10:29.
2. van der Leeuw G, Eggermont LH, Shi L, Milberg WP, Gross AL, Hausdorff JM, Bean JF, Leveille SG. Pain and cognitive function among older adults living in the community. J Gerontol A Biol Sci Med Sci. 2016;71(3):398–405. https://doi.org/10.1093/gerona/glv166.
3. M S, Njoo N, Hestermann M, Oster P, Hauer K. Acute and chronic pain in geriatrics: clinical characteristics of pain and the influence of cognition. Pain Med. 2004;5(3):253–62.
4. Smith TO, Purdy R, Latham SK, Kingsbury SR, Mulley G, Conaghan PG. The prevalence, impact and management of musculoskeletal disorders (MD) in older people living in care homes: a systematic review. Rheumatol Int. 2016;36(1):55–64. https://doi.org/10.1007/s00296-015-3322-1.
5. Stewart C, Leveille SG, Shmerling RH, Samelson EJ, Bean JF, Schofield P. Management of persistent pain in older adults: MOBILIZE Boston study. J Am Geriatr Soc. 2012;60(11):2081–6. https://doi.org/10.1111/j.1532-5415.2012.04197.x.
6. Takai Y, Yamamoto-Mitani N, Okamoto Y, Koyama K, Honda A. Literature review of pain prevalence among older residents of nursing homes. Pain Manag Nurs. 2010;11(4):209–23. https://doi.org/10.1016/j.pmn.2010.08.006.
7. Blyth FM, March LM, Brnabic AJ, Jorm LR, Williamson M, Cousins MJ. Chronic pain in Australia: a prevalence study. Pain. 2001;89(2–3):127–34.
8. Ligthart L, Visscher CM, van Houtem CM, Geels LM, Vink JM, de Jongh A, Boomsma DI. Comorbidity among multiple pain symptoms and anxious depression in a Dutch population sample. J Pain. 2014;15(9):945–55. https://doi.org/10.1016/j.jpain.2014.06.007.
9. Thomas E, Peat G, Harris L, Wilkie R, Croft PR. The prevalence of pain and pain interference in a general population of older adults: cross-sectional findings from the north Staffordshire osteoarthritis project (NorStOP). Pain. 2004;110(1–2):361–8.
10. Mehta RH, Rathore SS, Radford MJ, Wang Y, Wang Y, Krumholz HM. Acute myocardial infarction in the elderly: differences by age. J Am Coll Cardiol. 2001;38(3):736–41.
11. Andersson HI, Ejlertsson G, Leden I, Rosenberg C. Chronic pain in a geographically defined population: studies of differences in age, gender, social class and pain localization. Clin J Pain. 1993;9(3):174–82.
12. Inouye SK, Studenski S, Tinetti ME, Kuchel GA. Geriatric syndromes: clinical, research, and policy implications of a core geriatric concept. J Am Geriatr Soc. 2007;55(5):780–91.
13. Fox PL, Raina P, Jadad AR. Prevalence and Treatment of pain in older adults in nursing homes and other long-term care institutions: a systematic review. CMAJ. 1999 Feb 9;160(3):329–33.
14. Gagliese L. Pain and aging: the emergence of a new subfield of pain research. Critical Review J Pain. 2009;10(4):343–53. https://doi.org/10.1016/j.jpain.2008.10.013.
15. Alameddine M, Bauer JM, Richter M, Sousa-Poza A. Trends in job satisfaction among German nurses from 1990 to 2012. J Health Serv Res Policy. 2016; 21(2):101–8. https://doi.org/10.1177/1355819615614045.

16. Landi F, Russo A, Liperoti R, Danese P, Maiorana E, Pahor M, Bernabei R, Onder G. Daily pain and functional decline among old-old adults living in the community. J Pain Symptom Manag. 2009;38(3):350–7. https://doi.org/10.1016/j.jpainsymman.2008.10.005.
17. Cowan DT, Fitzpatrick JM, Roberts JD, While AE, Baldwin J. The assessment of pain and management of pain among older people in care homes: current status and future direction. Int J Nurs Stud. 2003;40(3):291–8.
18. Kölzsch M, Wulff I, Ellert S, Fischer T, Kopke K, Kalinowski S, Dräger D, Kreutz R. Deficits in pain treatment in nursing homes in Germany: a cross-sectional study. Eur J Pain. 2012;16(3):439–46. https://doi.org/10.1002/j.1532-2149.2011.00029.x.
19. Weyerer S, Eifflaender-Gorfer S, Köhler L, Jessen F, Maier W, Fuchs A, Pentzek M, Kaduszkiewicz H, Bachmann C, Angermeyer MC, Luppa M, Wiese B, Mösch E, Bickel H. German AgeCoDe Study group (German Study on Ageing, Cognition and Dementia in Primary Care Patients). Prevalence and risk factors for depression in non-demented primary care attenders aged 75 years and older. J Affect Disord. 2008;111(2–3):153–63.
20. Radbruch L, Loick G, Kiencke P, Lindena G, Sabatowski R, Grond S, Lehmann KA, Cleeland CS. Validation of the German version of the brief pain inventory. J Pain Symptom Manag. 1999;18(3):180–7. https://doi.org/10.1016/j.jad.2008.02.008.
21. König W, Lüttinger P, Müller W. A comparative analysis of the development and structure of educational systems. Methodological foundations and the construction of a comparative education scale. Munich: CASMIN working paper no.12; 1988.
22. Folstein MF, Folstein SE, McHugh PR. Mini-Mental State - A practical method for grading the cognitive state of patients for the clinician. J Psychiatr Res. 1975;12(3):189–98.
23. Yesavage JA. Psychopharmacol Bull. 1988;24(4):709–11.
24. Mahoney FI, Barthel D. Functional evaluation: the Barthel index. Md State Med J. 1965;14:61–5.
25. Zyczkowska J, Szczerbińska K, Jantzi MR, Hirdes JP. Pain among the oldest old in community and institutional settings. Pain. 2007;129(1–2):167–76.
26. Donald IP, Foy C. A longitudinal stusy of joint pain in older people. Rheumatology (Oxford). 2004;43(10):1256–60.
27. Turk DC, Okifuji A. Assessment of patients' reporting of pain: an integrated perspective. Lancet. 1999;353(9166):1784–8.
28. Keogh E. Sex differences in pain. Rev Pain. 2008;2:4–7. https://doi.org/10.1177/204946370800200203.
29. Savvas SM, Gibson SJ. Overview of pain Management in Older Adults. Clin Geriatr Med. 2016;32(4):635–50. https://doi.org/10.1016/j.cger.2016.06.005.
30. Eslami V, Katz MJ, White RS, Sundermann E, Jiang JM, Ezzati A, Lipton RB. Pain intensity and pain interference in older adults: role of gender, obesity and high-sensitivity c-reactive protein. Gerontology. 2016 Aug 4; [Epub ahead of print]
31. Bauer U, Pitzer S, Schreier MM, Osterbrink J, Alzner R, Iglseder B. Pain treatment for nursing home residents differs according to cognitive state – a cross-sectional study. BMC Geriatr. 2016;16:124. https://doi.org/10.1186/s12877-016-0295-1.
32. Maxwell CJ, et al. The prevalence and management of current daily pain among older home care clients. Pain. 2008;138(1):208–16. https://doi.org/10.1016/j.pain.2008.04.007.
33. Monroe TB, Misra SK, Habermann RC, Dietrich MS, Cowan RL, Simmons SF. Pain reports and pain medication treatment in nursing home residents with and without dementia. Geriatr Gerontol Int. 2014;14(3):541–8. https://doi.org/10.1111/ggi.12130.
34. Geerlings SW, Twisk JW, Beekman AT, Deeg DJ, van Tilburg W. Longitudinal relationship between pain and depression in older adults: sex, age and physical disability Soc Psychiatry Psychiatr Epidemiol 2002;37(1):23–30.
35. de Waal MW, Hegeman JM, Gussekloo J, Verhaak PF, van der Mast RC, Comijs HC. The effect of pain on presence and severity of depressive disorders in older persons: the role of perceived control as mediator. J Affect Disord. 2016;197:239–44. https://doi.org/10.1016/j.jad.2016.03.012.

2

Endometrial sampling in low-risk patients with abnormal uterine bleeding

Brenda F. Narice[1]* (iD), Brigitte Delaney[2] and Jon M. Dickson[2]

Abstract

Background: One million women per year seek medical advice for abnormal uterine bleeding (AUB) in the United Kingdom. Many low-risk patients who could be managed exclusively in primary care are referred to hospital based gynaecology services. Performing endometrial sampling (ES) in the community may improve care, reduce the rate of referrals and minimise costs. We aimed to search and synthesise the literature on the effectiveness of ES (Pipelle versus other devices) in managing AUB in low-risk patients.

Methods: We undertook an electronic literature search in MEDLINE via OvidSP, Scopus, and Web of Science for relevant English-language articles from 1984 to 2016 using a combination of MeSH and keywords. Two reviewers independently pre-selected 317 articles and agreed on 60 articles reporting data from over 7300 patients. Five themes were identified: sample adequacy, test performance, pain and discomfort, cost-effectiveness, and barriers and complications of office ES.

Results: Pipelle seems to perform as well as dilation and curettage and, as well or better than other ES devices in terms of sampling adequacy and sensitivity. It also seems to be better regarding pain/discomfort and costs. However, Pipelle can disrupt the sonographic appearance of the endometrium and may be limited by cervical stenosis, pelvic organ prolapse and endometrial atrophy.

Conclusions: The current evidence supports the use of Pipelle in the management of low-risk women presenting in the outpatient setting with symptomatic AUB when combined with clinical assessment and ultrasound scanning. However, the implications of its widespread use in primary care are uncertain and more research is required.

Keywords: Pipelle, Endometrial sampling, Abnormal uterine bleeding, Endometrial cancer, Endometrial hyperplasia, Premenopausal, Perimenopausal, Dilation and curettage

Background

Abnormal uterine bleeding (AUB), traditionally defined as uterine bleeding that is abnormal in volume, regularity, and/or timing [1] is common and affects 14–25% of women of reproductive age [2–4]. In the UK, approximately 1 million women seek medical advice for AUB every year, mostly in general practice [5, 6] and even though most cases could potentially be managed exclusively in primary care [7, 8], AUB is the fourth most common reason for referral to UK gynaecological services [6, 9, 10]. AUB has a major impact on quality of life [7], leads to 3.5 million days of work absence [11], and generates significant health care costs. Hospital referrals and hysterectomies are the major components of the £65 million/year treatment costs for AUB [10].

Most cases of AUB are benign and amenable to office-based treatments [12, 13]. However, patients often present with a myriad of symptoms, and their assessment requires training and expertise [13, 14]. The causes of AUB can be summarised using the PALM-COEIN acronym: polyps, adenomyosis, leiomyoma/fibroids, malignancy (and hyperplasia), coagulopathy, ovulatory disorders, endometrial, iatrogenic, and not otherwise classified [1].

* Correspondence: bnarice1@sheffield.ac.uk
[1]Clinical Research Fellow in Obstetrics & Gynaecology; Academic Unit of Reproductive and Developmental Unit, University of Sheffield, Sheffield S10 2SF, UK
Full list of author information is available at the end of the article

Some patients who present with AUB will have endometrial hyperplasia or cancer which is the commonest gynaecological malignancy in the Western world. Even though the incidence rises after menopause, it can occur at all ages and 7% of cases are under 50 [15, 16]. This percentage seems to be rising with increasing prevalence of obesity and diabetes [17, 18].

In the UK, women with AUB who are deemed at high risk of endometrial cancer such as those with postmenopausal bleeding (PMB) or family history of gynaecological neoplasms, should be referred to secondary care [19]. For low-risk premenopausal women the guidance is not as clear. Although urgent referral is not required [20], national guidelines recommend that endometrial sampling (ES) should be performed in women over 40–45 years to exclude cancer [21, 22], but they do not specify whether ES should be performed in primary or secondary care [22].

In the UK, ES for AUB patients has not been traditionally undertaken in primary care. For many years, the standard management was dilation and curettage (D&C) in hospital under general anaesthesia [23–25]. However, the need for admission and the risks of perforation and haemorrhage made D&C unpopular [23, 25] and various ES devices were developed such as the Novak (a silastic cannula with a bevelled lateral opening [26]), the Tis-u-Trap (a plastic curette with suction [27]), the Vabra Aspirator (a stainless steel cannula connected to a vacuum pump [28]), the Endorette (a plastic cannula with multiple openings [29]), the Tao Brush (a sheath brush device [30]), the Cytospat (a polypropylene cannula with a rhomboid head [31]), the Accurette (a quadrilateral-shaped curette with four cutting edges [32]) and the Pipelle, the most widely used device in the UK (a flexible plastic tube with a distal circular port [27]).

We conducted a systematic review of the literature to identify existing evidence about the effectiveness of Pipelle compared with other ES techniques for assessing low-risk women with AUB which could inform the development of new care pathways in primary care.

Why this study was necessary

Endometrial sampling is thought to be a safe and effective method for histological assessment of the endometrium. It is used as an alternative to the more invasive method of D&C. This is the first review to focus on AUB in low-risk pre- and perimenopausal women. We conclude that ES is a valuable tool in the assessment of these patients and that Pipelle is the best outpatient device available. The evidence supports the use of Pipelle in the outpatient setting but more research is required to assess its impact if introduced as routine management of AUB in the community.

Methods
Literature search

We used the PICO approach to develop a systematic search strategy [33]. We searched MEDLINE via OvidSP, Scopus, and Web of Science. For Medline, key concepts were identified (endometrial hyperplasia/cancer, abnormal uterine bleeding, endometrial sampling), a list of synonyms was generated for each concept and these lists were used to identify MeSH terms for the search (Additional file 1). Similar search strategies were used for Scopus and Web of Science (Additional file 1), always limited to papers from 1984 (when Pipelle was first introduced [34]) to 2016, written in English and involving humans.

We included papers investigating ES in women with AUB. We also considered studies in patients with known cancer; although these studies do not inform the indication of ES in primary care, they were an important source to evaluate test performance. We included review articles and opinion pieces. We excluded papers exclusively analysing postmenopausal patients, papers where the indication was assessment of fertility or recurrent miscarriage and papers where ES was assisted by hysteroscopy (unless this was used as a comparator to blind ES).

The initial search generated 173 results for Medline, 240 for Scopus, and 221 for Web of Science, totalling 634 search hits across all databases, 317 of which were excluded for duplication. The remaining 317 articles were assessed for inclusion using the titles and abstracts. The assessment was independently repeated by a second reviewer and a consensus was reached. After this process, 257 papers were excluded and the full text of 60 papers were read. Twenty-two further papers were excluded while another 22 papers were added from reference search, giving a final list of 60 papers. This selection included 16 randomized controlled trials (RCT), 26 prospective studies, 6 retrospective studies, 5 reviews, 2 meta-analyses, 1 survey, and 4 brief communications and letters to the editor, which were included in the final analysis providing data over 7300 women (Fig. 1).

Bias risk assessment

The quality of the RCTs was assessed using the standard Cochrane Risk of Bias tool [35], and the quality of observational studies was analysed with the modified Agency for Healthcare Research and Quality (AHRQ) quality assessment criteria [36].

Results
Risk of Bias / quality of studies

The overall quality of the RCTs was poor ($n = 4$) to moderate ($n = 12$), no high quality studies were identified. For observational studies, the risk of bias ranged from 31 to 79% with a mean weighted score 52.8% SD ± 11.8% which again suggests overall moderate quality [37]. See

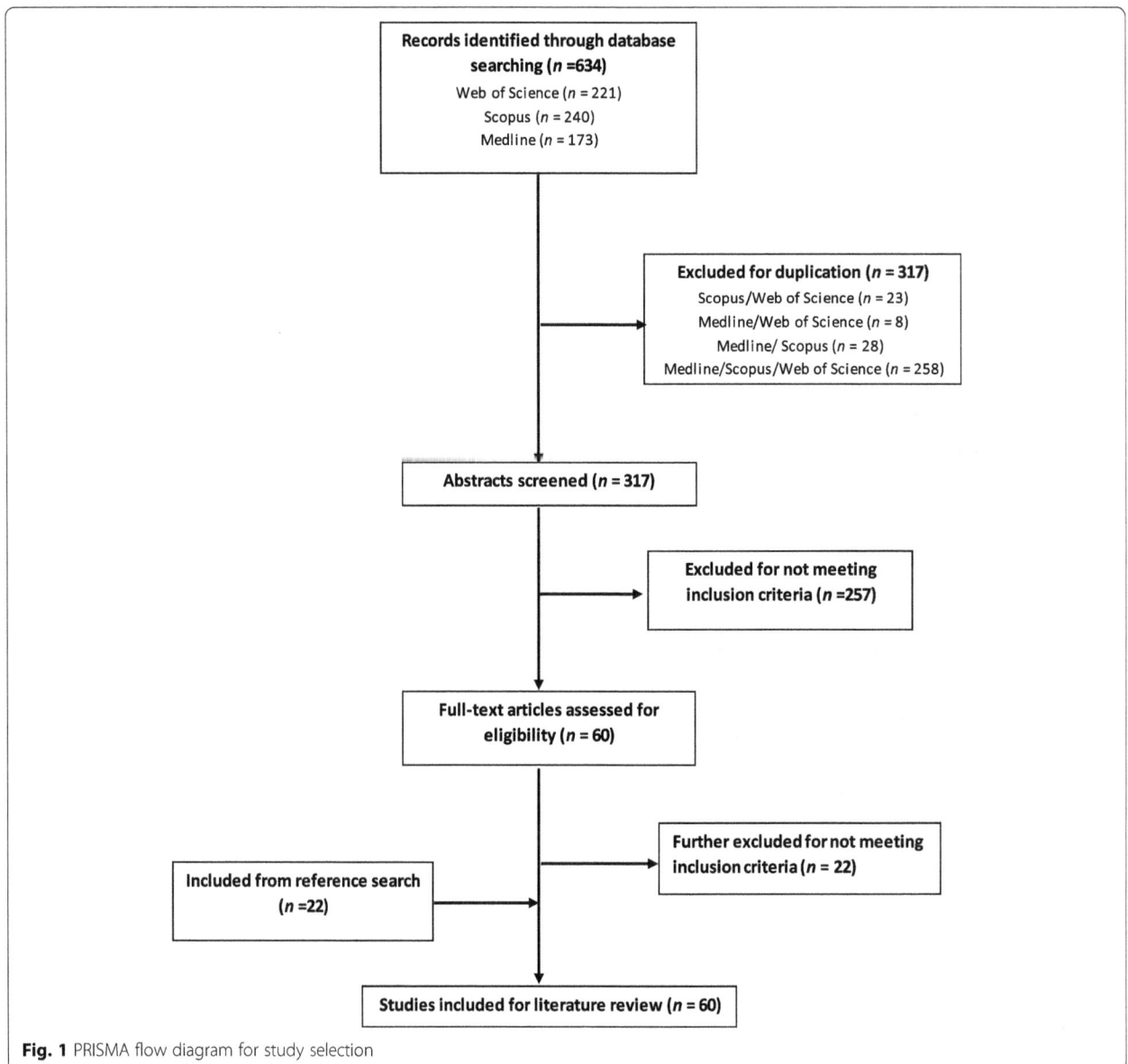

Fig. 1 PRISMA flow diagram for study selection

additional online content for tabulated assessments of individual studies (Additional file 2: TableS1 and 2, Additional file 2).

Five themes
We identified five major themes in the literature: (1) sample adequacy (defined as enough tissue to be analysed by pathologists [38]); (2) test performance when compared with hysterectomy and D&C; (3) acceptability by the patient in terms of pain experienced during sampling; (4) the costs of taking outpatient endometrial biopsies; and (5) the barriers and complications of performing office ES.

All studies, except for one, were carried out in specialised outpatient gynaecology clinics or hospital services (secondary care) [39]. Only one study looked exclusively at premenopausal women [40]. The rest reported on cohorts of

both pre- and post-menopausal women or they did not present results based on menopausal status. Most studies included women with symptomatic AUB and no risk of endometrial carcinoma. However, five studies targeted women with endometrial cancer to correlate pre-operative Pipelle with the hysterectomy histopathology [41–45]. Studies are summarised in Table 1.

Sample adequacy
Overall, the literature showed that the adequacy of material retrieved for histological analysis with Pipelle was comparable to D&C and superior to most of the other devices in pre-menopausal women. Ten studies [23, 24, 46–53] assessed Pipelle against D&C in premenopausal women, reporting rates of adequacy ranging from 89.74% [51] to 98% [23, 24] (Table 1).

Table 1 Comparison of the RCTs, prospective and retrospective studies included in this literature review. Papers have been grouped by intervention/ comparator

Study	Type of study	Age of participants (mean ± SD)	Intervention (n) vs Comparator (n)	Outcome	Pain	Cost
Pipelle versus D&C +/– Hysterectomy						
[23] Rauf et al. Pakistan 2014	RCT	46.3 ± 4.45	Pipelle (102) vs D&C (101)	Adequacy Pipelle 98% D&C 100%	Pipelle less painful	Pipelle cheaper
[46] Liu et al. China 2015	Prospective Sequential	43.6	Pipelle vs D&C (245)	Adequacy Pipelle 91.02% D&C 92.24%	Pipelle less painful	N/A
[47] Gungorduk et al. Turkey 2013	Prospective	Pipelle: 49.8 ± 6.1 D&C: 48.2 ± 6.5	Pipelle + hysterectomy (78) vs D&C + hysterectomy (189)	Adequacy Pipelle 95% D&C 96% Concordance Pipelle + hysterectomy 62% D&C + hysterectomy 67%	Pipelle less painful	Pipelle cheaper
[48] Kazandi et al. Turkey 2012	Prospective Sequential	48 ± 9.43	Pipelle + hysterectomy Vs D&C + hysterectomy (66)	Adequacy Pipelle 93% D&C 96% Concordance Pipelle and D&C 66% Pipelle & hysterectomy 64%	Pipelle less painful	Pipelle cheaper
[49] Demirkiran et al. Turkey 2012	Prospective	45.3	Pipelle + hysterectomy (212) vs D&C + hysterectomy (161)	Adequacy Pipelle 97% D&C98% Concordance Pipelle and D&C 84% Pipelle & hysterectomy 67% D&C and hysterectomy 80%	Pipelle less painful	Pipelle cheaper
[43] Sany et al. UK 2011	Retrospective	?	Pipelle + hysterectomy vs D&C + hysterectomy (total 191)	Concordance Both techniques 78%	N/A	N/A
[45] Daud et al. UK 2011	Retrospective	55.7 ± 11.4	Pipelle ± hysterectomy (75) vs D&C ± hysterectomy (220)	Concordance Pipelle + hysterectomy 76% D&C + hysterectomy 86%	N/A	N/A
[24] Fakhar et al. Pakistan 2008	Prospective Sequential	45.4 ± 7.2	Pipelle versus (D&C) (100)	Adequacy Pipelle 98% D&C 100% NPV for endometrial carcinoma Pipelle 100%	N/A (both techniques under GA)	Pipelle cheaper
[44] Huang	Retrospective	?	Pipelle +	Concordance	N/A	N/A

Table 1 Comparison of the RCTs, prospective and retrospective studies included in this literature review. Papers have been grouped by intervention/ comparator *(Continued)*

Study	Type of study	Age of participants (mean ± SD)	Intervention (n) vs Comparator (n)	Outcome	Pain	Cost
et al. USA 2006 [37] Macones et al. 2006	+ Letter		hysterectomy (253) vs D&C + hysterectomy (93)	Pipelle and hysterectomy 93.8% (low grade cancer) & 99.2% (high grade cancer) D&C and hysterectomy 97% (low grade cancer) & 100% (high grade cancer)		
[66] Machado et al. Spain 2002	Retrospective	Post-menopausal (68) Pre- or peri-menopausal (100)	Pipelle (168) vs D&C (92) ± Hysterectomy (76)	Accuracy Sensitivity 84.2% Specificity 99.1%	N/A	N/A
[51] Kavak et al. Turkey 1996	Prospective	50.8 ± 7.8	Pipelle ± TVS (78) vs D&C (78)	Concordance Sensitivity: 73% (increased to 90% with TVS) Specificity: 100%	N/A	N/A
[50] Ben-Baruch et al. Israel 1993	Prospective	Pre- and post-menopausal	Pipelle (172) vs D&C (97)	Adequacy Pipelle 90.6% D&C 68%	N/A	N/A
[68] Sanam et al. Iran 2015	Prospective	> 35	Pipelle (130) vs D&C (130)	Concordance Pipelle and D&C 94% Adequacy Pipelle 84.6% D&C 90%	N/A	Pipelle cheaper
[75] Gordon New Zealand 1999	Prospective	47.2 ± 1.8	Pipelle (100) vs D&C or hysterectomy (n =?)	Adequacy Pipelle 67%	N/A	N/A
[69] Goldchmit et al. Israel 1993	Prospective Sequential	48.1	Pipelle and TVS vs D&C (176)	Concordance Pipelle & D&C 90% (increased to 92% with TVS)	N/A	N/A
[52] Abdelazim et al. Turkey 2013	Prospective Sequential	44.5	Pipelle vs D&C (143)	Adequacy Pipelle 97.9% D&C 100% NPV for endometrial polyp Pipelle 89.6%	N/A	N/A
[72] Shams Pakistan 2012	Prospective Sequential	47.94	Pipelle vs D&C (50)	N/A	Pipelle less painful	Pipelle cheaper
[53] Rezk et al. Egypt 2016	Prospective	Pipelle: 47.2 ± 3.8 D&C: 46.9 ± 4.1	Pipelle (270) vs D&C (268)	Adequacy No difference (p'0.05)	D&C less painful	N/A
Pipelle versus Vabra +/− Hysterectomy						
[54] Eddowes et al. UK 1990	Prospective Sequential	41.6	Pipelle vs Vabra Aspirator (100)	Adequacy Pipelle 88% Vabra Aspirator 88%	Pipelle less painful	Pipelle cheaper
[55] Naim et al. Malaysia 2007	RCT	> 45	Pipelle (76) vs Vabra Aspirator	Adequacy Pipelle 73.3%	N/A	Pipellle cheaper

Table 1 Comparison of the RCTs, prospective and retrospective studies included in this literature review. Papers have been grouped by intervention/ comparator *(Continued)*

Study	Type of study	Age of participants (mean ± SD)	Intervention (n) vs Comparator (n)	Outcome	Pain	Cost
			(71)	Vabra 52.4%		
[28] Kaunitz et al. USA 1988	Prospective Sequential	46	Pipelle vs Vabra (56)	Adequacy Pipelle & Vabra 91% Concordance Pipelle & Vabra 89%	Pipelle less painful	Pipelle cheaper
[56] Rodriguez et al. USA 1993	RCT	?	Pipelle (12) vs Vabra (13) vs Hysterectomy (25)	Surface being sampled: Pipelle 4.2% Vabra 41.6%	N/A	N/A
Pipelle versus Tao Brush+/− Hysteroscopy						
[30] Williams et al. UK 2008	RCT Sequential	Moderate risk: 45.2 (SE 0.26)	For moderate risk Pipelle (34) Tao Brush (29)	Adequacy Both techniques 84% No significant difference for premenopausal	Tao Brush less painful	N/A
[57] Critchley et al. UK 2004	RCT	Moderate risk: pre-menopausal ˃40 or < 40 with risk for endometrial cancer Low risk	Pipelle vs Tao Brush Moderate risk (Total 326) Low risk (Total 157) ± hysteroscopy ± TVS	Successful completion of investigation: Pipelle 85% Adequacy of sample with Pipelle: Moderate risk 79%	Tao Brush less painful than Pipelle	Minimal difference
[58] Yang et al. USA 2003	Prospective Sequential	24–86	Pipelle (79) vs Tao Brush (79)	Factors affecting sensitivity: tumour size, type, location within the uterus, sampling mechanism and preparation method	N/A	N/A
[59] Del Priore et al. USA 2001	RCT Sequential	Pre-menopausal: 46 Post-menopausal: 61	Tao Brush vs Pipelle (50)	Sensitivity: Pipelle 86% Tao Brush 95.5% Specificity: Both 100%	N/A	Tao Brush cheaper than D&C
[60] Yang et al. USA 2000	Prospective Sequential	58	Tao Brush vs Tao Brush + Pipelle (25)	Adequacy Tao Brush 98% Pipelle 88%	Tao Brush less painful	Comparable
Pipelle versus Novak						
[40] Henig et al. USA 1989	RCT	Pre-menopausal	Pipelle (50) Vs Novak (50)	Adequacy Pipelle 94% Novak 98%	Better tolerance with Pipelle	N/A
[26] Stovall et al. USA 1991	RCT	Pipelle: 40 Novak: 44	Pipelle (149) vs Novak (126)	Adequacy Pipelle 87.2% Novak 90.5%	Pipelle less painful	Novak might be cheaper
[61] Silver et al. USA 1991	RCT Sequential	28–76	1st Pipelle then Novak (26) vs 1st Novak then Pipelle (29)	Adequacy Similar	Pipelle less painful	N/A
Pipelle versus Hysterectomy						

Table 1 Comparison of the RCTs, prospective and retrospective studies included in this literature review. Papers have been grouped by intervention/ comparator *(Continued)*

Study	Type of study	Age of participants (mean ± SD)	Intervention (n) vs Comparator (n)	Outcome	Pain	Cost
[67] Guido et al. USA 1995	Prospective Sequential	61	Pipelle vs Hysterectomy (71)	Adequacy Pipelle 97% Concordance Pipelle & hysterectomy 83%	N/A	N/A
[42] Ferry et al. UK 1993	Prospective Sequential	?	Pipelle vs Hysterectomy (37)	Concordance Pipelle & hysterectomy 67%	N/A	N/A
[41] G Zorlu et al. Turkey 1994	Prospective Sequential	51	Pipelle vs Hysterectomy (26)	Concordance Pipelle & hysterectomy 95%	Mild pain and discomfort with Pipelle	N/A
Pipelle versus Explora +/− Accurette						
[62] Leclair et al. USA 2011	RCT	Pipelle: 45.2 ± 7.3 Explora: 46.1 ± 7.7	Pipelle (37) vs Explora (32)	Adequacy Pipelle 91% Explora 97%	No differences seen	N/A
[32] Lipscomb et al. USA 1994	RCT	N/A Pre- and post-menopausal	Pipelle (85) vs Accurette (81) vs Explora (82)	Adequacy Pipelle 85.2% Accurette 72.5% Explora 85.4%	No significant difference in pain score	N/A
Pipelle versus Infant Feeding Tube (IFT)						
[63] Bhide et al. UK 2007	Prospective	?	Pipelle (29) vs IFT (31)	Adequacy Pipelle 73% IFT 71%	Less pain with IFT	N/A
Pipelle Mark 2 versus Pipelle Mark 2 + hysteroscopy						
[71] Polena et al. France 2006	Prospective Sequential	50	Pipelle Mark 2 vs Pipelle Mark 2 ± hysteroscopy (97)	Adequacy of Pipelle Mark 2 88.7%	No difference with conventional Pipelle	Slightly more expensive than conventional Pipelle
Pipelle versus Tis-u-Trap						
[27] Koonings et al. USA 1990	RCT	Pipelle: 42.9 Tis-u-trap: 42.3	Pipelle + hysterectomy (74) vs Tis-u-trap + hysterectomy (75)	Adequacy Pipelle 87.8% Tis-u-trap 84% Concordance Pipelle & hysterectomy 85% Tis-u-trap & hysterectomy 92%	N/A	Pipelle cheaper
Pipelle versus Endorette						
[29] Moberger et al. Sweden 1998	RCT Sequential	57.5 ± 11.5	Pipelle vs Endorette (152)	Adequacy and concordance No difference	No significant difference	N/A
Pipelle versus Cytospat +/−						

Table 1 Comparison of the RCTs, prospective and retrospective studies included in this literature review. Papers have been grouped by intervention/ comparator *(Continued)*

Study	Type of study	Age of participants (mean ± SD)	Intervention (n) vs Comparator (n)	Outcome	Pain	Cost
Hysterectomy						
[31] Antoni et al. Spain 1996	RCT	48.6 ± 9	Pipelle ± hysterectomy or D&C (191) vs Cytospat ± hysterectomy or D&C (174)	Adequacy Pipelle 75% Cytospat 76% Concordance Pipelle: Benign 84%, Hyperplasia 71%, Malignancy 60% Cytospat: Benign 82%, Hyperplasia 60%, Malignancy 60%	Better tolerance for Pipelle	Pipelle cheaper
Pipelle versus D&C +/– Hysteroscopy +/– TV US						
[85] Tahir et al. UK 1999	RCT	35	Inpatient: Hysteroscopy & D&C (200) vs Outpatient: Pipelle +/– TV US +/– Hysteroscpy (200)	Adequacy No difference Concordance Inpatient: 100& Outpatient: 82&	More pain in outpatient	N/A
Others						
[73] Trolice et al. USA 2000	RCT Anaesthesia for Pipelle	Lidocaine: 42.1 ± 11.9/ Saline: 44.9 ± 12.5	Lidocaine (19) vs Saline (22)	Significant reduction of pain with lidocaine	Less pain with intervention	N/A
[34] Cornier France 1984	Brief communication	Mostly pre-menopausal	Pipelle (250) No control	Useful for histologic dating of the endometrium	Little discomfort	Low cost
[74] Frishman USA 1990	Letter in response to study [27]	N/A	Pipelle versus Tis-u-Trap	N/A	N/A	Pipelle cheaper
[38] Mc Cluggage Northern Ireland 2006	Review	N/A	Pipelle versus other ES	Difficulties of processing outpatient ES samples	N/A	N/A
[79] Van Den Bosch Belgium 2005	Prospective sequential	Pre-menopausal: 41.6 ± 8.7 Post-menopausal: 59 ± 9.9	US before and after Pipelle (99)	Thickness of the endometrium ET on average 0.4 mm less after performing Pipelle	N/A	N/A
[76] Brandner et al. Germany 2000	Review	N/A	N/A	Progression of endometrial lesions (potential limitations for ES)	N/A	N/A
[80] Dijkhuizen et al. The Netherlands 2000	Meta-analysis	39 studies including 7914 patients	Different ES	Pipelle is superior to other ES for diagnosing cancer/ hyperplasia	N/A	N/A
[25] Cooper et al. USA 2000	Review	N/A	N/A	Directed biopsy with Hysteroscopy: most accurate ES (not for primary care)	N/A	N/A

Table 1 Comparison of the RCTs, prospective and retrospective studies included in this literature review. Papers have been grouped by intervention/ comparator *(Continued)*

Study	Type of study	Age of participants (mean ± SD)	Intervention (n) vs Comparator (n)	Outcome	Pain	Cost
[14] Farquhar et al. New Zealand 1996	Survey	68 replies from O&G consultants (48% of all contestants)	N/A	Management of menorrhagia in primary care	N/A	N/A
[78] Youssif et al. Australia 1995	Review	N/A	N/A	Effectiveness and safety of Pipelle	N/A	N/A
[77] Dantas et al. Brazil 1994	Letter	Nurses vs doctors performing Pipelle	N/A	Adequacy No difference	N/A	N/A
[82] Clark et al. UK 2002	Systematic review and meta-analysis	Mixed pre- (21%) and pos-tmenopausal (79%)	Pipelle vs other outpatient techniques	Likelihood ratio of endometrial cancer when Pipelle is: -ve: 0.1 +ve: 64.6	N/A	N/A
[86] Ahonkallio et al. Finland 2009	Prospective	Range 47–52 Post ablation	Pipelle (57)	Adequacy 29% failure If endometrium < 5 mm 5% failure if endometrium > 5 mm	N/A	N/A
[81] Du et al. China 2016	Review	N/A	N/A	Most appropriate ES devices for endometrial lesions	Little discomfort	N/A
[64] Masood et al. Pakistan 2015	Cross sectional	Pre- and post-menopausal 35–48	Pipelle (126) vs no comparator	Adequacy Pipelle 96.82%	N/A	Cost-effective
[39] Seamark UK 1998	Prospective	≥40 42–74 Primary care population	Pipelle (38) vs no comparator	Adequacy Pipelle 76%	N/A	N/A
[70]Seto UK 2016	Retrospective	Pre-menopausal 46.1 ± 4.6 Post-menopausal 57.2 ± 8.1	Pipelle against hysteroscopy	Positive predictive value for endometrial polyp Pipelle (pre-menopausal) 53.7%	N/A	N/A
[65] Piatek et al. Poland 2016	Retrospective	Pre- and post-menopausal	Pipelle (312) vs no comparator	Adequacy 83.01%	N/A	N/A

ES Endometrial sampling, *AUB* Abnormal uterine bleeding, *RCT* Randomized controlled trials, *US* Transvaginal ultrasound, *N/A* Non-applicable,*?* Unknown

Three studies compared the sample adequacy of Pipelle and Vabra Aspirator [28, 54, 55]. One of these studies [55] showed better rates for Pipelle (73.3% versus 52.4%, *P* = 0.02) whereas the remaining two could not identify any significant difference between both techniques (one study reported 91% for both techniques [28] whereas the other showed 89.79% for Vabra versus 88% for Pipelle [54], no *P* values provided) (Table 1). We also found a RCT which reported that Pipelle despite being equal or superior to Vabra in terms of sample adequacy only assesses 4.2% of the endometrium versus 41.6% with Vabra [56].

Five studies including mixed cohorts of pre- and post-menopausal women compared sample adequacy between Pipelle and Tao Brush [30, 57–60]. Despite one study

suggesting that Tao Brush bendable wire should improve sampling of the uterine lateral walls when compared to Pipelle more rigid structure, none of the studies showed significant differences in premenopausal populations [58] (Table 1).

Two studies [40, 61] also compared Pipelle to Novak and found no statistically significant difference in terms of adequacy of sample, which varied from 83 to 94% for Pipelle and from 85 to 98% for Novak [40, 61] (Table 1). Six additional studies did not find a significant difference when comparing Pipelle with other less popular ES techniques such as Explora [32, 62] (85.4–97% for Explora versus 85.2–91% for Pipelle), Tis-u-trap [27] (88% for Pipelle versus 84% for Tis-u-Trap *P* = 0.5), Endorette

[29] (56% for Endorette versus 43% for Pipelle), infant feeding tube [63] (73% for Pipelle versus 71% for IFT) and Cytospat [31] (Pipelle 74.9% versus 75.9% for Cytospat).

Three studies [39, 64, 65] assessed the ability of Pipelle to retrieve enough tissue for histological analysis without comparing it to other devices, and reported a success rate of 76% in GP practices [39], and a range from 83.01 to 96.82% in secondary care [64, 65] (Table 1).

Test performance
Nine studies compared the histopathological diagnosis of pre-operative Pipelle and D&C with the final results from hysterectomy (the gold standard diagnostic technique for uterine disorders) [41, 43–45, 47–49, 66, 67]. For Pipelle, the sensitivity ranged from 62% [47] to 99.2% [44] and for D&C sensitivity varied from 67% [47] to 100% [44]. One of these studies applied Pipelle and D&C sequentially before hysterectomy [48], while the rest were multi-arm studies [41, 43–45, 47, 49, 66, 67] (Table 1).

At least 5 studies [43, 48, 49, 68, 69] also reported on the concordance between Pipelle and D&C with values that ranged from 66% [48] to 94% [68].

One retrospective study which compared Pipelle samples suggestive of endometrial polyps with subsequent hysteroscopically-guided polypectomies reported Pipelle had a positive predictive value of 55.3% for sampling polyps in premenopausal women [70]. Pipelle has also been reported to have 100% negative predictive value (NPV) for endometrial carcinoma and hyperplasia [24] and up to 99.2% NPV for endometritis and 89.6% for endometrial polyps [52] (Table 1).

Pain / discomfort
Most studies included in this review performed ES on awake patients, but only 23 studies formally assessed patients' pain using visual pain analogue scales and questionnaires (Table 1). A total of 15 studies reported that most patients experienced minimal discomfort with Pipelle [23, 26, 28, 31, 34, 40, 41, 46–49, 54, 61, 71, 72], three did not find any significant difference between Pipelle and Explora [32, 62] and Pipelle and Endorette [29], three concluded that Tao Brush was better tolerated than Pipelle [30, 57, 60] and one study showed less discomfort when using an infant feeding tube as a prototype [63]. A RCT also reported that paracervical lidocaine during Pipelle may decrease pain when compared to placebo [73] (Table 1).

Costs of outpatient endometrial sampling
A total of 17 studies assessed the cost-effectiveness of Pipelle though none formally provided a health economic analysis [23, 24, 26–28, 31, 47–49, 54, 55, 57, 60, 68, 71, 72, 74]. Some of the factors they considered when assessing the total cost of ES were the need for general anaesthesia and hospital admission [23, 72] and the cost of operative hysteroscopy/ D&C following a failed office ES or an inadequate sample [55]. Fifteen studies showed Pipelle was cheaper than the alternative ES [23, 24, 26–28, 31, 47–49, 54, 55, 57, 68, 72, 74] and two did not find significant differences between Pipelle and Pipelle Mark 2 [71], and Pipelle and Tao Brush [60]. Two studies concluded that the Vabra was cheaper than Pipelle given its multiple use [26] but when all costs were considered including the need for follow-up for failed procedures, the average cost of Pipelle per patient was approximately 30% cheaper than the Vabra aspirator [55] (Table 1).

Barriers and complications to endometrial sampling in primary care
Several limitations to successful ES were reported including cervical stenosis and pelvic organ prolapse which hindered the access to the uterine cavity [24, 75] as well as focal endometrial pathology (e.g. endometrial polyps and sub-mucosal fibroids) and endometrial atrophy which reduces sample adequacy [30, 46, 69, 75, 76]. Lack of experience was also linked to inadequate sampling with higher failure rates seen in registrars (39%) than in consultants (25%), ($P = 0.13$)) [75]. However, a study which compared sample adequacy between nurses (83.3%) and doctors (80%), $P > 0.05$, concluded that with the right training the ability to perform successful Pipelle is independent of professional category [77].

While few complications have been associated with Pipelle [73]. [78], mainly discomfort and false negative results, a study showed that Pipelle makes the endometrium approximately 0.4 mm thinner and creates echogenic spots which can be misinterpreted as sonographic lesions if the ultrasound is not performed prior to ES [79] (Table 1).

Discussion
Our aim was to search and synthesise the whole range of literature on ES in AUB in low-risk patients to guide further research and develop new evidence-based care pathways in primary care. Overall, the evidence that we have identified supports the use of ES in the outpatient setting and is a valuable source for the development of new care pathways in primary care.

To the best of our knowledge, this study is the first systematic review to primarily focus on the role of ES in assessing and managing AUB in low-risk women in the outpatient setting [25, 78, 80–82]. The available evidence shows that when Pipelle is combined with clinical assessment and ultrasound findings, it becomes a valuable tool for investigating AUB in low-risk women. Pipelle seems to perform as well or better than any other ES device in terms of sampling adequacy and sensitivity, with comparable results to D&C which for years was the standard technique for obtaining endometrial tissue in patients with AUB [78]. Furthermore, Pipelle seems to be cost-effective and better tolerated in terms of pain/discomfort [83]. However, its use has shown to be limited by cervical stenosis, pelvic organ prolapse and endometrial atrophy [24, 75]. Since Pipelle causes changes in the endometrium, it should not be performed before USS [79], and if the ultrasound reports localised lesions, a hospital referral for a hysteroscopy-guided biopsy may prove more useful than performing a blind Pipelle [84] given its limited sensitivity for focal lesions [47, 70].

Despite our robust and thorough literature search, we have noted some limitations in the available evidence. We only identified one study which was conducted on a primary care population by general practitioners [39] and one study which looked exclusively at premenopausal patients [40] and therefore, our conclusions are mainly based on studies which were carried out in either outpatient specialised clinics or hospital departments on a mixed cohort of pre- and postmenopausal women. Many of the studies that we identified were of poor or moderate methodological quality with wide-ranging inclusion and exclusion criteria (see Additional file 2). This heterogeneity may partly be responsible for the significant variability seen in terms of the sensitivity and specificity of Pipelle for detecting endometrial hyperplasia/cancer.

A meta-analysis was beyond the scope of this paper but critical appraisal and analysis of pooled data from diagnostic studies is an important next step in establishing the utility of ES. Given the limited information about the true test performance of ES in the community, it is not possible for clinicians to quantify the risk of hyperplasia/cancer (or other pathology) based only on ES. This is especially pertinent when the sample result is normal but the patient is still symptomatic; clinicians should then continue to consider the possibility of false negative results e.g. undiagnosed cancer/hyperplasia in these patients.

Conclusions

The evidence we analysed suggests that performing ES in the outpatient setting may allow effective management of low-risk women with AUB in primary care without referral to a hospital. But the false negative rate, health economics and implications of such a change in practice are still unknown and more research is required.

Abbreviations

AUB: Abnormal uterine bleeding; D&C: Dilation and curettage; ES: Endometrial sampling; PMB: Postmenopausal bleeding; RCT: Randomised controlled trial; USS: Ultrasound scan

Acknowledgements

We would like to thank Dr. Mary Connor and Dr. Mauro A Rinaldi for their valuable comments.

Authors' contributions

JMD proposed the review and created the original search strategy. BD undertook the initial literature search and retrieved the manuscripts. BN revised the initial search, executed the final searches, compiled the results and undertook the quality assessments. BN and JMD wrote the manuscript, with contributions from BD, which all authors approved. All authors read and approved the final manuscript.

Competing interests

The authors declare that they have no competing interests.

Author details

[1]Clinical Research Fellow in Obstetrics & Gynaecology; Academic Unit of Reproductive and Developmental Unit, University of Sheffield, Sheffield S10 2SF, UK. [2]Academic Unit of Primary Medical Care, University of Sheffield, Sheffield S5 7AU, UK.

References

1. Munro M, Critchley H, Broder M, Fraser ID. ftFWGoM. FIGO classification system (FIGO-COEIN) for causes of abnormal uterine bleeding in nongravid women of reproductive age. Int J Gynaecol Obstet. 2011;113(1):3-13.
2. Fraser I, Langham SU-HK. Health-related quality of life and economic burden of abnormal uterine bleeding. Expert Rev Obstet Gynecol. 2009;4:179–89.
3. Shapley M, Jordan KCP. An epidemiological survey of symptoms of menstrual loss in the community. Br J Gen Pract. 2004;54:359–63.
4. Garside R, Stein K, Wyatt K, Round APA. The effectiveness and cost-effectiveness of microwave and thermal balloon endometrial ablation for heavy menstrual bleeding: a systematic review and economic modelling. Health Technol Assess (Rockv). 2004;8ii:155.
5. McCormick A, Fleming D, Charlton J, Royal College of General Practitioners GB S. OoPCa. Morbidity statistics from general practice: fourth national study. 1995.
6. Royal college of Obstetrics and Gynaecology. Heavy menstrual bleeding audit second annual report. 2012.
7. Kai J, Middleton L, Daniels J, Pattison H, Tryposkiadis K, Gupta J, et al. Usual medical treatments or levonorgestrel-IUS for women with heavy menstrual bleeding: long-term randomised pragmatic trial in primary care. Br J Gen Pract. 2016;66(653):e861-e70. Epub 2016 Oct 10.
8. Dickson J, Delaney B, Connor M. Primary care endometrial sampling for abnormal uterine bleeding: a pilot study. J Fam Plan Reprod Heal Care. 2017;43:247–8.
9. Lethaby A, Cooke IRM. Progesterone or progestogen-releasing intrauterine systems for heavy menstrual bleeding. Cochrane Database Syst Rev. 2005;19:CD002126.

10. Weeks A, Duffy SWJ. A double-blind randomised trial of leuprorelin acetate prior to hysterectomy for dysfunctional uterine bleeding. Br J Obstet Gynaecol. 2000;107:323–8.

11. Maresh M, Metcalfe M, McPherson K, Overton C, Hall V, Hargreaves J, et al. The VALUE national hysterectomy study: description of the patients and their surgery. Br J Obstet Gynaecol. 2002;109:302–12.

12. Pitkin J. Dysfunctional uterine bleeding. BMJ. 2007;334(7603):1110–1.

13. Warner P, Critchey H, Lumsden M, Cambell-Brown M, Dougas AMG. Referral for menstrual problems: cross sectional survey of symptoms, reasons for referral and management. BMJ. 2001;323:24–8.

14. Farquhar CM, Kimble RMN. How do New Zealand Gynaecologists treat menorrhagia? Aust New Zeal J Obstet Gynaecol. 1996;36:444–7. https://doi.org/10.1111/j.1479-828X.1996.tb02190.x.

15. Lumsden M, Gebbie AHC. Managing unscheduled bleeding in non-pregnant premenopausal women. BMJ. 2013;346. https://doi.org/10.1136/bmj.f3251.

16. Bignardi T, Van den Bosch T, Condous G. Abnormal uterine and post-menopausal bleeding in the acute gynaecology unit. Best Pract Res Clin Obstet Gynaecol. 2009;595-607. https://doi.org/10.1016/j.bpobgyn.2009.05.001.

17. Cancer Research UK. Uterine Cancer incidence statistics: uterine cancer incidence trends over time 2014. http://www.cancerresearchuk.org/health-professional/cancer-statistics/statistics-by-cancer-type/uterine-cancer/incidence#ref-2. (accessed 19 Jan 2017).

18. Wise MR, Gill P, Lensen S, Thompson JMD, Farquhar CM. Body mass index trumps age in decision for endometrial biopsy: cohort study of symptomatic premenopausal women. Am J Obstet Gynecol. 2016;215:598. e1–8. https://doi.org/10.1016/j.ajog.2016.06.006.

19. Cooper N, Barton P, Breijer M, Caffrey O, Opmeer B, Timmermans A, Cooper NA, Barton PM, Breijer M, Caffrey O, Opmeer BC. et al. Cost-effectiveness of diagnostic strategies for the management of abnormal uterine bleeding (heavy menstrual bleeding and post-menopausal bleeding): a decision analysis 2014;18. doi:https://doi.org/10.3310/hta18240.

20. National Insititute for Health and Care Excellence. Suspected cancer: recognition and referra. 2015.

21. Julian S, Naftalin N, Clark M, Szczepura A, Rashid A, Baker R, et al. An integrated care pathway for menorrhagia across the primary–secondary interface: patients' experience, clinical outcomes, and service utilisation. BMJ Qual Saf. 2007;16(2):110–5.

22. Royal College of Obstetrics and Gynaecology. Standards for Gynaecology. 2008.

23. Rauf RSA, Sadia S, Waqar F, Zafar S, Sultana SWS. Outpatient endometrial biopsy with Pipelle vs diagnostic dilatation and curettage. J Ayub Med Coll Abbottabad. 2004;26:145–8.

24. Fakhar S, Saeed G, Khan AH, Alam AY. Validity of pipelle endometrial sampling in patients with abnormal uterine bleeding. Ann Saudi Med. 2008;28:188–91.

25. Cooper JM, Erickson ML. Endometrial sampling techniques in the diagnosis of abnormal uterine bleeding. Obstet Gynecol Clin North Am. 2000;27:235–44. https://doi.org/10.1016/S0889-8545(00)80018-2.

26. Stovall TG, Ling FW, Morgan PL. A prospective, randomized comparison of the Pipelle endometrial sampling device with the Novak curette. Am J Obstet Gynecol. 1991;165:1287–90. https://doi.org/10.1016/0002-9378(91)90351-Q.

27. Koonings P, Moyer DL, Grimes DA. A randomised clinical trial comparing Pipelle and tis-u-trap for endometrial biopsy. Obstet Gynecol. 1990;75:293.

28. Kaunitz AM, Masciello A, Ostrowski M, Rovira EZ. Comparison of endometrial biopsy with the endometrial Pipelle and Vabra aspirator. J Reprod Med. 1988;33:427–31.

29. Moberger B, Nilsson S, Palmstierna S, Redvall L, Sternby N. A multicenter study comparing two endometrial sampling devices - Medscand Endorette TM and Pipelle De cornier R. Acta Obstet Gynecol Scand. 1998;77:764–9. https://doi.org/10.1034/j.1600-0412.1998.770712.x.

30. Williams ARW, Brechin S, Porter AJL, Warner P, Critchley HOD. Factors affecting adequacy of Pipelle and Tao brush endometrial sampling. BJOG An Int J Obstet Gynaecol. 2008;115:1028–36. https://doi.org/10.1111/j.1471-0528.2008.01773.x.

31. Antoni J, Folch E, Costa J, Foradada CM, Cayuela E, Comballa N, et al. Comparison of cytospat and pipelle endometrial biopsy instruments. Eur J Obstet Gynecol Reprod Biol. 1997;72:57–61. https://doi.org/10.1016/S0301-2115(96)02658-9.

32. Lipscomb GH, Lopatine SM, Stovall TG, Ling FW. A randomized comparison of the Pipelle, Accurette, and Explora endometrial sampling devices. Am J Obstet Gynecol. 1994;170:591–4. https://doi.org/10.1016/S0002-9378(94)70234-9.

33. Glasziou P, Irwig L, Bain CCG. The question. In: Systematic Reviews in Health Care: a Practical Guide. New York: Cambridge University Press; 2001. p. 9.

34. Cornier E. The Pipelle: a disposable device for endometrial biopsy. Am J Obs Gynecol. 1984;148:109–10.

35. Cochrane Handbook for Systematic Reviews of Interventions | Cochrane Training n.d. http://training.cochrane.org/handbook (accessed 12 July 2017).

36. West S, King V, Carey TS, et al. Systems to Rate the Strength of Scientific Evidence: Summary. In: AHRQ Evidence Report Summaries. Rockville (MD): Agency for Healthcare Research and Quality (US); 1998-2005. 2002;47. Available from: https://www.ncbi.nlm.nih.gov/books/NBK11930/.

37. Macones G. How accurate if Pipelle sampling: a study by Huang et al. Am J Obstet Gynecol 2007;196(3):280-1.

38. McCluggage WG. My approach to the interpretation of endometrial biopsies and curettings. J Clin Pathol. 2006;59:801–12. https://doi.org/10.1136/jcp.2005.029702.

39. Seamark CJ. Endometrial sampling in general practice. Br J Gen Pract [Internet]. 1998;48:434. Available from: http://bjgp.org/content/48/434/1597/tab-pdf.

40. Henig I, Tredway DR, Maw GM, Gullett AJ, Cheatwood M, C P. Evaluation of the Pipelle curette for endometrial biopsy. J Reprod Med. 1989;34:786–9.

41. Zorlu CG, Cobanoglu O, Işik AZ, Kutluay L, Kuşçu E. Accuracy of Pipelle endometrial sampling in endometrial carcinoma. Gynecol Obstet Investig. 1994;38:272–5.

42. Ferry J, Farnsworth A, Webster M, Wren B. The efficacy of the Pipelle endometrial biopsy in detecting endometrial carcinoma. Aust New Zeal J Obstet Gynaecol. 1993;33:76–8. https://doi.org/10.1111/j.1479-828X.1993.tb02060.x.

43. Sany O, Singh K, Jha S. Correlation between preoperative endometrial sampling and final endometrial cancer histology. Eur J Gynaecol Oncol. 2012;33:142–4.

44. Huang GS, Gebb JS, Einstein MH, Shahabi S, Novetsky AP, Goldberg GL. Accuracy of preoperative endometrial sampling for the detection of high-grade endometrial tumors. Am J Obstet Gynecol. 2007;196:243.e1–5. https://doi.org/10.1016/j.ajog.2006.09.035.

45. Daud S, Jalil SSA, Griffin M, Ewies AAA. Endometrial hyperplasia – the dilemma of management remains: a retrospective observational study of 280 women. Eur J Obstet Gynecol Reprod Biol. 2011;159:172–5. https://doi.org/10.1016/j.ejogrb.2011.06.023.

46. Liu H, Wang FL, Zhao YM, Yao YQ, Li YL. Comparison of Pipelle sampler with conventional dilatation and curettage (D&C) for Chinese endometrial biopsy. J Obstet Gynaecol. 2015;35:508–11.

47. Gungorduk K, Asicioglu O, Ertas IE, Ozdemir LA, Ulker MM, Yildirim G, et al. Comparison of the histopathological diagnoses of preoperative dilatation and curettage and pipelle biopsy. Eur J Gynaecol Oncol. 2014;35:539–43. https://doi.org/10.12892/ejgot24972014.

48. Kazandi M, Okmen F, Ergenoglu AM, Yeniel AO, Zeybek B, Zekioglu O, et al. Comparison of the success of histopathological diagnosis with dilatation-curettage and Pipelle endometrial sampling. J Obstet Gynaecol. 2012;32:790–4. https://doi.org/10.3109/01443615.2012.719944.

49. Demirkiran F, Yavuz E, Erenel H, Bese T, Arvas M, Sanioglu C. Which is the best technique for endometrial sampling? Aspiration (pipelle) versus dilatation and curettage (D&C). Arch Gynecol Obstet. 2012;286:1277–82. https://doi.org/10.1007/s00404-012-2438-8.

50. Ben-Baruch G, Seidman DS, Schiff E, Moran O, Menczer J. Outpatient endometrial sampling with the Pipelle curette. Gynecol Obstet Investig. 1994;37:260–2.

51. Kavak Z, Ceyhan N, Pekin S. Combination of vaginal ultrasonography and pipelle sampling in the diagnosis of endometrial disease. Aust NZ Obs Gynaecol. 1996;36:63.

52. Abdelazim IA, Elezz AA, Abdelkarim AF. Pipelle endometrial sampling versus conventional dilatation & curettage in patients with abnormal uterine bleeding. Asian Pacific J Reprod. 2013;2:45–8. https://doi.org/10.1016/S2305-0500(13)60115-3.

53. Rezk M, Sayyed T, Dawood R. The effectiveness and acceptability of Pipelle endometrial sampling versus classical dilatation and curettage: a three-year observational study. Gynecol Obstet Investig. 2016;81:537–42. https://doi.org/10.1159/000444711.

54. Eddowes HA, Read MD, Codling BW. Pipelle: a more acceptable technique for outpatient endometrial biopsy. BJOG An Int J Obstet Gynaecol. 1990;97:961–2. https://doi.org/10.1111/j.1471-0528.1990.tb02458.x.

55. Naim NM, Ahmad S, Razi ZR, M ZA. The Vabra aspirator versus the Pipelle device for outpatient endometrial sampling. Aust N Z J Obs Gynaecol. 2007;47:132–6.

56. Rodriguez GC, Yaqub N, King ME. A comparison of the Pipelle device and the Vabra aspirator as measured by endometrial denudation in hysterectomy specimens: The Pipelle device samples significantly less of the endometrial surface than the Vabra aspirator. Am J Obstet Gynecol. 1993; 168:55–9. https://doi.org/10.1016/S0002-9378(12)90884-4.

57. Critchley HOD, Warner P, Lee AJ, Brechin S, Guise J, Graham B. Evaluation of abnormal uterine bleeding: comparison of three outpatient procedures within cohorts defined by age and menopausal status. Health Technol Assess. 2004;8(34):8.

58. Yang GC, Del Priore G, W LS. Factors influencing the detection of uterine cancer by suction curettage and endometrial brushing. J Reprod Med. 2003;47:1005–10.

59. Del Priore G, Willliams R, Harbatkin CB, Wan LS, Mittal K, Yang GCH. Endometrial brush biopsy for the diagnosis of endometrial Cancer. Obstet Gynecol Surv. 2001;56:548–9.

60. Yang GC, Wan LS. Endometrial biopsy using the Tao brush method. A study of 50 women in a general gynecologic practice. J Reprod Med. 2000;45:109–14.

61. Silver MM, Miles P, Rosa C. Comparison of Novak and Pipelle endometrial biopsy instruments. Obstet Gynecol. 1991;78:828–30.

62. Leclair CM, Zia JK, Doom CM, Morgan TK, Edelman AB. Pain experienced using two different methods of endometrial biopsy: a randomized controlled trial. Obstet Gynecol. 2011;117:636–41. https://doi.org/10.1097/AOG.0b013e31820ad45b.

63. Bhide A, Gangji A, Anyanwu L. Endometrial biopsy: A pilot study of instrument used; Pipelle vs infant feeding tube. J Obstet Gynaecol. 2007;27: 838–9. https://doi.org/10.1080/01443610701718941.

64. Masood H, Ashraf S, Masood MS. Frequency of positive endometrial pipelle biopsies in patients with abnormal uterine bleeding for detection of endometrial carcinoma Pak J Med Health Sci. 2015;9:256–8. https://pdfs.semanticscholar.org/c724/5b497b4f5771a8e4356db03be05fc8a0f760.pdf. Accessed Apr 2017.

65. Piatek S, Panek G, Wielgoś M. Assessment of the usefulness of pipelle biopsy in gynecological diagnostics. Ginekol Pol. 2016;87:559–64. https://doi.org/10.5603/GP.2016.0044.

66. Machado F, Moreno J, Carazo M, León J, Fiol G, Serna R. Accuracy of endometrial biopsy with the cornier pipelle for diagnosis of endometrial cancer and atypical hyperplasia. Eur J Gynaecol Oncol. 2003;24:279–81.

67. Guido RS, Kanbour-Shakir A, Rulin MC, Christopherson WA. Pipelle endometrial sampling. Sensitivity in the detection of endometrial cancer. J Reprod Med. 1995;40:553–5.

68. Sanam M, Majid M. Comparison the diagnostic value of dilatation and curettage versus endometrial biopsy by Pipelle--a clinical trial. Asian Pac J Cancer Prev. 2015;16:4971–5. https://doi.org/10.7314/APJCP.2015.16.12.4971.

69. Goldchmit R, Katz Z, Blickstein I, Caspi B, Dgani R. The accuracy of endometrial Pipelle sampling with and without sonographic measurement of endometrial thickness. Obstet Gynecol. 1993;82:727–30.

70. Seto MTY, Ip PPC, Ngu S-F, Cheung ANY, Pun T-C. Positive predictive value of endometrial polyps in Pipelle aspiration sampling: a histopathological study of 195 cases. Eur J Obstet Gynecol Reprod Biol. 2016;203:12–5. https://doi.org/10.1016/j.ejogrb.2016.04.027.

71. Polena V, Mergui J-L, Zerat L, Sananes S. The role of Pipelle® Mark II sampling in endometrial disease diagnosis. Eur J Obstet Gynecol Reprod Biol. 2007;134:233–7. https://doi.org/10.1016/j.ejogrb.2006.07.026.

72. Shams, G. Comparison of Pipelle de Cornier with conventional dilatation and curettage in terms of patients' acceptability. Journal of Postgraduate Medical Institute ;Peshawar. 2012; 26 (4) [cited 2017 Jun 22]. Available from: http://www.jpmi.org.pk/index.php/jpmi/article/view/1377

73. Trolice MP, Fishburne CJR, McGrady S. Anesthetic efficacy of intrauterine lidocaine for endometrial biopsy: a randomized double-masked trial. Obstet Gynecol. 2000;95:345–7.

74. Frishman G, Jacobs S. A randomized clinical trial comparing Pipelle and tis-U-trap for endometrial biopsy. Obstet Gynecol. 1990;76:315–6.

75. Gordon SJ, Westgate J. The incidence and Management of Failed Pipelle Sampling in a general outpatient clinic. Aust New Zeal J Obstet Gynaecol. 1999;39:115–8. https://doi.org/10.1111/j.1479-828X.1999.tb03460.x.

76. Brandner P, Neis KJ. Diagnosis of endometrial Cancer and its precursors. Contrib Gynecol Obstet. 2000;20:27–40.

77. Dantas MC, Hidalgo MM, Bahamondes L, Marchi NM. A comparison of the performance of endometrial biopsy with the Pipelle® by nurses and physicians. Int J Gynecol Obstet. 1994;45:164–5. https://doi.org/10.1016/0020-7292(94)90128-7.

78. Youssif SN, McMillan DL. Outpatient endometrial biopsy: the pipelle. Br J Hosp Med. 1995;54(5):198–201.

79. Van den Bosch T, Van Schoubroeck D, Ameye L, Van Huffel S, Timmerman D. Ultrasound examination of the endometrium before and after Pipelle endometrial sampling. Ultrasound Obstet Gynecol. 2005;26: 283–6. https://doi.org/10.1002/uog.1967.

80. Dijkhuizen FPHLJ, Mol BWJ, Brölmann HAM, Heintz APM. The accuracy of endometrial sampling in the diagnosis of patients with endometrial carcinoma and hyperplasia. Cancer. 2000;89:1765–72. https://doi.org/10.1002/1097-0142(20001015)89:8<1765::AID-CNCR17>3.0.CO;2-F.

81. Du J, Li Y, Lv S, Wang Q, Sun C, Dong X, et al. Endometrial sampling devices for early diagnosis of endometrial lesions. J Cancer Res Clin Oncol. 2016;142: 2515–22. https://doi.org/10.1007/s00432-016-2215-3.

82. Clark TJ, Mann CH, Shah N, Khan KS, Song F, Gupta JK. Accuracy of outpatient endometrial biopsy in the diagnosis of endometrial hyperplasia. Acta Obstet Gynecol Scand. 2001;80:784–93.

83. Chambers JT, Chambers SK. Endometrial sampling: when? Where? Why? With what? Clin Obstet Gynecol. 1992;35:28–39.

84. Kotdawala P, Kotdawala S, Nagar N. Evaluation of endometrium in peri-menopausal abnormal uterine bleeding. J Midlife Health. 2013;4:16–21. https://doi.org/10.4103/0976-7800.109628.

85. Tahir MM, Digrigg MA, Browning JJ, Brookes T, Smith PA. A randomised controlled trial comparing transvaginal ultrasound, outpatient hysteroscopy and endometrial biopsy with inpatient hysteroscopy and curettage. BJOG An Int J Obstet Gynaecol. 1999;106:1259–64. https://doi.org/10.1111/j.1471-0528.1999.tb08179.x.

86. Ahonkallio SJ, Liakka AK, Martikainen HK, Santala MJ. Feasibility of endometrial assessment after thermal ablation. Eur J Obstet Gynecol Reprod Biol. 2009;147:69–71. https://doi.org/10.1016/j.ejogrb.2009.06.014.

3

Using the CollaboraKTion framework to report on primary care practice recruitment and data collection: costs and successes in a cross-sectional practice-based survey in British Columbia, Ontario, and Nova Scotia, Canada

Sabrina T. Wong[1,2]* (ID), William Hogg[3,4], Fred Burge[5], Sharon Johnston[3,4], Ilisha French[4] and Stephanie Blackman[5]

Abstract

Background: Across Canada and internationally we have poor infrastructure to regularly collect survey data from primary care practices to supplement data from chart audits and physician billings. The purpose of this work is to: 1) examine the variable costs for carrying out primary care practice-based surveys and 2) share lessons learned about the level of engagement required for recruitment of practices in primary care.

Methods: This work was part of a larger study, TRANSFORMATION that collected data from three provincial study sites in Canada. We report here on practice-based engagement. Surveys were administered to providers, organizational practice leads, and up to 20 patients from each participating provider. We used the CollaboraKTion framework to report on our recruitment and engagement strategies for the survey work. Data were derived from qualitative sources, including study team meeting minutes, memos/notes from survey administrators regarding their interactions with practice staff, and patients and stakeholder meeting minutes. Quantitative data were derived from spreadsheets tracking numbers for participant eligibility, responses, and completions and from time and cost tracking for patient survey administration.

Results: A total of 87 practices participated in the study ($n = 22$ in BC; $n = 26$ in ON; $n = 39$ in NS). The first three of five CollaboraKTion activities, Contacting and Connecting, Deepening Understandings, and Adapting and Applying the Knowledge Base, and their associated processes were most pertinent to our recruitment and data collection. Practice participation rates were low but similar, averaging 36% across study sites, and completion rates were high (99%). Patient completion rates were similarly high (99%), though participation rates in BC were substantially lower than the other sites. Recruitment and data collection costs varied with the cost per practice ranging from $1503 to $1792.

(Continued on next page)

* Correspondence: sabrina.wong@nursing.ubc.ca
[1]School of Nursing, University of British Columbia, T201 2211 Westbrook Mall, Vancouver, BC V6T 2B5, Canada
[2]Centre for Health Services and Policy Research, University of British Columbia, 201-2206 East Mall, Vancouver, BC V6T 1Z3, Canada
Full list of author information is available at the end of the article

(Continued from previous page)

Conclusions: A comprehensive data collection system in primary care is possible to achieve with partnerships that balance researcher, clinical, and policy maker contexts. Engaging practices as valued community members and independent business owners requires significant time, and financial and human resources. An integrated knowledge translation and exchange approach provides a foundation for continued dialogue, exchange of ideas, use of the information produced, and recognises recruitment as part of an ongoing cycle.

Keywords: Waiting room, Patient experience, Provider, Engagement, Integrated knowledge translation

Background

High performing primary care is foundational to achieving the triple aim of health reform—better health, improved patient experience, and more affordable costs [1]. Bodenheimer and colleagues [2] suggest 10 building blocks of high-performing primary care; Data-driven improvement was one of four foundational building blocks necessary before achieving success in the higher order blocks. Yet, much of what we know about high performing primary care is based on analyses using health administrative data [3–6] and chart audits, [7, 8] not data from patients, clinicians, or the practices. Moreover, across Canada and internationally we have poor infrastructure to regularly collect survey data from primary care practices to supplement the administrative data. Primary health care clinicians in Canada have historically low (2–21%) and declining response rates for survey research [9–11], comparable to other countries [12]. Common barriers include time constraints, disruption to clinic flow, competing research, and a fear of performance evaluation and its consequences [13–15]. Additionally, the environment for collecting data from multiple sources (e.g. administrative, surveys) across different organizations and regions remains challenging given the diverse custodians of data, multiple ethics review committees and privacy impact assessments.

In order for practices and jurisdictions to achieve data driven improvement, data systems that track clinical (e.g. diabetes management), operational (e.g. continuity of care and access) and patient reported experiences and outcomes are needed [2]. If there is to be more routine and widespread practice-based data collection an integrated knowledge translation and exchange (KTE) strategy is needed in order to develop greater research capacity and goodwill in future projects by meaningfully engaging participants in primary care research [16]. Improvement towards high performing community-based primary health care (CBPHC) requires those who can influence change or take action on indicators have accurate and meaningful measurement information for reporting [17–31]. Involving patients [32], clinicians [33], and practices [33] in contributing to meaningful measurement in CBPHC is essential to driving improvement. As a guide for others interested in developing data systems that can drive improvement and to support the further development of these approaches, we present strategies for recruitment of practices using the CollaboraKTion Framework [34, 35]. The CollaboraKTion Framework is a KTE approach sensitive to context and is focused on establishing partnerships with organizations and individuals.

The purpose of this paper is to report on lessons learned in working with CBPHC practices to recruit and collect data. We add new information to the literature by: 1) examining the variable costs for carrying out primary care practice-based surveys; and 2) sharing lessons learned regarding the level of engagement required for recruitment of practices in primary care.

Methods

Given the historical difficulty of practice-based recruitment, we used an integrated (KTE) approach to engage with potential participants. While we did not explicitly use any one integrated KTE approach during practice recruitment and data collection, the CollaboraKTion framework provides a well-aligned approach to reporting our diverse recruitment strategies. The CollaboraKTion framework is an expansion of Kitson's CoKT framework, which accounts for researcher and community contexts that converge on a set of 5 iterative activities: 1) Contacting and Connecting; 2) Deepening Understandings; 3) Adapting and Applying the Knowledge Base; 4) Supporting and Evaluating Continued Action; and 5) Transitioning and Embedding (Fig. 1) [34, 35].

TRANSFORMATION is a cross-sectional study on improving the science and reporting of CBPHC performance in three Canadian geographic regions: Fraser East, British Columbia (BC); Eastern Ontario Health Unit, Ontario (ON), and Central Zone, Nova Scotia (NS). As part of the larger study, we carried out a practice-based survey. Since the study remains ongoing, we report here on practice recruitment activities. Physician, staff and patient participation in data collection for ongoing CBPHC performance measurement and reporting is critical, making the CollaboraKTion framework a useful roadmap for implementing a comprehensive data system that could be used to drive CBPHC performance.

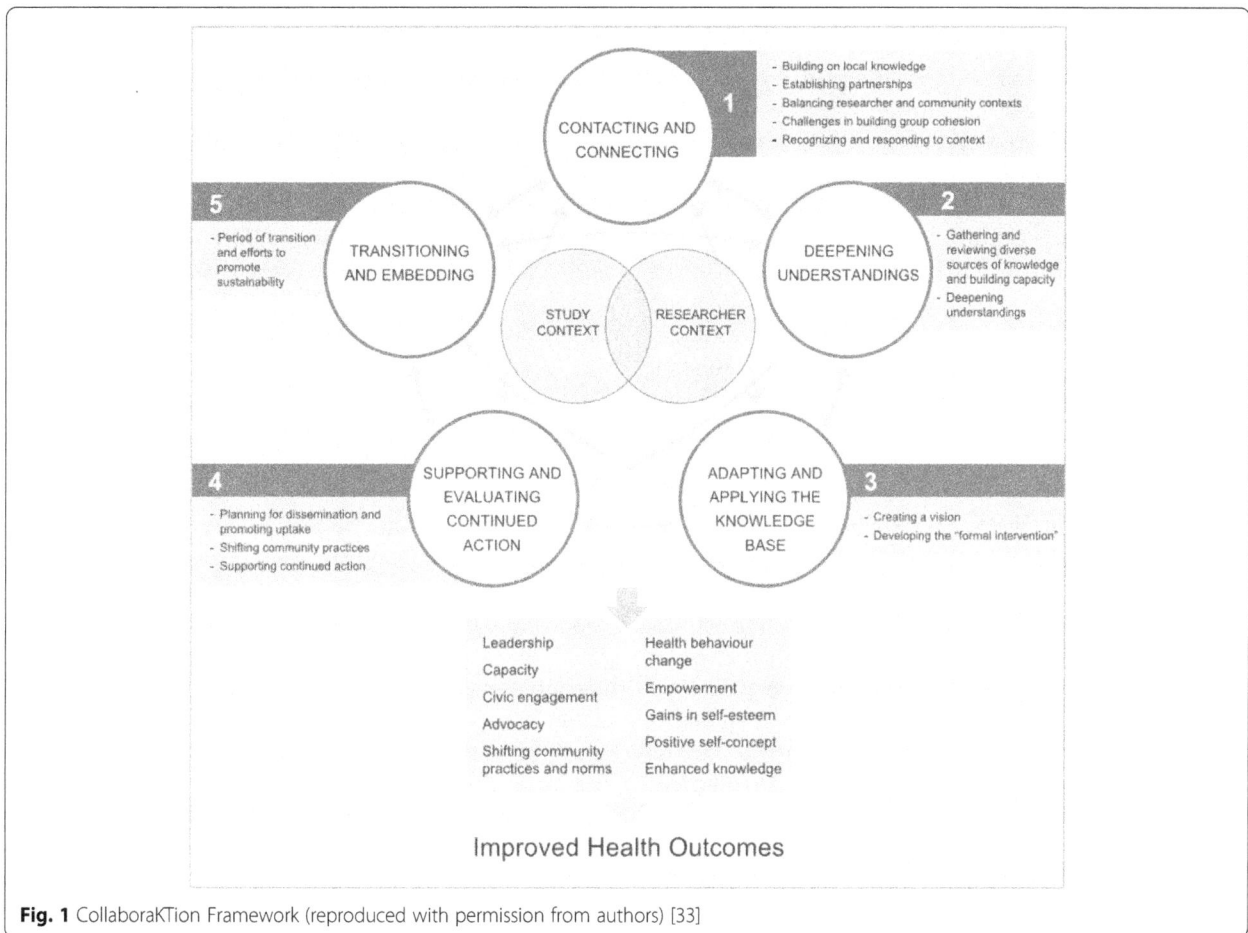

Fig. 1 CollaboraKTion Framework (reproduced with permission from authors) [33]

Participants

In Fraser East, BC, there were 164 providers (family physicians and nurse practitioners) working in 58 practices; in Eastern Ontario Health Unit, ON, there were 190 providers in 63 practices; and in Central Zone, NS, there were 190 providers in 123 practices. Once the list of practices and providers was verified by each region's stakeholder advisor group, we recruited between 22 and 39 eligible primary care practices via individual primary care providers within the region. Our sample size calculation required a minimum of 15 practices per region to detect minimal differences of 2–5% across jurisdictions in two main patient-level performance indicators, access and continuity of care, using a Bonferroni-corrected two sided alpha level of 0.017 to account for multiple pair-wise comparisons. For these calculations, we used estimated standard deviations and intraclass correlation coefficients from data collected in the Comparison of Primary Care Models in Ontario study [4]. These calculations take into account that patients who share the same provider may be more similar to each other and may have similar primary care experiences, and that different providers from the same practice may not practice

as independently from each other as providers in different practices. A maximum of five physicians/ nurse practitioners per *independent* practice were eligible to participate. Based on previous work [36], practices were considered independent if they did not share more than four of the following five criteria: 1) office space; 2) staff; 3) expenses; 4) patient records; and 5) on-call duties. Physicians and nurse practitioners were eligible to participate if they met the following criteria: 1) must be part of their current practice for at least 1 yr; 2) identify that practice as their "principal clinical practice"; and 3) practice comprehensive, all-ages primary care and not limit their practice to a special focus such as sports medicine, emergency medicine, palliative care, or psychotherapy (i.e., the special focus does not comprise more than 20% of their total practice time).

Recruitment

Providers were initially informed about the study through a letter or email sent by local decision-makers. Research coordinators in each region then mailed out a recruitment letter to physicians with an expression of interest mail-back card enclosed. Those who sent back expression of interest cards were contacted immediately by the research coordinators, whereas those practices who did not send back an expression of interest were contacted by phone after ten business days. We expected to send up to three follow-up reminder emails/phone calls but left our recruitment protocol open to more contacts if needed. For consenting practices, organizational leads were asked to complete one organizational survey, and one to five physicians or nurse practitioners completed a provider survey in each practice. To minimize burden on providers, this survey was kept as short as possible (e.g. number of years practicing, age range, gender). All staff were also asked to complete one Team Climate Survey [37, 38]. Once practices agreed to participate, we then recruited a consecutive sample of their patients (a minimum of 20 per practice) to fill out a paper-based patient experience survey. Patients were eligible to participate if the following criteria were met: 1) aged 18 years and over; 2) have been with their current provider for at least 1 yr; and 3) able to complete the survey in either English or French.

Data were collected between 2014 and 2016. Provider and organizational surveys were collected using REDCap (Research Electronic Data Capture) [39] or paper surveys. A survey administrator distributed patient surveys in primary care practice waiting rooms. Written informed consent was obtained from all clinicians and patients. Patients were specifically asked for written consent to: a) participate in the survey, b) have their survey data linked to the administrative data, c) be contacted again for further related studies. All procedures were approved by the Behavioural Research Ethics Boards at Fraser Health, University of British Columbia, Ottawa Health Science Network, Bruyère Continuing Care, and the Nova Scotia Health Authority.

Data sources & analysis
Data for this report of study recruitment methods were derived from qualitative sources including: study team meeting minutes; memos/notes from survey administrators regarding their interactions with practice staff, providers, and patient participants; and stakeholder meeting minutes. Data were also derived from spreadsheets with numbers for participant eligibility, responses, and survey completions and from time and cost tracking for recruitment and survey administration.

All notes were electronically documented. We used the CollaboraKTion framework steps to guide our analysis. Notes were read several times and coded by two members of the research team according to the first three steps: contacting and connecting; deepening understandings; and adapting and applying the knowledge base. Codes were then organized into themes; initial coding and author agreement was reached through an iterative process of discussion and returning to the data.

We calculated participation and completion rates for the patient surveys using the Wong et al. [12] approach to calculating the different rates for comparability with existing literature on CBPHC performance measurement. This method tracked the participation process, allowing the elucidation of "steps" and their respective attrition rates. The project had one research coordinator per region, which represents our fixed costs of carrying out this work. We also calculated a detailed breakdown of variable costs required for practice recruitment and survey implementation in each province.

Results
A total of 87 practices participated in the study ($n = 22$ in BC; $n = 26$ in ON; $n = 39$ in NS). Future analyses will be conducted using administrative health data to better understand how our sample compares to the larger population studied and how our sample compares to another practice-based survey sample conducted for the Quality and Costs of Primary Care Study [12].

Recruitment procedures
In recruiting practices, the first three CollaboraKTion activities, Contacting and Connecting, Deepening Understandings, and Adapting and Applying the Knowledge Base, and their associated processes were most pertinent to our participant and community engagement strategy. As CBPHC performance measurement and reporting continues beyond the end of the study and scales up in the study regions, the other two CollaboraKTion activities, Supporting and Evaluating Continued Action, and, Transitioning and Embedding, will become more relevant with continued re-iteration through the other three activities. Table 1 provides an overview of the specific actions we took in engagement during our recruitment and data collection phase. In keeping with the iterative nature of the CollaboraKTion framework, the described actions did not necessarily happen chronologically as presented. Extracting the qualitative data and our spreadsheets on recruitment training was key for our discussion of the costs associated with recruitment (Excel tracking sheets) and the different strategies for engagement in each region (meeting minutes and data collection notes).

Contacting and connecting
Building on local knowledge
Determining the landscape of CBPHC practices in each region was challenging due to a lack of centralized sources that describe regional primary care practice structures. We conducted an extensive investigation in each region on the number and types of practices present. For example, in Ontario, we worked with the regional health authority called the Champlain Local

Table 1 Variation in approaches across sites

	General approaches	Regional additions/variation		
		BC	ON	NS
Practice Recruitment	Regional study advisory stakeholder committee	Yes – comprised of lead physicians and executive directors from the Chilliwack, Abbotsford and Hope Divisions of Family Practice[a], other health professionals, patients, and policy makers (n = 12)	No - Email correspondence with local physicians and policy makers for advice (n = 6)	Yes – comprised of local physicians, other health professionals, patients, and policy makers (n = 12)
	Engagement with local organizations	Partnership with Divisions of Family Practice. Meetings with Doctors of BC and General Practice Service Committee	Presentations to the Association of Family Health Teams, Health Quality Ontario, and the Ministry of Health and Long-Term Care	Meetings with the Nova Scotia Health Authority Department of Family Practice, Department of Health and Wellness, Provincial Primary Health Care Teams Operations Networking Group
	Presence at physician-attended events	Standalone TRANSFORMATION events hosted by each Division of Family Practice in the study region Billing Workshop for physicians	Local Health Integration Network (LHIN) conference[a]	Health authority's Career Development Event Health authority's Department of Family Practice Forum
	Peer-to-peer practice recruitment	Three peer-to-peer recruiters.	Four geographically-dispersed peer-to-peer recruiters	One peer-to-peer recruiter
	Demonstrate study relevance	Offered practice-based portrait of study findings 1-page brief created, with preliminary data as it is available, for peer-to-peer recruiters to use Standalone TRANFORMATION catered dinner to share preliminary data	Practices already receive practice-based feedback from provincial organization	Offered practice-based portrait of study findings
Patient Recruitment	Localized survey implementation	Hired localized survey administrators (SAs) Hired Punjabi-speaking SA for practices with high proportion (> 50%) of Punjabi-speaking patients	Did not hire localized SAs because researchers did not have sufficient ties to research assistants in the study region Surveys available in both English and French	Hired localized SAs Surveys only available in English
	Token of appreciation	$10 coffee gift card to patients	No gift card offered	$5 coffee gift cards to patients

[a]Divisions of Family Practice are groups of family physicians that work to achieve common health care goals within communities [49]; Local Integrated Health Networks (LHINs) are community-based health authorities that plan and coordinate local health care services [50]

Health Integration Network (LHIN) to identify practicing family physicians and nurse practitioners. In all regions, we used other publicly available sources such as information from the College of Family Physicians of Canada, provincial Colleges, local health authorities, and Google.

We hired survey administrators, who had local knowledge of the communities within each region to administer the patient surveys at each participating clinic. Their presence allowed the research team to work directly with the practice staff and patients. In NS and BC, Regional Stakeholder Advisory Committees were formed to advise on all aspects of the study, including tailoring recruitment approaches in each region. These committees included local experts who held a variety of roles, including patients, physicians and decision-makers, in a variety of clinical, academic, policy, and other decision-making contexts. Ontario took a different approach by individually engaging physician opinion leaders representative of their study region. Together, team members and clinicians strategized how to avoid overwhelming practices by being aware of potentially competing "asks" on their time. For example, in NS, we were mindful not to recruit during times when several other local asks for practice participation in research were in progress. When the study team noted enrollment of new practices coming to a standstill, all regions employed local physician peer-to-peer practice recruiters. These paid physician recruiters were identified through existing relationships with the research team and were chosen largely based on their connections to the local physician community.

Establishing partnerships
Having previous experience in physician and patient recruitment but minimal or modest existing networks of relationships within the study regions, the team devoted substantial resources to engage practices in recruitment.

Over a series of regional advisory meetings, 13 in BC and 7 in NS, we listened and learned about how primary care was delivered in each jurisdiction and the political tensions in conducting research or trying to measure performance of primary care. In addition, we established and held meetings of an International Stakeholder Advisory Group consisting of international experts in primary care research, utilizing one of the meetings to learn from the expertise of the committee to better understand recruitment issues. To foster ongoing relationships, we invited several local and provincial decision-makers from each study region to annual face-to-face full team meetings and to other team meetings within the region. In BC, we partnered closely with three Divisions of Family Practice, who provided guidance for tailored recruitment in each Division. In exchange, we provided the option to give data back to the Divisions (with participants' consent). We also made presentations to other relevant physician-attended community organizations and initiatives, locally and beyond (See Table 1).

Balancing researcher and community (clinical) contexts

The divide between academic and clinical contexts emerged early in our recruitment over the use of the term "independent" practices. For clinicians, the term independent was tied to notions of being independently responsible for their medical practice, whereas for the purposes of our study, an independent physician shares up to four of the following features: space, staff, on-call duties, records, and finances [36]. In BC, decision makers and clinicians had particular challenges with this definition as it didn't fit with their conceptualization or realities of practice (physicians who had independent panels of patients but were working in large groups). However, we had designed and funded recruitment based on assumptions of how family physicians were practicing (mostly single providers) [36]. Given our mutual authentic engagement on this grant, clinicians, health authority partners and researchers were able to appreciate each other's contexts and carry on with recruitment and data collection. Scientific rigor and recruitment according to our eligibility was maintained. It was also agreed that the research team provide participating practices with a report on their individual performance, if requested.

The research team was able to recruit some practices on their own. However, there were competing demands for time by clinicians on our team. For example, one clinician on our team also was a senior administrator in ON. He was enthusiastic about the goal of our study (CBPHC performance measurement and reporting) and originally agreed to help recruit practices and promote the study and its objectives but was unable to commit the time to fulfill his role due to ongoing and emerging priorities in his regular position.

In order to balance research and clinical contexts we used two additional recruitment strategies. First, we employed physician recruiters, 3 in BC, 4 in ON, and 1 in NS, who were more likely to understand the day-to-day practice reality and connect directly with potential physician participants. Physician peer recruiters were successful in recruiting "harder to reach" CBPHC practices. These were practices in which the research coordinator had made three follow-up phone calls but still had no answer from the practice. Research coordinators spent approximately 30% or more of their time on recruitment for three to 4 mos before the peer-to-peer recruiters were employed to assist with practice recruitment. All recruiters, except for one, were selected largely based on their pre-existing relationships with many of the practices in each region. Second, in order to keep data collection minimally disruptive for practices, we hired survey administrators who could work with each practice's population. Survey administrators worked in English (all regions), Punjabi (BC), and French (ON).

To address the known barriers regarding provider compensation for participation in research, we offered a number of incentives for participation. Upon completion of the provider and organizational surveys, practices received an honorarium in recognition for their time ($250 in NS and BC; $500 in ON). Offering additional funds to providers in ON was a local strategy developed after the initial protocol. Family physicians were also offered Continuing Medical Education credits. In BC and NS, the practice staff who worked with our survey administrator, as well as patients who completed the patient survey, were provided with coffee cards (e.g. Tim Horton's, Starbucks) as a token of appreciation.

In order to balance the clinical contexts, researchers built relationships with each consenting practice in order to find dates and times for recruiting potential patients. On practices' requests, a poster for the lunch or staff room was provided to each practice to inform and/or remind staff when patient recruitment will take place. On the date set by practices, a survey administrator from TRANSFORMATION recruited up to 20 consecutive patients for each participating physician/nurse practitioner. A key relationship was between the survey administrator and the office staff. Together, they went over procedures for recruitment and data collection. Practice staff were provided with a script to introduce patients to our on-site survey administrator. The survey administrator then explained the study, assessed eligibility, and obtained informed consent from participants. Patients were also asked if they would like to participate in related studies (e.g. focus groups and/or deliberative dialogues), consent to link their survey data to health administrative data via patient health card numbers, and consent to a follow-up phone or email survey of approximately five questions.

Challenges in building group cohesion

Our recruitment and engagement strategy was diverse. It did not require all stakeholders to totally agree on our processes across or within the regions. We did, however, encounter challenges with group cohesion when it was desired. Neither ON nor NS had purposeful organizations of CBPHC practices such as divisions of family practice in BC (See Table 1). In ON, the large geography of the study region paired with the concentration of the investigators and study staff in a single metropolitan area outside of the study region prohibited the formation of a cohesive regional stakeholder advisory committee. Instead, ON had 6 study advisors whom we consulted on an ad hoc basis. In the other regions, we struggled to sustain committee participation and had particular trouble finding meaningful ways to engage patient members. For example, in NS, we sent out an open call for patient representatives through a local volunteer recruitment website. We recruited three patient representatives to the committee. While the study team did not expect the patient representatives to have very much knowledge of the study topic prior to committee participation, we had hoped that orientation to the topic over multiple meetings would spur interest, but inconsistent attendance at meetings and the prioritization of personal agendas only tangentially related to the study topic were barriers to meaningful and productive involvement. More targeted patient recruitment approaches in BC, through an existing patient engagement organization, yielded representatives better equipped to engage with our study topic, as this organization matches patient representatives to opportunities suited to their interests.

Deepening understandings
Gathering and reviewing diverse sources of knowledge and building capacity

We aimed to build our own skills in the contexts of our study regions and share our learnings with the broader community to raise awareness and capacity for CBPHC performance measurement and reporting. We began the study with an understanding of the challenges of provider and patient recruitment from several previous studies and initially drafted our recruitment strategies using best practices found in the literature. We looked to our regional committees and advisors to help amend and contextualize our procedures and to communicate back out with their communities. Similarly, we met with a number of provincial organizations, which allowed for a two-way dialogue. We also met with several other provincial, national, and international stakeholders, including our international

scientific advisory committee, to gather advice and share our own findings to the international community. In several of these engagements, we shared our surveys to inform tool development for other performance measurement and related initiatives.

Deepening understandings

Meeting recruitment targets hinged on making our work relevant to potential participants and deepening their knowledge of CBPHC performance measurement and reporting. We presented to a large number of national, provincial, and regional stakeholders to spread the word about performance measurement and the value of our study. Our regional advisory committees identified the need for practice feedback and advised us on how to proceed. In the spirit of reciprocity, we offered to produce Practice Portraits for participating practices that would contain practice-level information from the suite of surveys, linked to health administrative data.

Adapting and applying the knowledge base
Creating a vision

Unlike the prescribed use of Co-KT and CollaboraKTion frameworks, our vision to create conditions conducive to comprehensive CBPHC performance measurement with sufficient response rates in the study regions was determined a priori. However, through extensive engagement with relevant communities in each region, we integrated their knowledge to iteratively refine the vision. We identified and posited solutions to barriers we faced specifically in the recruitment and engagement strategy and generally in promoting CBPHC performance measurement and reporting.

Developing the information system

In our study, we introduced CBPHC performance measurement and reporting approaches, and through our iterative recruitment strategies, tested their sustainability and acceptance in the study regions. Our methods manifested differently in each study region in reaction to contacting and connecting with local stakeholders and reciprocally deepening understandings of the local researcher and clinical realities. To overcome challenges in recruiting practices and patients, we implemented a "learning system" approach, using a variety of strategies with localized, contextual variations. A core set of the research team (co-principal investigators and staff) met weekly to deal with any issues arising during the course of recruitment and data collection; we continuously revised our methods, within the protocol limits, by learning from our sample.

Practice recruitment

Practice participation and completion rates for all three study regions are presented in Fig. 2. Participation rates was similar (average was 36%) across the study sites and completion rates were high (99%) once practices agreed to participate.

Patient recruitment

Patient participation and completion rates for all three study regions are presented in Fig. 3. Participation rates in BC were substantially lower than in the ON or NS sites. In part, this may have been due to the involvement of front office staff. In BC, the receptionist only introduced patients to the survey administrator (SA) if the patients were both interested and eligible, whereas the front office staff in the other provinces were encouraged to send all interested patients to the SA so that the SA could directly screen the patients for eligibility. While all provinces had intended on the receptionist screening for patient eligibility, we found that the staff in ON and NS were too busy to do this additional step. It is possible that the BC front office staff may have informally screened patients for eligibility in a way that some patients who could have been eligible and interested in participating were not told about the study. We learned that the front office staff appreciated being as minimally disrupted as possible, and in cases such as ours where there was an opportunity for research staff to be on site during patient survey recruitment and data collection, it may be advantageous to screen for patient eligibility directly.

Time and variable costs of practice recruitment and data collection

The variable costs required to recruit practices and administer the patient surveys ranged from $1503 to $1792 and are summarized in Table 2. In BC and NS, the survey administrator was embedded within the community so less time (and expenses) was spent on travel. In ON, the survey administrator was based at the university and spent more time in travel. The lower practice recruitment costs in the areas of peer recruiter and community engagement in NS are likely due to the fact that they had the highest number of eligible practices in their study region and they were able to recruit more practices. Researchers in NS also had strong ties to decision maker leads and existing research relationships with many of the physicians in the region and the peer recruiter for NS stood out in that they were particularly capable of quickly recruiting practices, largely due to pre-existing relationships with physicians in the community.

Each region strategized practice recruitment expenditures differently. Although recruiting practices was the main concern for success of our study and was also the largest recruitment expense, we did funnel some funds into patient recruitment. BC and NS offered coffee cards to front office staff and participating patients. Given the lack of existing relationships between researchers and potential practice participants and the known time conflicts of providers in the ON study region, the research team in ON decided to offer practices a higher honorarium amount than the other provinces ($500 vs. $250). This meant that they did not have the funds to offer gift cards to patients. BC also used funds for community engagement and peer recruiters. Across all sites, recruitment funds were targeted in ways most appropriate to their given contexts.

Discussion

Recruiting primary care practices and gathering data from clinicians, staff, and patients, who are considered to be in the best position to report on specific core attributes of primary care, is feasible. We outlined our

	BC	ON	NS	TOTAL
Eligible practices in study region	58	63	123	244
Participation rate of practices n(%)	22 (37.9%)	26 (41.3%)	39 (31.7%)	87 (35.7%)
Completion rate of practices n(%)	22 (100.0%)	26 (100.0%)	38 (97.4%)	86 (98.8%)

Fig. 2 Participation rates of practices. Participation rates were calculated as the number of practices that were recruited to the study divided by the number of eligible practices in the region, all of which were invited to participate. Completion rates were calculated as the number of practices that returned completed (at least 85% of questions answered) organizational surveys divided by the total number of participating practices. British Columbia (BC), Ontario (ON), Nova Scotia (NS)

	BC	ON	NS	TOTAL
Total number of patients seen by participating physician/nurse practitioner	1848	1562	3311	**6721**
Number of patients who received a consent discussion (i.e., both interested AND eligible)	887	669	1077	**2633**
Participation rate of patients n(%)	504 (56.8%)	572 (85.5%)	878 (81.5%)	**1954 (74.2%)**
Completion rate of patients n(%)	490 (97.2%)	539 (94.2%)	807 (91.9%)	**1836 (94.0%)**

Fig. 3 Participation and completion rates for patient recruitment. Participation rates were calculated as the number of patients who consented to participate divided by the number of interested and eligible patients. Completion rates were calculated as the number of patients who completed 85% or more of the survey questions divided by the total number of patients who consented to participate. British Columbia (BC), Ontario (ON), Nova Scotia (NS)

challenges and successes in practice recruitment, as well as the variable costs associated with recruitment and data collection, taking local contexts into account and engaging the community through a KTE approach. Across the study we also had fixed costs of a research coordinator per region. The generalizability of our results is enhanced in that we took our findings from three different Canadian health regions across BC, ON, and NS. As part of our KTE approach, we emphasize the necessity to arrive at a tailored approach to recruitment, through a process of community engagement and adapting to the needs of each region. Much time was spent within the three jurisdictions on 1) contacting and connecting with primary care practices; 2) deepening understandings of each other as service delivery clinicians and researchers; and 3) adapting and applying our common and distinct knowledge bases to create a common vision and develop a primary care information system.

Insights from our study show that multijurisdictional research initiatives may require different strategies in each region to achieve similar recruitment rates. Flexibility of protocols and recruitment budgets are key, and researchers should seek local inputs throughout research processes. Researchers should note that tailoring approaches may result in project delays when navigating the complexities of multijurisdictional research (e.g. multiple research ethics boards, different requirements for data privacy, etc). Through strategies such as partnering with local advisors and decision makers and hiring peer-to-peer recruiters, the 'contacting and connecting' theme was the most immediately integral of the three themes to recruiting practices. However, each

Table 2 Time and variable costs for practice-based survey data collection

	BC	ON	NS	All sites
Number of practices	22	26	39	87
Mean number of data collection days per practice (SD)	2.32 (1.86)	3.50 (1.50)	4.95 (2.89)	3.89 (2.43)
Honoraria for practices/providers	$5500	$13,000	$9750	$28,250
Tokens of appreciation for staff and patients	$5240	$0	$5645	$10,885
Physician peer recruiters	$5916	$3360	$2145	$11,421
Community engagement for implementation	$7886	$3805	$3641	$15,332
Survey administrators for patient survey implementation	$14,894	$25,938	$37,441	$78,273
Total	$39,436	$46,103	$58,622	$144,161
Average costs per practice	$1793	$1773	$1503	$1657

The cost of Survey Administrators includes travel time and mileage ($25 CAD/hour, $0.40 CAD/km), time spent in practice, meals, and accommodation. Cost of community engagement includes honoraria for committee participants, meeting costs, travel for external presentations, and bringing decision makers to full team face-to-face meetings of the three integrated KTE themes were integral to our current and future success in the long term by furthering buy-in to our study's objective in a way that was meaningful and useful to participants. Using this multi-pronged approach to recruitment, we were able to recruit 32–41% of all eligible practices in a region. This is an achievement, particularly considering we were asking a lot out of practices (four different types of surveys, patient data collection over multiple days, etc.). Reasons given for not participating were similar to what has been reported in past work: time constraints, disruption to clinic flow, fear of performance evaluation and its consequences [13–15] and that survey administration with their specific patient panels (e.g. high number who were Indigenous) was not appropriate.

A comprehensive data collection system in primary care that can drive improvement is possible to achieve with partnerships that balance researcher, clinical and policy maker contexts. There are challenges building group cohesion and recruiting independently owned and operated primary care practices. Working with practices ought to take a two-way learning approach. Engaging with practices and building relationships between researchers and clinicians take time. Importantly, implementation of findings requires capturing their minds, hearts and attention with the significance of the work being proposed. By re-orienting our approach from project-based – entering practices only to collect data once and then leaving – to a KTE approach for recruitment, we can engage with practices and other stakeholders iteratively over time. Our approach is likely too expensive for widespread use throughout primary care. However, we suggest this framework could be used more broadly in primary care in thinking about how to create ongoing relationships for purposes of healthcare learning at the health authority level. In particular, it is helpful for considering front-end strategy development, relationship building, and flexible recruitment implementation. Primary care practices are an essential part of each community. Engaging them as valued community members and independent business owners requires significant time and resources.

Indeed, several strategies have proven successful in improving physician response rates to survey research, which embed elements of a KTE strategy. In addition to modified versions of the proven Dillman approach [40], many recruitment protocols focus on engagement strategies targeted to local contexts. Regional factors vary, requiring recruiters to adapt tailored and iterative recruitment approaches [41]. Clinician-to-clinician recruitment has been used successfully to improve physician response rates [13, 41, 42], where familiarity between the recruiter and participant improves rapport [43]. In particular, using recruiters who are known to

prospective participants allows them to be cognizant of and responsive to local conditions that may affect participation [44]. Similarly, endorsement from professional organizations synchronized with that from local champions have also been shown to assist in recruitment [41, 42, 45]. These strategies align with our peer-to-peer approach, which had variable success across the study regions.

A lesson learned from our work is the value of budgeting for flexibility in recruitment approaches and that some regions may need more time and resources than others. We show how we flexibly use recruitment funds, channeling them differently in the three regional contexts to achieve similar response rates. Ontario had the highest recruitment rate for both practices and patients. This region offered more funds to the physician than the other regions and did not offer patients or practice staff a gift card. Given that the practices, not the patients, were the most challenging to recruit, ON's strategy for higher physician compensation may have contributed to the better responses. Another lesson learned is to be mindful and understand the interplay of relationships within each local context. For example, some of the providers in our regions expressed disinterest in our study due to tensions with our local partners (provincial ministries and regional health authorities). It is helpful to keep these types of tensions in mind when working with local partners.

The literature on recruitment strategies is focused on pre-data collection recruitment and does not capture post-study engagement. Steps four and five of the CollaboraKTion framework [34], supporting and evaluating continued action, and, transitioning and embedding, describe continued engagement throughout intervention development, implementation, and beyond. In the context of our study's research topic, CBPHC performance measurement and reporting, recruitment was conceptualized as an ongoing and iterative KTE activity. Building a learning research environment, where practices' participation comes with access to expertise and opportunities to learn about and shape performance reports useful to them and recruitment for subsequent studies facilitated by the involvement of past participants, could be a solution to historically low primary care participation.

The recruitment and data collection strategy of TRANSFORMATION adds to the existing literature on practice-based engagement, above and beyond physician recruitment. The regional stakeholder advisory committees in BC and NS are an important component of the integrated KTE approach. These committees will assist in carrying out the CollaboraKTion framework steps of supporting and evaluating continued action and transitioning and embedding knowledge. Our model of connecting with community partners and stakeholders will also continue as the study progresses through presentations, meetings, and stakeholder feedback on the products of our study.

This work is limited in that we worked with three geographic areas within three provinces. While these learnings may not apply to all jurisdictions, those with similar contexts may find this information useful. Our "intervention" of performance measurement and reporting was researcher driven and not as participatory in some respects, such as how a practice was defined. Ideally, the community and researchers would jointly agree on all aspects of the research project, including the intervention, before undertaking the study. Also, given the tendency of practice-based surveys to have certain response biases [46, 47], an important part of our future analysis will be to assess for the representativeness of our survey sample.

A community-based engagement approach can be expensive. Developing trust and lasting relationships requires time, energy, and financial resources. Managing the regional budgets required localized approaches and trade-offs. For example, in ON, higher per-practice honoraria were offered instead of tokens of appreciation for patients. In addition to the added costs of the intensive hands-on recruitment and survey administration strategies, such as community engagement, hiring peer recruiters, and hiring local highly qualified survey administrators, practices still expect to be compensated for their participation in research activities [13, 14, 48]. One place to decrease costs and potentially increase the recruitment rate of practices may be to administer patient surveys using electronic approaches and automation of patient recruitment. Automating patient, provider, and organizational survey administration could assist if CBPHC practices routinely need to collect data or if there was demand for a more widespread (e.g. multiple health authorities, provinces, etc.) practice-based survey to inform delivery of primary care.

Conclusions

The CollaboraKTion framework was a good match for our study in that we were able to use the framework to more comprehensibly organize our discussion of our recruitment activities. There are some key lessons which could assist in future primary care work. First, collecting data from patients, clinicians, and teams requires community-based engagement strategies as early as possible. The roles of the office staff (receptionist, office manager) are important to successful recruitment and data collection. While some automated extraction of data from primary care is possible (e.g. via electronic medical records or telephone robots), the need to engage practices and patients will continue to be necessary. Second, our practice recruitment rate (36%) remained

similarly low, and therefore likely lacks external generalizability to the regions, across the three sites despite context-specific strategies and working with different primary care organizations such as the Divisions of Family Practice in BC. Without a clear need to participate in practice-based surveys (e.g. requirement to report on patient experiences in order to receive funding), working with CBPHC practices remains challenging. More work is needed to increase participation rates of CBPHC practices within regions. Third, engaged CBPHC practices, however, play an important role in developing, contributing to and implementing research, quality initiatives and system change. Co-created recruitment and data collection strategies in addition to a feedback loop between researchers, clinicians, policy makers and patients can move us in the direction of a learning health system in primary care. Finally, an integrated KTE approach provides a foundation for continued dialogue, exchange of ideas, use of the information produced, and recognises recruitment as part of an ongoing cycle that supports the need to develop our culture of learning in CBPHC.

Abbreviations
BC: British Columbia; CBPHC: Community-based primary health care; KTE: Knowledge translation and exchange; LHIN: Local Health Integration Network; NS: Nova Scotia; ON: Ontario; SA: Survey administrator

Acknowledgements
The authors wish to acknowledge Sara Wuite, Jackie Schultz, the survey administrators and practices for their help in developing this work.

Funding
This research was funded by the Canadian Institutes of Health Research (grant number TTF-128265) and Michael Smith Foundation (grant number PT-CPH-00001-134).

Authors' contributions
Contributions to the conception of the manuscript –all authors. Involved in critically revising manuscript for intellectual content – all authors. Given final approval of the version to be published – all authors. Accountable for the integrity of the work – all authors.

Competing interests
The authors declare that they have no competing interests.

Author details

[1]School of Nursing, University of British Columbia, T201 2211 Westbrook Mall, Vancouver, BC V6T 2B5, Canada. [2]Centre for Health Services and Policy Research, University of British Columbia, 201-2206 East Mall, Vancouver, BC V6T 1Z3, Canada. [3]Department of Family Medicine, University of Ottawa, 201-600 Peter Morand Cresc, Ottawa, ON K1G 5Z3, Canada. [4]Montfort Hospital Research Institute 713 Montreal Rd, Ottawa, ON K1K 0T2, Canada. [5]Department of Family Medicine, Dalhousie University, 5909 Veterans' Memorial Lane, Abbie J. Lane Building, Halifax, NS B3H 2E2, Canada.

References

1. Berwick DM, Nolan TW, Whittington J. The triple aim: care, health, and cost. Health Aff. 2008;27:759–69.

2. Bodenheimer T, Ghorob A, Willard-Grace R, Grumbach K. The 10 building blocks of high-performing primary care. Ann Fam Med. 2014;12:166–71. https://doi.org/10.1370/afm.1616.

3. Hogg W, Johnston S, Russell G, Dahrouge S, Gyorfi-Dyke E, Kristjanssonn E. Conducting waiting room surveys in practice-based primary care research: a user's guide. Can Fam Physician. 2010;56:1375–6. http://www.ncbi.nlm.nih.gov/pubmed/21156900. Accessed 23 Feb 2017

4. Dahrouge S, Hogg W, Russell G, Geneau R, Kristjansson E, Muldoon L, et al. The comparison of models of primary Care in Ontario (COMP-PC) study: methodology of a multifaceted cross-sectional practice-based study. Open Med. 2009;3:149–64. https://www.ncbi.nlm.nih.gov/pmc/articles/PMC3090123/. Accessed 15 Jan 2015

5. Jaakkimainen L, Klein-Geltink JE, Guttman A, Barnsley J, Zagorski BN, Kopp A, et al. Indicators of primary care based on administrative data. In: Jaakimanian L, Upshur R, Klein-Geltink J, Leong A, Maaten S, Schultz S, et al., editors. Primary care in Ontario: ICES atlas. Toronto, Inst for Clinical Evaluative Sci; 2006. p. 207–50.

6. Stukel TA, Croxford R, Rahman F, Bierman AS, Glazier RH. Variations in quality indicators across Ontario physician networks. Toronto: Institute for Clinical Evaluative Sciences; 2016. https://www.ices.on.ca/Publications/Atlases-and-Reports/2016/Variations-in-Quality-Indicators-Across-Ontario-Physician-Networks. Accessed 7 Dec 2017

7. Tu K, Mitiku TF, Ivers NM, Guo H, Lu H, Jaakkimainen L, et al. Evaluation of electronic medical record administrative data linked database (EMRALD). Am J Manag Care. 2014;20:e15–21.

8. Green ME, Hogg W, Savage C, Johnston S, Russell G, Jaakkimainen RL, et al. Assessing methods for measurement of clinical outcomes and quality of care in primary care practices. BMC Health Serv Res. 2012;12:214. https://doi.org/10.1186/1472-6963-12-214.

9. Cook JV, Dickinson HO, Eccles MP. Response rates in postal surveys of healthcare professionals between 1996 and 2005: an observational study. BMC Health Serv Res. 2009;9:160. https://doi.org/10.1186/1472-6963-9-160.

10. The College of Family Physicians of Canada, Canadian Medical Association, The Royal College of Physicians and Surgeons of Canada. 2010 National Physician Survey (NPS): National Demographics. 2010. http://nationalphysiciansurvey.ca/wp-content/uploads/2012/05/2010-NationalDemographics.pdf. Accessed 27 Feb 2017.

11. The College of Family Physicians of Canada, Canadian Medical Association, The Royal College of Physicians and Surgeons of Canada. 2014 National Physician Survey (NPS): National Demographics. 2014. http://nationalphysiciansurvey.ca/wp-content/uploads/2014/10/NPS-2014-National-Demographics-EN.pdf. Accessed 27 Feb 2017.

12. Wong ST, Chau LW, Hogg W, Teare GF, Miedema B, Breton M, et al. An international cross-sectional survey on the Quality and Costs of Primary Care (QUALICO-PC): recruitment and data collection of places delivering primary care across Canada. BMC Fam Pract. 2015;16:20. https://doi.org/10.1186/s12875-015-0236-7.

13. Cave A, Ahmadi E, Makarowski C. Recruiting issues in community-based studies: some advice from lessons learned. Can Fam Physician. 2009;55:557–8. http://www.ncbi.nlm.nih.gov/pubmed/19439712. Accessed 23 Feb 2017

14. Shelton BJ, Wofford JL, Gosselink CA, McClatchey MW, Brekke K, Conry C, et al. Recruitment and retention of physicians for primary care research. J Community Health. 2002;27:79–89. http://www.ncbi.nlm.nih.gov/pubmed/11936759. Accessed 23 Feb 2017

15. Robitaille H, Légaré F, Tre G. A systematic process for recruiting physician-patient dyads in practice-based research networks (PBRNs). J Am Board Fam Med. 2014;27:740–9. https://doi.org/10.3122/jabfm.2014.06.140035.

16. Armstrong K, Kendall E. Translating knowledge into practice and policy: the role of knowledge networks in primary health care. Heal Inf Manag J. 2010;39:9–17.

17. Health Quality Ontario. Quality matters: realizing excellent care for all. 2017. http://www.hqontario.ca/Portals/0/documents/health-quality/realizing-excellent-care-for-all-1704-en.pdf. Accessed 12 Jun 2017.

18. The Commonwealth Fund. 2011 Commonwealth Fund international health policy survey. New York, NY: The Commonwealth Fund; 2011. http://www.commonwealthfund.org/interactives-and-data/surveys/international-health-policy-surveys/2011/2011-international-survey. Accessed 7 Dec 2017

19. Faber M, Bosch M, Wollersheim H, Leatherman S, Grol R. Public reporting in health care: how do consumers use quality-of-care information? A systematic review. Med Care. 2009;47:1–8. https://www.ncbi.nlm.nih.gov/pubmed/19106724

20. Watson DE. For discussion: a roadmap for population-based information systems to enhance primary healthcare in Canada. Healthc Policy. 2009;5(Special Issue):105–20. http://www.pubmedcentral.nih.gov/articlerender.fcgi?artid=2906208&tool=pmcentrez&rendertype=abstract. Accessed 23 Aug 2013

21. Hibbard JH, Greene J, Sofaer S, Firminger K, Hirsh J. An experiment shows that a well-designed report on costs and quality can help consumers choose high-value health care. Health Aff. 2012;31:560–8. https://www.ncbi.nlm.nih.gov/pubmed/22392666

22. Smith MA, Wright A, Queram C, Lamb GC. Public reporting helped drive quality improvement in outpatient diabetes care among Wisconsin physician groups. Health Aff. 2012;31:570–7. https://www.ncbi.nlm.nih.gov/pmc/articles/PMC3329125/

23. Young GJ. Multistakeholder regional collaboratives have been key drivers of public reporting, but now face challenges. Health Aff. 2012;31:578–84. https://www.ncbi.nlm.nih.gov/pubmed/22392669

24. Tu JV, Donovan LR, Lee DS, Wang JT, Austin PC, Alter DA, et al. Effectiveness of public report cards for improving the quality of cardiac care: the EFFECT study: a randomized trial. J Am Med Assoc. 2009;302:2330–7.

25. Campanella P, Vukovic V, Parente P, Sulejmani A, Ricciardi W, Specchia ML. The impact of public reporting on clinical outcomes: a systematic review and meta-analysis. BMC Health Serv Res. 2016;16:296. https://doi.org/10.1186/s12913-016-1543-y.

26. Lamb GC, Smith MA, Weeks WB, Queram C. Publicly reported quality-of-care measures influenced Wisconsin physician groups to improve performance. Health Aff. 2013;32:536–43. https://doi.org/10.1377/hlthaff.2012.1275.

27. Powell AE, Davies HT, Thomson RG. Using routine comparative data to assess the quality of health care: understanding and avoiding common pitfalls. Qual Saf Heal Care. 2003;12:122–8.

28. Oxman AD, Lewin S, Lavis JN, Fretheim A. SUPPORT tools for evidence-informed health policymaking (STP) 15: engaging the public in evidence-informed policymaking. Heal Res Policy Syst. 2009;7(Suppl 1):1–9. https://doi.org/10.1186/1478-4505-7-S1-S15.

29. Oxman AD, Lavis JN, Lewin S, Fretheim A. SUPPORT Tools for evidence-informed health Policymaking (STP) 1: what is evidence-informed policymaking? Heal Res Policy Syst. 2009;7(Suppl 1):S1.

30. Ellins J, McIver S. Supporting patients to make informed choices in primary care: what works? Birmingham: University of Birmingham Health Services Management Centre; 2009. http://epapers.bham.ac.uk/747/. Accessed 7 Dec 2017

31. van Walraven C, Dhalla IA, Bell C, Etchells E, Stiell IG, Zarnke K, et al. Derivation and validation of an index to predict early death or unplanned readmission after discharge from hospital to the community. Can Med Assoc J. 2010;182:551–7. http://www.cmaj.ca/content/182/6/551.abstract

32. Wong ST, Langton JM. Harnessing patients' voices for improving the healthcare system. In: Carson AS, Nossal KR, editors. Managing a Canadian healthcare strategy. Kingston, ON: McGill-Queen's University Press; 2016. p. 103–23.

33. Haggerty J, Burge F, Lévesque J-F, Gass D, Pineault R, Beaulieu M-D, et al. Operational definitions of attributes of primary health care: consensus among Canadian experts. Ann Fam Med. 2007;5:336–44. https://doi.org/10.1370/afm.682.

34. Jenkins EK, Kothari A, Bungay V, Johnson JL, Oliffe JL. Strengthening population health interventions: developing the CollaboraKTion framework for community-based knowledge translation. Heal Res Policy Syst. 2016;14:65. https://doi.org/10.1186/s12961-016-0138-8.

35. Kitson A, Powell K, Hoon E, Newbury J, Wilson A, Beilby J. Knowledge translation within a population health study: how do you do it? Implement Sci. 2013;8:54. https://doi.org/10.1186/1748-5908-8-54.

36. Hogg WE, Wong ST, Burge F. Statistical research: lost in translation? If you want to get doctors onside, speak their language. Can Fam Physician. 2016;62:524. http://www.ncbi.nlm.nih.gov/pubmed/27303011. Accessed 16 Mar 2017

37. Anderson NR, West MA. Measuring climate for work group innovation: development and validation of the team. J Organ Behav. 1998;19:235–58. https://doi.org/10.1002/(SICI)1099-1379(199805)19:3<235::AID-JOB837>3.0.CO;2-C.

38. Beaulieu M-D, Dragieva N, Del Grande C, Dawson J, Haggerty JL, Barnsley J. The team climate inventory as a measure of primary care teams' processes: validation of the French version. Healthc Policy. 2014;9:40–54.

39. Harris PA, Taylor R, Thielke R, Payne J, Gonzalez N, Conde JG. Research electronic data capture (REDCap): a metadata-driven methodology and workflow process for providing translational research informatics support. J Biomed Inform. 2009;42:377–81. https://doi.org/10.1016/j.jbi.2008.08.010.

40. Hoddinott SN, Bass MJ. The dillman total design survey method. Can Fam Physician. 1986;32:2366–8. http://www.ncbi.nlm.nih.gov/pubmed/21267217. Accessed 23 Feb 2017

41. Johnston S, Liddy C, Hogg W, Donskov M, Russell G, Gyorfi-Dyke E, et al. Barriers and facilitators to recruitment of physicians and practices for primary care health services research at one Centre. BMC Med Res Methodol. 2010;10:109. https://doi.org/10.1186/1471-2288-10-109.

42. Goodyear-Smith F, York D, Petousis-Harris H, Turner N, Copp J, Kerse N, et al. Recruitment of practices in primary care research: the long and the short of it. Fam Pract. 2009;26:128–36. https://doi.org/10.1093/fampra/cmp015.

43. Levinson W, Dull VT, Roter DL, Chaumeton N, Frankel RM. Recruiting physicians for office-based research. Med Care. 1998;36:934–7. http://www.ncbi.nlm.nih.gov/pubmed/9630134. Accessed 23 Feb 2017

44. National Institute of Mental Health. Points to consider about recruitment and retention while preparing a clinical research study; 2005. p. 1–9. https://www.nimh.nih.gov/funding/grant-writing-and-application-process/points-to-consider-about-recruitment-and-retention-while-preparing-a-clinical-research-study.shtml. Accessed 23 Feb 2017

45. McIntosh S, Ossip-Klein D, Hazel-Fernandez L, Spada J, McDonald P, Klein J. Recruitment of physician offices for an office-based adolescent smoking cessation study. Nicotine Tob Res. 2005;7:405–12. https://doi.org/10.1080/14622200500125567.

46. McFarlane E, Olmsted MG, Murphy J, Hill CA. Nonresponse bias in a mail survey of physicians. Eval Health Prof. 2007;30:170–85. https://doi.org/10.1177/0163278707300632.

47. Mazor KM, Clauser BE, Field T, Yood RA, Gurwitz JH. A demonstration of the impact of response bias on the results of patient satisfaction surveys. Health Serv Res. 2000;37:1403–17.

48. Johnston S, Wong ST, Blackman S, Chau LW, Grool AM, Hogg W. Can a customer relationship management program improve recruitment for primary care research studies? Prim Health Care Res Dev. 2017:1–5.

49. Divisions of Family Practice. About us. 2014. https://www.divisionsbc.ca/provincial/aboutus. Accessed 7 Dec 2017.

50. Ontario's LHINs. Local health integration network (LHIN). 2014. http://www.lhins.on.ca/. Accessed 7 Dec 2017.

4

Patient safety and safety culture in primary health care

Muna Habib AL. Lawati[1,2]* (iD), Sarah Dennis[3,4], Stephanie D. Short[1] and Nadia Noor Abdulhadi[5]

Abstract

Background: Patient safety in primary care is an emerging field of research with a growing evidence base in western countries but little has been explored in the Gulf Cooperation Council Countries (GCC) including the Sultanate of Oman. This study aimed to review the literature on the safety culture and patient safety measures used globally to inform the development of safety culture among health care workers in primary care with a particular focus on the Middle East.

Methods: A systematic review of the literature. Searches were undertaken using Medline, EMBASE, CINAHL and Scopus from the year 2000 to 2014. Terms defining safety culture were combined with terms identifying patient safety and primary care.

Results: The database searches identified 3072 papers that were screened for inclusion in the review. After the screening and verification, data were extracted from 28 papers that described safety culture in primary care. The global distribution of the articles is as follows: the Netherlands (7), the United States (5), Germany (4), the United Kingdom (1), Australia, Canada and Brazil (two for each country), and with one each from Turkey, Iran, Saudi Arabia and Kuwait. The characteristics of the included studies were grouped under the following themes: safety culture in primary care, incident reporting, safety climate and adverse events. The most common theme from 2011 onwards was the assessment of safety culture in primary care (13 studies, 46%). The most commonly used safety culture assessment tool is the Hospital survey on patient safety culture (HSOPSC) which has been used in developing countries in the Middle East.

Conclusions: This systematic review reveals that the most important first step is the assessment of safety culture in primary care which will provide a basic understanding to safety-related perceptions of health care providers. The HSOPSC has been commonly used in Kuwait, Turkey, and Iran.

Keywords: Patent safety, Safety culture, Primary care, Gulf countries, Oman

Background

The World Health Organization (WHO) defines patient safety as "the prevention of errors and adverse effects to patients associated with health care" and "to do no harm to patients" [1, 2]. There are millions of patients globally who suffer disabilities, injuries or death each year due to unsafe medical practices [3]. This has led to the wider recognition of the importance of patient safety, the incorporation of patient safety approaches into the strategic plans of health care organizations and a growing body of research in this field [4]. "To Err is Human: Building a Safer Health System" was published in 1999 by the Institute of Medicine (IOM), it emphasized that safety was the key fundamental concern. This was a landmark publication for patient safety and warned of errors in health care and the potential for patient harm [5]. Patient safety in primary care has not been explored to the same extent as in the hospital settings [6] however more recently there has been more research emerging in primary care [7–10]. Achieving a culture of safety requires an understanding of the values, attitudes, beliefs and norms that are important to health care organization and what attitudes and behaviors are appropriate and expected for patient safety [10].

* Correspondence: drmunali@gmail.com
[1]Faculty of Health Sciences, Discipline of Behavioral and Social Sciences in Health, The University of Sydney, Science Road, Sydney, NSW 2006, Australia
[2]Department of Quality Assurance and Patient Safety, Ministry of Health, P.O.Box, 626, Wadi Al Kabir, 117 Muscat, PC, Oman
Full list of author information is available at the end of the article

This systematic review aimed to identify the patient safety measures used globally to assess the effectiveness of safety culture in primary care. The outcome of this study will help to inform strategies for patient safety for primary care in Oman in order to accomplish the 2050 vision. The specific research questions for this review were:

1. What processes or systems are in place to facilitate a safety culture in in primary care?
2. What are the measures used globally to assess the effectiveness of safety culture in primary care?
3. What is the impact of safety culture in primary care?

Methods

A systematic review of the published literature from 2000 to 2014 was conducted. This date range was chosen because it followed the publication of "To Err is Human" in 1999 [5]. The databases used to identify the articles were Medline, Embase, CINAHL and Scopus. The terms used in Medline search were *Health System, Safety Culture, Patient Safety, Primary Health care, Adverse Event, Health Care Professionals and Health Care Managers*.

There were several key definitions used to scope the review and inform the inclusion and exclusion criteria:

1. Patient Safety: WHO defines patient safety "as the absence of preventable harm to a patient during the process of health care" [1].
2. Safety Culture: Defined "as shared values, attitudes, perceptions, competencies and patterns of behaviors".
3. Primary Care: WHO defined primary care "as socially appropriate, universally accessible, scientifically sound first level care provided by a suitably trained workforce supported by integrated referral systems (to secondary care or tertiary care) and in a way that gives priority to those most needed, maximizes community and individual self-reliance and participation and involves collaboration with other sectors. It includes the following: health promotion, illness prevention, care of the sick, advocacy and community development" [11].

Articles were included in the review if they were published in the year 2000 or later and met the following four inclusion criteria:

1. They reported on the use of patient safety tools or approaches or mechanisms or procedures used in primary health care with an impact on patient care (outcome) measured.
2. If they were contained any of the following methodologies; systematic review, intervention study (randomized controlled trials), descriptive study or qualitative design.

3. They discussed patient safety in primary care, or safety culture in primary care.
4. Published in English.

Articles were excluded if they were opinion papers/essays, editorial reviews, interviews, comments or narrative reviews.

After removal of the duplicates and papers with no abstracts, the titles and abstracts of 61 papers were screened by two researchers (MA and NN). The full text of all articles remaining were obtained and reviewed by two researchers (MA and NN). The full text articles were read and those that met the inclusion criteria were included in the review. The flow chart in Additional file 1 illustrates the selection process by using Preferred Reporting Items for Systematic Reviews and Meta-Analyses (PRISMA) flowchart [12].

The following information was extracted from the included articles: authors, year of publication, title and aims, objectives, methods, country and key findings. To assess the quality three different tools were used according to study design. Systematic reviews were evaluated by Assessing Methodological Quality of Systematic Review (AMSTAR), quantitative studies were assessed by Effective Public Health Practice Project (EPHPP) and cross sectional studies were evaluated by using Strengthening the Reporting of Observational studies in Epidemiology (STROBE) [13].

Results

The database searches identified 3072 papers that were screened for inclusion in the review. After title and abstract screening there were 61 remaining papers that described interventions in safety culture in primary care. Following verification and data extraction there were a total number of 28 articles included in the systematic review (Additional file 1). The global distribution of the articles are as follows: the Netherlands (7), the United States (5), Germany (4), Australia, Canada and Brazil (two for each country), the United Kingdom (1), and with one each from Turkey, Iran, Saudi Arabia and Kuwait. The characteristics of the included studies grouped under the following themes: safety culture in primary care, incident reporting, safety climate and adverse events are specified in Table 1.

Safety culture in primary care

Thirteen studies addressed safety culture and tools to assess safety culture in general practice and most (9/13) were cross sectional studies [7, 8, 10, 14–19], the other studies were qualitative interviews [20], a systematic review [21], a retrospective audit [22], randomized control trial [22], mixed methods [23] and a case study [24].

The definition of patient safety culture varied among the articles. A common definition of safety culture was

Table 1 Characteristics of the selected studies in the systematic review (studies categorized by themes)

Author and year	Title	Study design	Study Results and significant conclusions	Quality assessments
Safety Culture in primary care setting				
Kirk S [26] 2007	Patient safety culture in primary care; developing a theoretical framework for practical use.	Literature review followed by semi-structured interviews.	Study details development of the Manchester Patient Safety Framework	
Bodur S [8] 2009	A survey on patient safety in primary healthcare services in Turkey	Cross sectional study	Hospital survey on patient safety survey was adapted with modification to fit the Turkish primary care context. Positive responses were highest for teamwork within the units (76%) and lowest for events reporting (59%) and non-punitive response to errors (18%). Health center administrator must focus on improving patient safety culture and encourage staff to report errors without fear.	All items of STROBE statement covered
Dorien LM Zwart [22] 2011	Patient safety culture measurement in general practice. Clinimetric properties of 'SCOPE'	Descriptive Cross sectional study	88.8% completed the questionnaire, out of which 25% were GPs, 60% medical administrative assistants and 15% nurses. SCOPE seems a suitable tool to measure safety culture in general practice	All items of STROBE statement covered
Nargis T [7] 2012	The first study of patient safety culture in the Iranian primary health care.	Cross sectional study	Teamwork across the units scored the highest 77.7%, continuous organization learning scored 72% and the lowest was non-punitive response to error 17%.	All items of STROBE statement covered
Jacobs L [27] 2012	Creating a culture of patient safety in primary care physicians group.	Proactive approach Case study	Study based on adaptation of medical risk management strategy to help create a culture of safety in primary care. This led to reduction of malpractice claims and enhanced learning experience among physicians.	All items of STROBE statement covered
Benjamin H [20] 2012	Better medical office safety culture is not associated with better scores on quality measures.	Cross section study	Response rate was 79%, significate variations on safety culture scores and quality scores. There was no association between safety culture and quality outcome measures.	All items of STROBE statement covered
Yahia M [21] 2013	Attitude of primary care physicians toward safety in Aseer region, Saudi Arabia	Cross sectional study	Highest score was given to reduction of medical errors (6.2 points). Followed by training and learning on patient safety (6 and 5.9). Undergraduate training was given the least score and participants did not agree that errors were due to nurses or doctor's carelessness.	All items of STROBE statement covered
Lucine M [29] 2013	Is health professional's perception of patient safety related to figures on safety incidents?	Retrospective Observational study	Communication breakdown inside or outside the practice are threats to patient safety. The study indicates that assessments of professional's perception are complementary to observed safety incidents.	All items of STROBE statement covered

Table 1 Characteristics of the selected studies in the systematic review (studies categorized by themes) *(Continued)*

Author and year	Title	Study design	Study Results and significant conclusions	Quality assessments
Fernando P [18] 2013	Patient safety culture in primary health care.	Cross sectional study	Working conditions, teamwork climate, communication and management of healthcare were significate with patient safety culture.	All items of STROBE statement covered
Maha G [10] 2014	Assessment of patient safety culture in primary health care setting in Kuwait.	Cross sectional studies	Hospital survey on patient safety survey was adapted with modification to fit the Kuwaiti primary care context. Dimensions with low positivity were: the non-punitive response to errors, frequency to error reporting, staffing, communication openness and center handoffs. High positivity was teamwork within the unit and organizational learning. Overall the safety culture is not strong in Kuwait.	All items of STROBE statement covered
Natasha J [24] 2014	Improving patient safety in primary care: a systematic review.	Systematic review	2 articles selected which provide basic understanding of improvement strategies in primary care, low level of evidence	9/11 using AMSTAR
Hoffmann B [25] 2014	Effects of a team based assessment and intervention on patient safety culture in general practice: an open randomized controlled trail.	Randomized control trail	FraTrix, which was derived from MaPSaf, was applied over a period of 9 months in the intervention practice. Fratrix didn't lead to measurable improvements in error managements but lead to better reporting of patient safety incidents.	(EPHPP Statement used for assessment) A strong study which highlighted limitations and implications.
Palacios D [23] 2010	Dimensions of patient safety culture in family practice.	Qualitative case study	Explores the dimensions of patient safety culture related to family practice in UK, USA and Canada.	Global rating of this paper was moderate (Effective Public Health Practice Project)

Incident reporting in primary care setting

Douglas H [35] 2004	Event reporting to a primary care patient safety reporting system: A report from the ASIPS collaborative.	Incident report analysis	Highest number of events was reported due to communication errors 71% followed by diagnostic and medication errors. A safe reporting system, which relies on voluntary reporting, can be adapted in primary care settings.	All items of STROBE statement covered
Singh R [34] 2006	"Chance favors only the prepared mind". Preparing minds to systematically reduce hazards in the testing process in primary care.	Prospective study	A proposed approach called as systematic appraisal of risk and its management for error reduction for test process (SARAIMER) was used. Successfully used in medication safety in primary care.	All items of STROBE statement covered
Makeham M [33] 2007	Patient safety events reported in general practice: taxonomy.	Taxonomy	The outline taxonomy of events in general practice provides a complete tool for clinicians describing threats to patient safety and can build an error reporting system.	All items of STROBE statement covered
Marleen S [38] 2010	Patient safety in out-of-hour's primary care: a review of patient records.	Retrospective	Most frequent incidents occur in out-of- hours primary care were incidents on treatment (56%). Incidents did not result in patient harm. Improved understanding in clinical reason and adherence to guidelines will enhance patient safety.	All items of STROBE statement covered

Table 1 Characteristics of the selected studies in the systematic review (studies categorized by themes) *(Continued)*

Author and year	Title	Study design	Study Results and significant conclusions	Quality assessments
Zwart D [6] 2011	Central or local incident reporting? A comparative study in Dutch GP out of hour's services.	Quasi experimental study	Local incident reporting facilitates the willingness to report and faster implementation of improvements. In contrast, central reporting seems better at addressing generic and recurring safety issues. Both approaches should be combined.	All items of STROBE statement covered
Dorien LM Zwart [37] 2011	Feasibility of center-based incident reporting in primary healthcare: The SPIEGEL study	Prospective Observational study	476 incidents reported in 9 months, 62% incidents reported in the reporting week and majority were process oriented. All involved centers initiated improvement strategies due to reported incidents. Locally implemented incident reporting procedure as a tool for managing patient safety is feasible in general practice.	All items of STROBE statement covered
Zwart D [36] 2013	Introducing incident reporting in primary care: a translation from safety science into medical practice	Prospective Observational study	The aim of the study was to understand and describe particular ways primary care physicians make incident reporting procedure part of dealing with safety issues.	All items of STROBE statement covered
Marchon SG [39] 2014	Patient safety in primary health care: a systematic review.	Systematic review	33 articles were selected from 2007 to 2012: 26% on retrospective studies, 44% prospective studies. Frequent method used was incident reporting system 45% and the most relevant contributing factor was communication failure.	8/11 using AMSTAR

Safety climate in primary care setting

Author and year	Title	Study design	Study Results and significant conclusions	Quality assessments
Hoffmann B [35] 2011	The Frankfurt patient safety climate questionnaire for general practice (FraSik): analysis of psychometric properties.	Cross sectional studies	Questionnaire was modified in order to be applicable for general practice. The tool can be used for assessment of the safety climate of general practice.	All items of STROBE statement covered
De Wet C [37] 2012	Measuring perception of safety climate in primary care: a cross- sectional study.	Cross sectional study	Perception of safety climate in the UK primary care with a validated tool specifically designed for it. Measuring safety climate has various benefits at the individual, practice and regional level.	All items of STROBE statement covered
Hoffmann B [36] 2013	Impact of individual and team features of patient safety climate: A survey in family practice.	Cross section studies	FraSik was used to identify potential predictors of the safety climate in family practice in Germany. The overall climate was positive but the health professional's use of incident reporting and systems approach to errors was fairly rare.	All items of STROBE statement covered

Adverse events in primary care setting

Author and year	Title	Study design	Study Results and significant conclusions	Quality assessments
Sweidan M [41] 2010	Identification of features of electronic prescribing systems to support quality and safety in primary care using a modified Delphi process.	Modified Delphi process.	114 software features were developed which relate to recording and use of patient data, the medication selection process, prescribing decision-making support, monitoring drug therapy and clinical reports. This feature supports safety and quality of pre-scription of medication in general practice.	Modified Delphi process.

Table 1 Characteristics of the selected studies in the systematic review (studies categorized by themes) *(Continued)*

Author and year	Title	Study design	Study Results and significant conclusions	Quality assessments
Wong K [40] 2010	A systematic review of medication safety outcomes related to drug interaction software.	Systematic review	No study addressed the benefits and harms or cost effectiveness of drug interactions. The evidence does not support a benefit of software on medication safety or support any practice in this policy.	7/11 using AMSTAR
Singh R [42] 2004	Estimation impacts on safety caused by the introduction of the electronic medical records in primary care.	FMEA	Hazard score was calculated for each error before and 1 year after implementation of electronic medical records. Hazards perceived by staffs decreased in domains of physician –nurses and physicians –chart. But increase in physician- patient and nurse-chart domain.	All items of STROBE statement covered
Joachim S [43] 2011	Effectiveness of a quality improvement program in improving management of primary care practices	Cross sectional study	Primary care practices that completed the European Practice assessments twice over a period of 3 yrs showed overall improvements in practice management, quality and safety and complaint management.	All items of STROBE statement covered

utilized in eight studies, which referred to shared values, perceptions, attitudes, competencies and behaviors within an organization [8, 10, 14, 15, 19–23]. The definition of safety culture was lacking in two articles but they defined patient safety and patient safety incidents respectively [18]. There was one study where patient safety culture was defined as acceptance and actions of patient safety as the first priority in the organization [7] and four articles did not define safety culture [17, 24–26].

Two studies of safety culture utilized a qualitative approach, followed by a survey or an audit. The other eleven studies utililized quantitative tools to assess safety culture. The systematic review included a study by Gaal et al. in the Netherlands that explored the views of primary care doctors and nurses to identify aspects of care linked to patient safety in a qualitative study [16]. Medication safety was most frequently mentioned with incidents occurring in diagnosis and treatment, errors in communication and poor patient doctor relationship were the most common errors in primary care [25]. The aspects that were considered essential for patient safety were; the availability of medical instruments, telephone accessibility and safe electric sockets. General practitioners relied on the skills and knowledge of the practice nurses since most of the patients were seen by them. The GPs did not supervise the practice nurses when providing advice to patients over the phone which they felt was a threat to patient safety. The results of this qualitative study were used to develop a web-based survey, which was one of the first to assess the views of general practitioners (GPs) on patient safety [16] in the Netherlands. They found that GPs were concerned about

the maintenance of medical records, prescription and monitoring of medication.

Another Dutch study identified that health care professionals who had a perception and understanding of patient safety had more incidents recorded [26]. All the health professionals surveyed felt that communication breakdown inside and outside the practice was a threat to patient safety and was associated with more incidents [26].

A systematic review on the use of interventions of patient safety that affect safety culture in primary care only included two studies [21]. One of the included studies described the implementation of an electronic medical records system in general practice using the safety attribute questionnaire as a part of patient safety improvements [21]. The authors facilitated two workshops for general practice on risk management and significant audit analysis. The authors concluded that further research was required to assess the effect of interventions on safety culture in primary care [21].

Two main tools were used to measure safety culture; the Manchester Patient Safety Framework (MaPSaF) and the Hospital Survey on Patient Safety Culture (HSOPSC). The Manchester Patient Safety Framework (MaPSaF) [23] was developed to measure the multidimensional and dynamic nature of safety culture and enabled recognition of subcultures within a single organization because subcultures act as a powerful influence on error detection and learning. In addition, the tool provided insights into patient safety culture, facilitated interactive self-reflection about safety culture of an organization, explored differences in perception among different staff categories, helped understand how mature an organization was in terms of safety culture and evaluated interventions which were aimed at improving safety culture. The MaPSaF is founded on Westrum's typology of organizational communication from 1992, which defined how different types of organizations process information. This typology was expanded upon by Parker and Hudson to describe five levels of progressively maturing organizational safety culture. The MaPSaF measures ten dimensions of safety culture, derived from a literature review on patient safety in primary care and in-depth interviews and focus group discussions with health care professionals and managers. The dimensions are commitment to overall safety, priority given to safety; system errors and individual responsibility; recording incidents and best practice; evaluation incidents and best practice; learning and effecting change; communication about safety issues; staff education and training and team work approach. The tool helped to acknowledge that patient safety was multidimensional and complex, offered insights and demonstrated strengths and weaknesses of a patient safety culture, provided differences in perception among and helped the organization to understand what a mature safety culture in health care might look like. It should not be used to conduct performance management nor to divide or attribute blame when the organization's safety culture is not sufficiently mature [27]. This tool is best used as a facilitative educational tool for health care providers and managers.

The Manchester Patient Safety Framework (MaPSaF) [14, 22] has been adapted for use in different health systems. The MaPSaF was modified and tested in the New Zealand context to facilitate learning about safety culture and facilitate team communication mentioned in the systematic review [15]. The MaPSaF has been modified for use in the German health system and was renamed the Frankfurt Patient Safety Matrix (FraTix) [22]. This tool was validated and used in a randomized control trial of 60 general practices to determine safety culture at different levels. There were no differences between the general practice physicians' groups but the intervention group showed improved reporting and management of patient safety incidents than the control group. FraTix appeared to be a good tool for self-assessments aimed at improving safety culture but did not lead to measurable improvements in error management.

The Hospital Survey on Patient Safety Culture (HSOPSC) was developed by the Agency of Health Care and Research for Hospitals in 2004, and has been adapted and modified for other health care settings. It measures healthcare professional's perspectives towards safety culture at the individual, unit and organizational level. It was pilot tested with more than 1400 hospital employees from 21 hospitals across the USA [28]. The tool was developed after an extensive literature review on safety, accidents, medical errors, safety climate and

culture and organizational climate and culture. There were also interviews with hospital staff and surveys. The instrument includes fourteen dimensions, twelve are multiple item dimensions (two safety culture dimensions and two outcome dimensions) and the last two are single item dimensions used to check the validity. This tool has a broad spectrum of applicability has been completed by all types of hospital staff from security guards to nurses, paramedical staff and physicians employed by the organization. In terms of reliability and validity the HSOPSC was found to be "psychometrically sound at the individual, unit and hospital level analysis" [29] in primary care settings. It has since been used in Kuwait, Turkey, the Netherlands and Iran [7, 8, 10, 19]. The dimension most commonly scored among Kuwait, Turkey and Iran was teamwork within the units and the least was non-punitive response to errors. Similarly, the HSOPSC has since been adapted and validated for use in Dutch general practice, and was renamed SCOPE [19], a Dutch abbreviation for systematic culture on patient safety in primary care. Table 2 compares the characteristics of the MaPSaF and HSOPSC.

Paese [15] used the Safety Attitudes Questionnaire (SAQ) to assess attitudes to safety culture in Brazilian primary care. The survey was conducted among community health agents, nursing technicians and nurses. The SAQ assesses the quality of safety and teamwork standards in a given time in a health care organization. Nine attributes are assessed which are: job satisfaction, teamwork climate, perception of work environment, communication, patient safety, ongoing education, management of the healthcare center, recognition of stress, error prevention by using preventive measures. Patient safety attribute was considered to be an important attribute among the respondents whereas prevention measures to avoid errors were viewed as being a less important attribute.

A case study in a primary care physician practice in the USA explored the impact of a comprehensive risk management program from 2003 to 2009. The program resulted in fewer insurance claims and considerable cost savings thereby enhancing patient safety culture in primary care by implementing risk management program, the program further provided the physicians' a sense of control over the treatment of malpractice and encouraged them to provide the best care for their patients [24].

Incident reporting in primary care

Incident reporting to assess patient safety in primary care has grown in importance. There were two types of study under this theme; 1) studies that explored different approaches to incident reporting [6, 30–34] and 2) different mechanism to report incidents [35, 36].

Table 2 Comparision of Manchester Patient Safety Framework (MaPSaF) and Hospital Survey on Patient Safety Culture (HSOPSC)

The Manchester Patient Safety Framework (MaPSaF)	The Hospital Survey on Patient Safety Culture (HSOPSC)
Developed by University of Manchester	Developed by the US agency for Healthcare and Research
Defined patient safety culture according to 10 dimensions: • Continuous improvement • Priority given to staff • System errors and individual responsibility • Recording incidents • Evaluation incidents • Learning and effecting change • Communication personnel management • Staff education • teamwork	Defined patient safety culture according to 12 dimensions: • Frequency of error reporting • Number or error reporting • Supervisors expectations and actions • Organizational learning • Teamwork within units • Communication openness • Feedback and communication about errors\ • Non-punitive response to errors • Staffing • Management support • Teamwork across units • Handoffs and transitions
Reflects on safety culture, highlights differences in perception between staff groups help understand what a mature safety culture might look like and monitor changes over time	The tool can assess safety culture at individual, unit and organizational level.
Deigned to be used in the UK context	Designed to be used globally

A number of studies have looked at incident reporting mechanisms and no one method was found to be superior. A mixture of methods was required to identify adverse events in primary care. The feasibility of a locally implemented incident reporting procedure (IRP) in primary health centers was evaluated [33]. Introducing IRP in primary care to manage patient safety seemed to be less suitable for dealing with serious adverse events since it neglected the emotional needs of the healthcare workers involved in the medical error [33]. This study further compared the number and the nature of incident reports collected locally (IRP) and from the existing centralized incident reporting procedure. They found that the local incident reporting procedure enabled the health care professionals to control the assessments of their incident reports since the reports remained within the health center. This facilitated organizational learning and in turn increased the willingness to report and facilitated quicker implementation of improvement. The central procedure that collected reports from many settings, appeared to address common and recurrent safety issues more effectively. Therefore, they concluded that both approaches were necessary and should be combined [37].

A systematic review reported on the methodologies to evaluate incidents in primary care, types of incidents, contributing factors and solutions to make a safer primary care. There were 33 included articles and the most universally used method was incident analysis from incident reports (45%). The review did not report on the effectiveness of any specific method for incident reporting nor were specific tools mentioned. The most frequent types of incident were associated with medication and diagnosis errors and the most relevant contributing factor was communication failure among healthcare team [15]. Reviewing medical reports as an approach to

incident reporting in primary healthcare was examined in a Dutch study mentioned in the systematic review. This retrospective review identified records with evidence of a potential patient safety incident in out-of-hours primary care and reviewed the type, causes and consequences of the incident. They found that incidents did occur in out-of-hours primary care but that most (70%) did not result in patient harm. The most frequent incident was treatment errors (56%). All incidents were attributed to failures in clinical reasoning because of lack of access to the patient's medical history, insufficient medical knowledge, high workload, age and being high risk (patients with one or more conditions such as cardiac and vascular disease, asthma/COPD, diabetes, pregnancy, malignancy and immune disease). The mean age for patients with incidents was 52 years compared to 36 years for patients without incidents. Logistic regression analysis identified that the likelihood of an incident increased by 1.03 (95% confidence interval: 1.01 to 1.04) for each year increase in patient age the baseline age used was less or more then 50 [15].

Safety climate in primary care

Safety climate was assessed in three cross sectional studies using similar definitions of safety climate and safety culture [38–40]. Safety climate was defined as "shared employee perceptions of the priority of safety at their unit and organization at large" [38]. The safety climate was referred to as what was happening in an organization whereas; safety culture explained why it was happening [41].

There was no tool to assess safety climate so Hoffman et al. evaluated the use of the existing Safety Attribute Questionnaire, Ambulatory version which was piloted and modified to be used in general practice. It was renamed the Frankfurt patient safety climate questionnaire for general practice (FraSik) and was used to assess the safety climate in German general practice [38]. FraSik was further assessed in a survey which recognises strengths and weaknesses of the safety climate of general practice and in addition too, individual and practical features that affect the safety climate perception of health care professionals in primary care [39]. Doctors and health care assistants perceived that safety climate in German general practice was positive and highlighted areas for improvement in patient safety, reporting incidents and cause of errors. A limitation of the study was a low response rate because those that responded to the survey might have an interest in patient safety and therefore more positive response and may not reflect the views other health professionals working in the system [39].

Interestingly, the terms safety climate and safety culture in the studies mentioned above have been used interchangeably although they mean different things. Safety climate is defined as "surface features of the safety culture from attitudes and perceptions of individuals at a given point in time" and "the measurable components of safety culture" [42]. Whereas, a safety culture is the "product of individual and group values, attitudes, competencies and patterns of behavior that determine the commitment to, and the style and proficiency of an organization's health and safety programs" [14].

Adverse events in primary care

Two papers reported on adverse events with a focus on medication error [43, 44]. Both the papers related to information technology to improve patient safety and quality of care. A systematic review, which reviewed literature on the use of drug interaction detection software (DIS) [43]. Only four studies met the inclusion criteria and they were not able to address the benefits and harms of drug interaction software for medication safety. There was no published evidence to supports these systems or policies.

An Australian study aimed to identify the features of e-prescribing software that best supported patient safety and quality of care in primary care. A list of 114 features was identified by literature review, key informant and expert groups (Delphi Process). These features could be used to develop software standards by policy makers and could be adapted in other settings and countries, but were not evaluated [44]. Another paper discussed the introduction of an electronic medical record system into primary care because of its impact to improve health care quality. The electronic medical system further includes current practice knowledge, which can support decision making, eventually leading to reduction to practice expenses and further increasing revenues by accurate billing and customer satisfaction [45].

The European Practice Assessment tool was used in a German study to assess the primary care practice focusing on the five domains in primary care practice (infrastructure, people, finance, quality and safety). Two groups where selected, the intervention group is the one which had a previous training in the tool and showed improvement in all the five domains compared to the comparative group which group which didn't have any previous trainings. This highlighted that there is a benefit to quality improvement when accreditation tools are introduced as a benchmark assessment to improve the health care professional's performance [46].

Discussion

Patient safety is critical to health care quality and remains a developmental challenge in primary care in many countries. In addition interventions addressing patient safety culture in primary care are limited compared to secondary care [21].

To improve patient safety, an important first step is to address and understand the safety culture of an organization. Similarly assessment of safety culture helps health care organizations to assess areas for improvement and analyze changes over time [9]. This systematic review has recognized that the most common theme emerging from 2011 onwards was the assessment of safety culture in primary care. An important first strategy to improve all aspects of health care quality is creating a culture of safety within health care organizations [47].

An understanding of the safety culture is vital to improve the problematic practices or attitudes such as miscommunication, adverse events and a non-punitive response to errors, which can lead to an improvement in the safety culture of primary care. Likewise, the measurement of safety culture in primary care can help in the identification of areas for improvement which might cause adverse events and errors. Patient care follow-up, communication openness and work pressure were essential to improve patient safety in primary care [2]. Secondly, another key area for improvement seen in the systematic review was the issue of inadequate numbers of staff and providers to handle patients in primary care, highlighting this as an area that requires attention [7, 8, 10].

Communication breakdown, which affects both safety culture and acts as a contributing factor for incidents, needs to be emphasized and addressed to help strengthen patient safety culture in primary care [19]. Communication openness was seen in the Kuwaiti and Turkey studies as an area of concern [8, 10] unlike in the Iranian and the Dutch studies [7, 19]. The inconsistency between outcomes regarding communication openness might be associated with differences in cultural background where disparagement and disagreement is regarded as blame and thus can lead to loss of occupation or personal relationships among staff and therefore staff tend to avoid it. In general communication openness was found to be a problem in developing and Middle Eastern countries due to the blame culture [9]. Organizations with a positive safety culture constituted a communication policy, established the importance of safety in health care and developed preventive measures.

This systematic review brings to light an emerging literature on patient safety culture in primary care from middle to low income countries. As health care organizations attempt to improve, there is a need to establish a culture of safety an example seen in primary care in Oman.To to achive that, its essential to understand the culture of safety which requires an understanding of the values, beliefs, and norms about what is significant in an organization and what attitudes and behaviors related to patient safety are important and suitable. Establishing an environment for patient safety may be challenging in Oman because no studies on patient safety have been undertaken in primary care, only hospital care. A further complication is that the health centers are scattered unlike hospitals which is a single unit and in addition the health care workforce includes many nationalities and backgrounds with varying understandings of patient safety from different health care systems.

The insight one may draw from the literature is that, the most reliable and effective strategy for improving the quality of care is in changing the perception of the frontline health care professionals towards patient safety which in-turn will result in reduced adverse events and communication breakdown [47].

The safety of the staff and patients in a health care organization was affected by the extent of safety perceived across the organization. This concept was assessed by two frequently used tools in the systematic review which assessed safety culture in primary care: the Manchester Patient Safety Framework (MaPSAF) and Hospital Survey on Patient Safety Culture (HSOPSC). The HSOPSC tool emerged as the most likely tool to be used in the GCC to assess the safety culture in primary care for the following reasons; firstly, it was used successfully in Kuwait and more recently in Yemen and both countries have a similar GCC primary health systems. Secondly, the same questionnaire has been used to assess the hospital safety culture in other countries in the GCC [48].

Incident reporting is an important aspect for achieving patient safety [6]. There is a need to develop an incident reporting system in primary care in the Middle East within the health centers, similar to hospitals, which is computerized and helps in tracking and following up the incidents. The findings from this systematic review suggest that the system developed should include a local incident reporting system which will record and monitor incidents within the health center along with a centralized reporting system at the ministry of health which can address and monitor incidents which are recurrent and common in primary care [49]. A local approach aids in willingness to report and facilitate quicker implementation whereas a central approach addresses the common and recurrent safety issues [49].

Patient safety in primary care is an emerging field of research in western countries but little has been published from Oman and the other Gulf Cooperation Council Countries (GCC). The Ministry of Health (MOH) in Oman has been working for many years at different levels to improve the quality of health care services and its safety.

Patient safety in primary care can be enhanced in the GCC by introducing 5 yrs plans across primary care. This such example was seen in Oman where they developed a "Vision 2050" which is updated every 5 yrs. Potential areas for improvement are introduced for the next 2020–2025 five-year plan for patient safety in primary care across all the regions of Oman. With the aid of these plans the Ministry of Health, in partnership with the Ministry of Information Technology, are working together to achieve information transfer, linkage of patient information between health centers, secondary care and hospitals so that the civil identification number can be used as a single identification number to access all patient health information across the health institutions.

Conclusion

This systematic review reveals that the most important first step is the assessment of safety culture in primary care which will provide basic understanding to safetyrelated perceptions of the health care providers. The most commonly used safety culture assessment tool is the HSOPSC which aids in identifying areas for improvement at the individual, unit and organizational level. This review recognized that safety culture in primary care should be assessed on a regular basis to evaluate the effectiveness of safety in health institutions.

Furthermore, results from this review will be used to inform an empirical study of safety culture in primary care in Oman using the Hospital Survey on Patient Safety Culture (HSOPSC) tool, with a view to developing a template for the development of safety culture in primary care in the context of rapid economic growth.

Abbreviations
AMSTAR: Assessing Methodological Quality of Systematic Review; EPHPP: Quantitative studies were assessed by Effective Public Health Practice Project; GCC: Gulf Cooperation Council; HSOPSC: Hospital survey on patient safety culture; IOM: International Institute of Medicine; MOH: Ministry of Health; PRISMA: Preferred Reporting Items for Systematic Reviews and Meta-Analyses; SAQ: Safety attribute questionnaire; STROBE: Cross sectional studies were evaluated by using Strengthening the Reporting of Observational studies in Epidemiology; WHO: World Health Organization

Authors' contributions

MA and NN screened the titles and abstracts of all remaining papers and the full text of all articles remaining were obtained and reviewed by two researchers MA and NN. All Authors participated in developing study method, definitions and criteria. All authors participated in the sequence in drafting the manuscript. All authors read and approved the final manuscript.

Authors information

PhD Student at the University of Sydney, Head of Quality and Patient Safety at the Directorate General of Health Services, Ministry of Health, Muscat, Oman.

Competing interests

The authors declare that they have no competing interests.

Author details

[1]Faculty of Health Sciences, Discipline of Behavioral and Social Sciences in Health, The University of Sydney, Science Road, Sydney, NSW 2006, Australia. [2]Department of Quality Assurance and Patient Safety, Ministry of Health, P.O.Box, 626, Wadi Al Kabir, 117 Muscat, PC, Oman. [3]Ingham Institute for Applied Medical Research, Campbell Street, Liverpool, NSW 2170, Australia. [4]Faculty of Health Sciences, Discipline of Physiotherapy, The University of Sydney, 71 East Street, Lidcombe, NSW 2141, Australia. [5]Directorate General of Planning and Studies, Ministry of Health, Muscat, Oman.

References

1. World Health Organization, G. Conceptual framework for the international classification for patient safety. In: Version 1.1 final technical report January 2009; 2009.
2. Gaal S, Verstappen W, Wensing M. What do primary care physicians and researchers consider the most important patient safety improvement strategies? BMC Health Serv Res. 2011;11:102.
3. Sorra J, Nieva VF. A tool for improving patient safety in healthcare organizations. Qual Saf Health Care. 2003;12(Suppl II):ii17–23.
4. Gonzalez-Formoso C, et al. Adverse events analysis as an educational tool to improve patient safety culture in primary care: a randomized trial. BMC Fam Pract. 2011;12:50.
5. Linda TK, Corrigan JM, Donaldson MS. To err is human: building a safer health system. Washington DC: National Academy Press; 1999.
6. Zwart DL, Van Rensel EL, Kalkman CJ, Verheij TJ. Central or local incident reporting? A comparative study in Dutch GP out-of-hours services. Br J Gen Pract. 2011;61(584):183–7. https://doi.org/10.3399/bjgp11X561168.
7. Tabrizchi N, Sedaghat M. The first study of patient safety culture in Iranian primary health centers. Acta Med Iran. 2012;50(7):505–10.
8. Bodur S, Filiz E. A survey on patient safety culture in primary healthcare services in Turkey. Int J Qual Health Care. 2009;21(5):348–55.
9. Webair HH, Al-Assani SS. Reema H. Al-Haddad, Wafa H. Al-Shaeeb, Manal A. Selm, and A.S. Alyamani. Assessment of patient safety culture in primary care setting, Al-Mukala, Yemen. BMC Fam Pract. 2015;16:136.
10. Ghobashi MM, et al. Assessment of patient safety culture in primary health care settings in Kuwait. Epidemiol Biostat Public Health. 2014;11(3):e9101–9.
11. World Health Organization. Conceptual Framework for the International Classification for Patient Safety. GENEVA: WHO; 2009. Contract No.: WHO/IER/PSP/2010.2.
12. Liberati A, Altman DG, Tetzlaff J, Mulrow C, Gotzsche PC, JPA I, et al. The PRISMA statement for reporting systematic reviews and meta-analyses of studies that evaluate healthcare interventions: explanation and elaboration. BMJ. 2009;339(1):b2700.
13. STROBE. Strengthening the Reporting of OBservational studies in Epidemiology (STROBE). 2009; Available from: http://www.strobe-statement.org/.
14. Wallis K, Dovey S. Assessing patient safety culture in New Zealand primary care: a pilot study using a modified Manchester patient safety framework in Dunedin general practices. J Prim Health Care. 2011;3(1):35–40.
15. Paese F, Sasso GT. Patient safety culture in primary health care [Portuguese]. Texto & Contexto Enfermagem. 2013;22(2):302–10.
16. Gaal S, Verstappen W, Wensing M. Patient safety in primary care: a survey of general practitioners in the Netherlands. BMC Health Serv Res. 2010;10:21.
17. Hagopian B, et al. Better medical office safety culture is not associated with better scores on quality measures. J Patient Saf. 2012;8(1):15–21.
18. Al-Khaldi YM. Attitude of primary care physicians toward patient safety in Aseer region, Saudi Arabia. Journal of Family & Community Medicine. 2013;20(3):153–8.
19. Zwart DLM, et al. Patient safety culture measurement in general practice. Clinimetric properties of 'SCOPE'. BMC Fam Pract. 2011;12(1):117.
20. Palacios-Derflingher L, et al. Dimensions of patient safety culture in family practice. Healthc Q. 2010;13:121–7.
21. Verbakel NJ LM, Verheij TJ, Wagner C, Zwart DL. Improving Patient Safety Culture in Primary Care: A Systematic Review. PubMed. 2014;00(00).
22. Hoffmann B, et al. Effects of a team-based assessment and intervention on patient safety culture in general practice: an open randomised controlled trial. BMJ Qual Saf. 2014;23(1):35–46.
23. Kirk S, et al. Patient safety culture in primary care: developing a theoretical framework for practical use. Qual Saf Health Care. 2007;16(4):313–20.
24. Jacobs L, et al. Creating a culture of patient safety in a primary-care physician group. Conn Med. 2012;76(5):291–7.
25. Gaal S, et al. Patient safety in primary care has many aspects: an interview study in primary care doctors and nurses. J Eval Clin Pract. 2010;16(3):639–43.
26. Martijn L, et al. Are health professionals' perceptions of patient safety related to figures on safety incidents? J Eval Clin Pract. 2013;19(5):944–7.
27. Parker D, Kirk S, Claridge T, Lawrie M, Ashcroft DM. The Manchester Patient Safety Framework (MaPSaF). In Patient Safety Research: shaping the European agenda - International Conference Porto, Portugal. 2007.
28. Westat R, Joann Sorra, and Veronica Nieva, Hospital Survey on Patient Safety Culture. 2004.
29. Sorra JS, Dyer N, Multilevel psychometric properties of the AHRQ hospital survey on patient safety culture. BMC Health Serv Res. 2011;10(199).
30. Makeham MA, et al. Patient safety events reported in general practice: a taxonomy. Qual Saf Health Care. 2008;17(1):53–7.
31. Singh R, et al. "Chance favors only the prepared mind": preparing minds to systematically reduce hazards in the testing process in primary care. J Patient Saf. 2014;10(1):20–8.
32. Fernald DH, et al. Event reporting to a primary care patient safety reporting system: a report from the ASIPS collaborative. Ann Fam Med. 2004;2(4):327–32.
33. Zwart DLM, de Bont AA. Introducing incident reporting in primary care: a translation from safety science into medical practice. Health. Risk and Society. 2013;15(3):265–78.
34. Zwart DLM, et al. Feasibility of Centre-based incident reporting in primary healthcare: the SPIEGEL study. BMJ Qual Saf. 2011;20(2):121–7.
35. Smits M, et al. Patient safety in out-of-hours primary care: a review of patient records. BMC Health Serv Res. 2010;10:335.
36. Marchon SG, Mendes Junior WV. Patient safety in primary health care: a systematic review. Cadernos de Saúde Pública. 2014;30:1815–35.
37. De Wet C, Johnson P, Mash R, McConnachie A, Bowie P. Measuring perceptions of safety climate in primary care: A cross-sectional study. J Eval Clin Pract. 2012;18(1):135–42.
38. Hoffmann B, et al. The Frankfurt patient safety climate questionnaire for general practices (FraSiK): analysis of psychometric properties. BMJ Qual Saf. 2011;20(9):797–805.
39. Hoffmann B, et al. Impact of individual and team features of patient safety climate: a survey in family practices. Ann Fam Med. 2013;11(4):355–62.
40. De Wet C, et al. Measuring perceptions of safety climate in primary care: a cross-sectional study. J Eval Clin Pract. 2012;18(1):135–42.
41. Ellis Hadyn, N Macrae., Validation in psychology: research Perspectives 2001.
42. Gaba David M, Singer SJ, Sinaiko Anna D, Bowen Jennie D, Ciavarelli Anthony P. Differences in safety climate between hospital personnel and naval aviators. Hum factors. 2003;45(2):173–85.
43. Wong K, Yu SKH, Holbrook A. A systematic review of medication safety outcomes related to drug interaction software. Canadian Journal of Clinical Pharmacology. 2010;17(2):e243–55.
44. Sweidan M, et al. Identification of features of electronic prescribing systems to support quality and safety in primary care using a modified Delphi process. BMC Med Inform Decis Mak. 2010;10:21.
45. Singh R, et al. Estimating impacts on safety caused by the introduction of electronic medical records in primary care. Inform Prim Care. 2004;12(4):235–42.
46. Szecsenyi J, et al. Effectiveness of a quality-improvement program in improving management of primary care practices. CMAJ. 2011;183(18):E1326–33.

5

Mental well-being and job satisfaction among general practitioners: a nationwide cross-sectional survey in Denmark

Karen Busk Nørøxe[1]* ⓘ, Anette Fischer Pedersen[2], Flemming Bro[1] and Peter Vedsted[1]

Abstract

Background: Poor mental well-being and low job satisfaction among physicians can have significant negative implications for the physicians and their patients and may also reduce the cost efficiency in health care. Mental distress is increasingly common in physicians, including general practitioners (GPs). This study aimed to examine mental well-being and job satisfaction among Danish GPs and potential associations with age, gender and practice organisation.

Methods: Data was collected in a nationwide questionnaire survey among Danish GPs in 2016. Register data on GPs and their patient populations was used to explore differences between respondents and non-respondents. Associations were estimated using multivariate logistic regression analysis.

Results: Of 3350 eligible GPs, 1697 (50.7%) responded. Lower response rate was associated with increasing numbers of comorbid, aging or deprived patients. About half of participating GPs presented with at least one burnout symptom; 30.6% had high emotional exhaustion, 21.0% high depersonalisation and 36.6% low personal accomplishment. About a quarter (26.2%) experienced more than one of these symptoms, and 10.4% experienced all of them. Poor work-life balance was reported by 16.2%, low job satisfaction by 22.1%, high perceived stress by 20.6% and poor general well-being by 18.6%. Constructs were overlapping; 8.4% had poor overall mental health, which was characterized by poor general well-being, high stress and ≥ 2 burnout symptoms. In contrast, 24.6% had no burnout symptoms and reported high levels of general well-being and job satisfaction. Male GPs more often than female GPs reported low job satisfaction, depersonalisation, complete burnout and poor overall mental health. Middle-aged (46–59 years) GPs had higher risk of low job satisfaction, burnout and suboptimal self-rated health than GPs in other age groups. GPs in solo practices more often assessed the work-life balance as poor than GPs in group practices.

Conclusion: The prevalence of poor mental well-being and low job satisfaction was generally high, particularly among mid-career GPs and male GPs. Approximately 8% was substantially distressed, and approximately 25% reported positive mental well-being and job satisfaction, which shows huge variation in the mental well-being among Danish GPs. The results call for targeted interventions to improve mental well-being and job satisfaction among GPs.

Keywords: General practitioner, Primary care, Burnout, Job satisfaction, Mental health, Work-life balance, Denmark

* Correspondence: karen.bn@ph.au.dk
[1]Research Unit for General Practice, Department of Public Health, Aarhus University, Bartholins Allé 2, 8000 Aarhus C, Denmark
Full list of author information is available at the end of the article

Background

Mental distress such as perceived stress and burnout is common in physicians. It seems to be an escalating problem, also among general practitioners (GPs) [1–7]. The negative implications of dissatisfaction and mental distress are far-reaching for the affected physicians, but they may also influence the quality of patient care and the cost-efficiency in health care [8–10].

Physicians experience continuous changes in their working conditions. These are caused by the changing needs and demands of the population, expansion of the medical knowledge, new health technology and reorganisation of the healthcare systems. The transfer of medical care from secondary to primary care, more administrative tasks, an aging population and the growing prevalence of people with chronic conditions have increased the workload in primary care. Together with workforce concerns, these changes may have affected the mental well-being and the job satisfaction among GPs [11–13].

The positive aspects of the clinical work among GPs are generally related to the close relationship with the patients and the provision of high-quality and continuous patient care [13–16]. However, such positive aspects may be eroded by time constraints and organizational changes aiming to cope with increasing workloads [17–19].

The past decade has seen a rise in the clinical workload in primary care when measured as number of patient contacts per GP [20, 21]. A further increase in the clinical workload is expected as the elderly population continues to grow, and more people live with chronic disease. Patients with multiple diagnoses often consult their GP and have several contacts to specialised care; these consultations are often complex, time-consuming and perceived as demanding by GPs [22–24]. In line with this, caring for a practice population with a high share of deprived patients has been shown to be associated with GP burnout [25].

Burnout is considered a prolonged response to work-related distress that evolves gradually over time. It has been described as an erosion of engagement; energy turns into exhaustion, involvement into cynicism and efficacy into perceived ineffectiveness [26, 27].

Motivated by concerns of increasing prevalence of mental distress among Danish GPs and potential implications thereof, we conducted a nationwide study aiming to explore changes in mental well-being and job satisfaction among Danish GPs and potential associations with age, gender and practice organisation.

Methods

Setting

Danish GPs work as independent contractors for the regional health authorities. GPs working under this tax-financed public reimbursement system are organised in the Organisation of General Practitioners in Denmark (PLO).

Almost all citizens (99%) are listed with a specific general practice, which they must consult (free of charge) for medical advice. Danish GPs act as gatekeepers to the rest of the health care system (except for emergencies), and the GPs provide comprehensive primary care (including preventive maternal and child care) with high levels of continuity [28]. Listed patients on average consult the general practice nearly seven times annually, and the average list size is approximately 1600 patients per GP [21]. The GPs must provide medical care all weekdays from 8 am to 4 pm, and all acute situations must be dealt with on the same day. Many GPs are also obligated to participate in out-of-hours cooperatives.

Study population

We included only GPs who were independent contractors (owners) working with the regional health authorities (excluding locums and trainees) in practices with at least 500 listed patients. A total of 3350 GPs were eligible for inclusion (Fig. 1).

Data collection

All Danish GPs listed with a valid email address at PLO in May 2016 received an email with a link to an electronically administered questionnaire. The survey was announced 1 week before by email and in a newsletter on the PLO website. Non-respondents received a reminder after 2 weeks and after 4 weeks, and the data collection terminated on 1 July 2016. The link to the questionnaire was personal; it contained a unique serial number but no personal identifiers. The PLO distributed the link, and the research group collected the survey data. The PLO provided administrative data on the GPs. The data was transferred to Statistics Denmark separately; survey data by the research group and administrative data by the PLO. The data was linked at Statistics Denmark by the unique serial number, which was subsequently deleted and combined with register data by encrypted identifiers for anonymous analysis.

Questionnaire survey

The questionnaire was developed from themes identified in existing literature and interviews with experienced researchers and clinicians. The interviews included eight individual telephone interviews (with seven GPs and one social worker employed by the Danish Medical Association) and a focus-group interview involving a representative from the Collegial Network for Physicians in Denmark (an organisation offering support to physicians), an occupational psychologist employed by the Danish Medical Association and a GP.

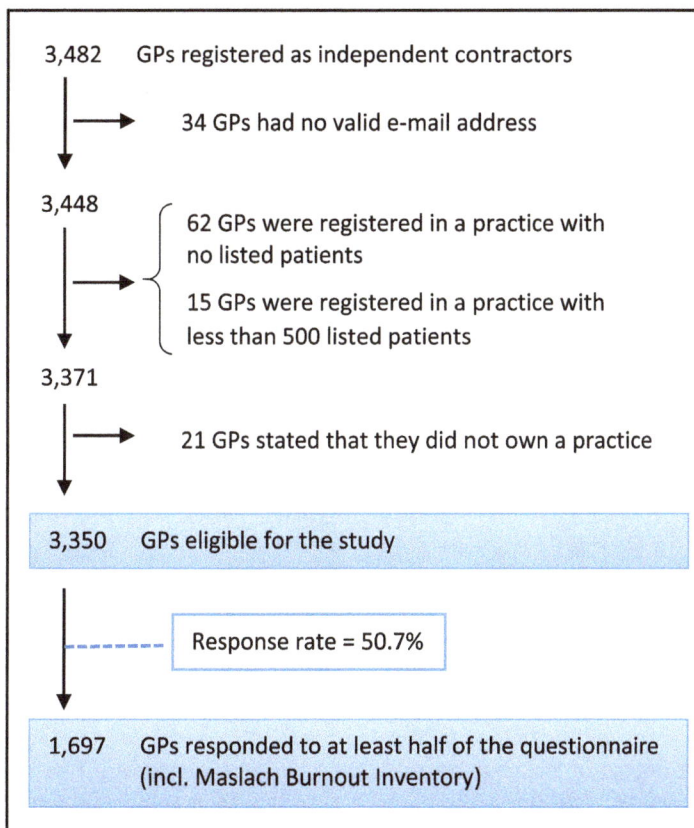

Fig. 1 Flowchart of GPs included in the study

We used validated scales whenever possible and constructed ad hoc items when validated scales were unavailable. Scales and items were discussed and agreed upon in the research group. A pilot test was conducted among 10 GPs to assess the relevance and comprehensiveness of the questionnaire battery. Only minor changes (deletion of a few ad hoc items) were made based on the pilot test.

The following scales were used in this study: the Maslach Burnout Inventory-Human Services Survey (MBI-HSS), the 10-item Danish version of Cohen's Perceived Stress Scale (PSS-10), the Warr-Cook-Wall Job Satisfaction Scale (WCW-JSS) and the World Health Organisation (Five) Well-Being Index (WHO-5). In addition, items concerning self-rated health (from the 12-item Short Form Health Survey (SF-12)), strains in private life and work-life balance were used.

Included scales have previously been translated for research use by standardised procedures; these generally include a forward translation carried out by researchers and a linguistic expert, backward translation by a native English-speaking person who was fluent in Danish, panel discussion and pilot test [29, 30].

Additional items concerned topics such as GP demographics, practice organisation, working hours, potential job-related strains, stress management, presentism and

self-rated quality of clinical work. A free-text field was also added at the end of the questionnaire.

The GPs were required to respond to all items in the specific scale in order to proceed; this setup ensured that no items were missing. Completing the questionnaire took approximately 25 min.

Other data
The administrative data on the GPs included civil registration number (CRN), age, gender, region and provider number. The number of GPs registered with each practice was categorised into: 1 GP, 2–3 GPs and > 3 GPs. Practices with one GP were defined as solo practices and practices with two or more GPs as group practices. GP age was categorised into three age groups: ≤ 45, 46–59 and ≥ 60 years.

Data on patients listed with each practice was collected from national registers. All Danish citizens are assigned a unique CRN, which allows accurate linkage of information from numerous different registers at the individual level [31].

The number of listed patients per GP was calculated as practice list size divided by the number of GPs. This was done for all listed patients, patients ≥70 years and patients with a score of ≥1 in Charlson's Comorbidity

Index (CCI). The CCI was computed based on all primary and secondary diagnoses in the Danish National Patient Register (both inpatient and outpatient hospital diagnoses) from 2006 to 2016 [32, 33].

The socio-economic burden within the practice population was measured by the Danish Deprivation Index (DADI) [25], which estimates the socio-economic burden based on eight key variables. Higher values indicate a higher proportion of deprived patients. The number of patients per GP (all patients and subgroups) and DADI scores were categorised into quartiles based on all eligible GPs and practices. Information on the practice population was collected at the end of 2015.

Outcome measures

Burnout and engagement was measured by the MBI-HSS. This instrument is considered a gold standard for assessment of burnout. It measures three burnout dimensions: (1) emotional exhaustion (EE), which is characterised by depletion of emotional resources, (2) depersonalisation (DP), which is characterised by emotional detachment from people related to work including patients, and (3) personal accomplishment (PA), which includes perceived value of work and self-efficacy. Subscale sum scores reflect the degree of burnout on each dimension. Based on predefined cut-off values for healthcare workers, each subscale score was defined as low, moderate or high [34]. Overlap between subscale scores that were indicative of burnout (high EE, high DP and low PA) was reported (Fig. 2). Complete burnout syndrome was defined as burnout-indicative scores on all MBI subscales. The opposite positive pole (low EE, low DP and high PA) was labelled 'engagement' [26, 27].

Job satisfaction was measured by the WCW-JSS. Nine job satisfaction facets and the overall job satisfaction were rated on a scale from 1 ('extreme dissatisfaction') to 7 ('extreme satisfaction') and added up to a sum score [35]. As no pre-determined cut-off values exist, respondents were divided into quartiles based on their sum score. For descriptive statistics, the GPs' own ratings of their overall job satisfaction (single item) were used: a score of ≤3 was categorised as low, 4–5 as moderate and ≥6 as high job satisfaction. The single item had high correlation with the full scale (Pearson's correlation coefficient: 0.89).

Perceived stress was measured by the PSS-10 [36, 37]. This widely used instrument consists of ten items about the frequency of stress-related feelings and thoughts. Each item is rated on a scale from 0 ('never') to 4 ('very often'). In accordance with previous research, a sum score of ≥18 was considered as high level of perceived stress [38].

General well-being was measured by the WHO-5, which consists of five positively phrased items about cheerfulness, calmness, energy and interest in day-to-day activities in the previous 14 days. Items are added up and multiplied by four to create a scale from 0 (worst quality of life possible) to 100 (best quality of life possible). In general populations, the mean WHO-5 score is 70. When screening for depression, a cut-off score of ≤50 is recommended [45]. We divided general well-being into three categories: 'high' for a score of > 70, 'poor' for a score of ≤50 and 'moderate' for a score in between.

Self-rated health was assessed by a single item from the SF-12 asking respondents to rate their general health as 'excellent', 'very good', 'good', 'fair' or 'poor' [39].

Work-life balance was assessed by one item: *'Do you generally experience a good balance between work and private life?'* Responses were categorised as 'good' (*'to a very high degree'* and *'to a high degree'*), 'moderate' (*'partly'*) or 'poor' (*'to a low degree'* and *'to a very low degree'*).

Strains in private life were assessed by one item: *'Do you feel burdened by factors related to your private life (economic issues, family problems, health conditions or similar)?'* Responses were categorised as *'No'*, *'Yes, but it burdens me only little'*, *'Yes, and it burdens me to some extent'*, *'Yes, and it burdens me a lot'* and *'I do not know/I do not wish to answer'*. The latter response category was classified as 'missing'.

Analysis

GPs who completed at least half of the questionnaire (including the WCW-JSS and the MBI-HSS) were classified as respondents. The response rate within subgroups and the corresponding 95% confidence interval (CI) were calculated. The response rate within subgroups was further adjusted for gender, age, GPs per practice, listed patients per GP and DADI score, and these estimates were presented as risk difference (RDs) with 95% CI.

For each scale, we computed mean sum score, standard deviation (SD), median sum score and interquartile interval (IQI). Within each category of well-being and satisfaction, the percentage of GPs was calculated with 95% CI.

Overlap of burnout symptoms (high EE, high DP and low PA) was visualised in an area-proportional Venn diagram. Likewise, we made Venn diagrams of negative mental health aspects (≥ 2 burnout symptoms, high perceived stress and poor general well-being) and of positive mental health aspects (no symptoms of burnout and high general well-being) and job satisfaction.

Associations between outcome measures and selected GP characteristics (age, gender and type of practice) were estimated as odds ratios (OR) with 95% CI using logistic regression while adjusting for the mentioned GP characteristics.

Scale performance was assessed by Cronbach's alpha, average inter-item correlation, and floor and ceiling effects. Analyses were performed in Stata, version 12. *P*-values of ≤0.05 were considered statistically significant.

Results

Out of 3350 eligible GPs, 1697 (50.7%) responded (Fig. 1). The response rate varied according to GP characteristics (Table 1). In the adjusted analyses, the response rate was lower among men than among women and lower among GPs aged ≥60 years than among GPs aged ≤45 years. Increasing number of elderly patients per GP, number of patients with morbidity per GP and higher deprivation index were all factors associated with lower response rate (Table 1).

The internal consistency of all included scales was adequate, with Cronbach's alpha coefficient ranging from 0.78 to 0.92. The mean sum scores of the WCW-JSS and the WHO-5 were 48.3 (SD: 13.2) and 65.7 (SD: 18.2), respectively (see the table in the Additional file 1).

Table 2 shows the prevalence of positive and negative mental health and of job satisfaction. When we combined high EE (30.6%), high DP (21.0%) and low PA (36.6%), 26.2% of GPs had high burnout scores on at least two subscales, and 10.4% experienced the complete burnout syndrome. A total of 48.5% reported no symptoms of burnout (Fig. 2). Low job satisfaction was reported by 22.1% of participants, high stress by 20.6% and poor general well-being by 18.6%.

Constructs were overlapping; 8.4% had poor overall mental health characterised by poor general well-being, high stress and substantial burnout (Fig. 3a), while 24.6%

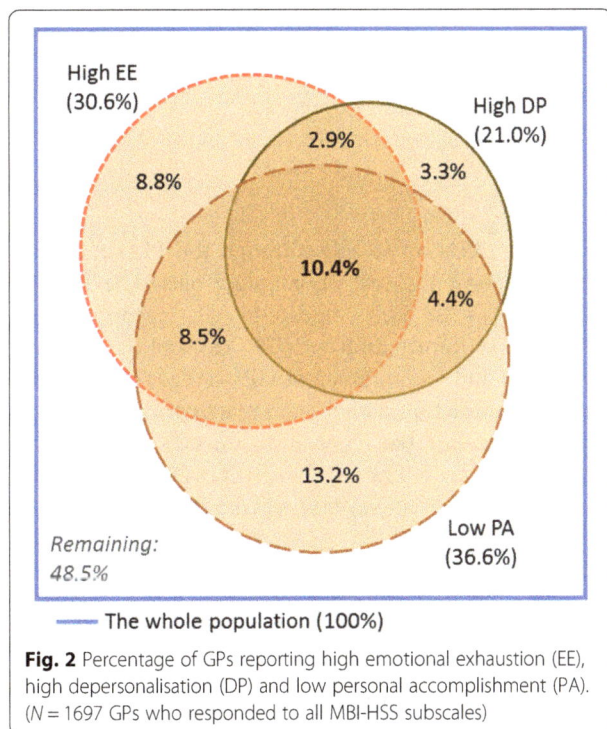

Fig. 2 Percentage of GPs reporting high emotional exhaustion (EE), high depersonalisation (DP) and low personal accomplishment (PA). (*N* = 1697 GPs who responded to all MBI-HSS subscales)

experienced positive mental health (high general well-being and no symptoms of burnout) and high job satisfaction (Fig. 3b).

The work-life balance was reported as good by 39.4% and poor by 16.2% (Table 2). Strains related to private life burdened 2.9% to a high degree. The general health was rated as just fair by 7.7% and outright poor by 0.4%.

Table 3 shows adjusted associations between mental well-being and GP characteristics. Male GPs were more likely than female GPs to experience low job satisfaction (OR = 1.55 (95% CI: 1.23–1.95)) and poor mental well-being, including complete burnout syndrome (OR = 1.50 (95% CI: 1.08–2.07)) and poor overall mental health (OR = 1.65 (95% CI: 1.16–2.36)). In contrast, male GPs were more likely to experience a good work-life balance (OR = 1.31 (95% CI: 1.07–1.62)).

Middle-aged GPs (45–59 years) more often reported burnout on all dimensions (OR = 1.45 (95% CI: 1.01–2.08), age ≤ 45 years as reference), low job satisfaction (OR = 1.44 (95% CI: 1.10–1.90)) and suboptimal self-rated health (OR = 1.55 (95% CI: 1.00–2.40)). In contrast, GPs aged ≥60 years less often reported poor overall mental health (OR = 0.39 (95% CI: 0.22–0.70)) and high perceived stress (OR = 0.49 (95% CI: 0.34–0.71)). This group also had higher likelihood of engagement (OR = 1.70 (95% CI: 1.07–2.70)), high general well-being (OR = 2.57 (95% CI: 1.93–3.40)) and good work-life balance (OR = 2.11 (95% CI: 1.58–2.79)) than their younger colleagues. GPs in group practices were significantly less likely to report poor work-life balance than GPs in solo practices (OR = 0.72 (95% CI: 0.53–0.97)).

Discussion

Main findings

Negative mental well-being and low job satisfaction were common among Danish GPs. One in ten met the criteria for complete burnout syndrome, one in five met the criterion for high perceived stress, and one in five reported poor general well-being. These bleak aspects overlapped, and 8% of GPs experienced poor overall mental health as a combination of poor general well-being, high stress and substantial burnout.

Still, about 25% of the GPs reported no symptoms of burnout along with high job satisfaction and general well-being. Furthermore, most GPs rated their general health as good, and only few reported to feel much burdened by strains in private life. However, the majority of GPs assessed the work-life balance as only moderate or poor.

The highest frequency of low job satisfaction and complete burnout syndrome was seen among GPs aged 45–59 years and male GPs. Male GPs also had higher risk of depersonalisation and poor overall mental health than women. Yet, female GPs more

Table 1 Characteristics of eligible GPs and survey respondents

		Eligible GPs N (%)	Respondents N (%)	Response rate % (95% CI)	Risk difference, adjusted[a] PP[b] (95% CI)
Total		3350 (100)	1697 (100)	50.7 (48.9–52.4)	
Gender	Female	1670 (49.9)	941 (55.5)	56.3 (53.9–58.7)	ref.
	Male	1680 (50.1)	756 (44.5)	45.0 (42.6–47.4)	**-8.2 (-11.7; -4.7)**
Age (years)	≤ 45	934 (27.9)	501 (29.5)	53.6 (50.4–56.9)	ref.
	46–59	1404 (41.9)	771 (45.4)	54.9 (52.2–57.5)	1.7 (-2.4–5.9)
	≥ 60	1012 (30.2)	425 (25.0)	42.0 (38.9–45.1)	**-8.0 (-12.7; -3.3)**
GPs per practice	1	965 (28.8)	439 (25.9)	45.5 (42.3–48.7)	ref.
	2–3	1515 (45.2)	786 (46.3)	51.9 (49.4–54.5)	1.3 (-3.0–5.6)
	> 3	871 (26.0)	472 (27.8)	54.2 (50.8–57.5)	2.4 (-2.6–7.3)
Listed patients per GP (number):					
All patients	< 1400	841 (25.1)	442 (26.1)	52.6 (49.1–56.0)	ref.
	1400–1589	836 (25.0)	456 (26.9)	54.5 (51.1–58.0)	2.1 (-2.7–6.9)
	1590–1779	836 (25.0)	416 (24.5)	49.8 (46.3–53.2)	− 2.4 (-7.2–2.4)
	> 1779	837 (25.0)	383 (22.6)	45.8 (42.3–49.2)	**-5.4 (-10.3; -0.5)**
Patients with CCI score of ≥1	< 224	846 (25.3)	471 (27.8)	55.7 (52.3–59.1)	ref.
	224–263	837 (25.0)	446 (26.3)	53.3 (49.8–56.7)	-2.9 (-7.9–2.0)
	264–311	836 (25.0)	416 (24.5)	49.8 (46.3–53.2)	**-5.0 (-10.3; -0.5)**
	> 311	831 (24.8)	364 (21.5)	43.8 (40.4–47.3)	**-7.6 (-13.5; -1.6)**
Patients aged ≥70 years	< 152	839 (25.0)	468 (27.6)	55.8 (52.3–59.2)	ref.
	152–200	840 (25.1)	433 (25.5)	51.5 (48.1–55.0)	**-4.8 (-9.6–0.0)**
	201–250	839 (25.0)	426 (25.1)	50.8 (47.3–54.2)	**-5.2 (-10.2; -0.3)**
	> 250	832 (24.8)	370 (21.8)	44.4 (41.1–47.9)	**-7.0 (-12.2; -1.8)**
DADI[c] score	≤ 22.75	842 (25.2)	469 (27.7)	55.7 (52.3–59.1)	ref.
(missing information: n = 6)	23–27.25	837 (25.0)	439 (25.9)	52.5 (49.0–55.9)	-2.6 (-7.4–2.1)
	27.5–31.75	834 (24.9)	404 (23.8)	48.9 (45.0–51.9)	**-5.5 (-10.3; -0.8)**
	≥ 32	831 (24.9)	381 (22.5)	45.8 (42.4–49.3)	**-6.4 (-11.3; -1.5)**

[a]Adjusted for gender, age, GPs per practice, number of listed patients per GP and DADI score in categories as presented in the table
[b]PP percentage points
[c]DADI Danish deprivation index
Bold indicates statistically significant difference in adjusted response rate ($p ≤ 0.05$)

often than male GPs reported a poor work-life balance. Likewise, GPs in solo practices more often than GPs in group practices reported a poor work-life balance.

Strengths and limitations
This nationwide survey is among the largest surveys worldwide of mental health and job satisfaction among GPs. Both the number of respondents ($N = 1697$) and the range of information retrieved are substantial. Furthermore, the unique Danish registers allowed for precise linkage of information on listed patients. Another major strength is the use of validated scales that have shown adequate internal consistency within the study population. The validity of single items constructed for the survey was investigated in a small-scale pilot test.

The identification of GPs through the PLO membership minimised the risk of sampling bias. The list was valid and adequately updated; the recorded and self-reported information on GP age and gender was consistent, and the number of GPs categorised as independent contractors within each practice was in accordance with the number reported by the GPs in 96% of the cases. However, a few of the invited GPs ($n = 21$) reported not to be active; this was mainly due to recent retirement.

The response rate was comparable to those reported in similar GP studies. In consideration of the significant size of the questionnaire, we consider this satisfactory. This study allowed for comparison of respondents and non-respondents, and response bias was present. Caring for a higher number of elderly patients, a higher number

Table 2 Reported well-being and job satisfaction among participating GPs

	n	% (95% CI)
Burnout/engagement (MBI)		
Emotional exhaustion (EE)		
High (indicative of burnout)	519	30.6 (28.4–32.8)
Medium	501	29.5 (27.4–31.8)
Low	677	39.9 (37.6–42.3)
Depersonalisation (DP)		
High (indicative of burnout)	357	21.0 (19.1–23.1)
Medium	505	29.8 (27.6–32.0)
Low	835	49.2 (46.8–51.6)
Personal accomplishment (PA)		
Low (indicative of burnout)	621	36.6 (34.3–38.9)
Medium	810	47.7 (45.3–50.1)
High	266	15.7 (13.9–17.5)
Overall job satisfaction (WCW-JSS, single item)		
Low (score ≤ 3)	375	22.1 (20.1–24.1)
Moderate (score 4–5)	564	33.2 (31.0–35.5)
High (score ≥ 6)	758	44.7 (42.3–47.1)
Perceived stress (PSS-10)		
Score ≥ 18 (indicative of high stress)	345	20.6 (18.7–22.6)
General well-being (WHO-5)		
Poor (score ≤ 50)	312	18.6 (16.8–20.6)
Moderate	506	30.3 (28.1–32.5)
Good (score > 70)	855	51.1 (48.7–53.5)
Self-rated health (SF-12, single item)		
Poor	6	0.4 (0.1–0.8)
Fair	129	7.7 (6.5–9.1)
Good	545	32.6 (30.3–34.9)
Very good or excellent	994	59.4 (57.0–61.7)
Work-life balance		
Poor	272	16.2 (14.5–18.1)
Moderate	743	44.4 (42.0–46.8)
Good	660	39.4 (37.1–41.8)
Strains in private life		
No	935	56.6 (54.2–59.0)
A little	419	25.4 (23.3–27.5)
Some	250	15.1 (13.4–17.0)
A lot	48	2.9 (2.1–3.8)

of patients with comorbidity and a more deprived patient population were all factors associated with non-response. This supports the assumption that GPs facing greater practice demands may be less likely to take out time to respond to questionnaire surveys. Thus, the proportion of GPs experiencing high levels of burnout and stress may be underestimated. The lower response rate among the oldest GPs corresponds to the findings in other GP studies [40] .

The cross-sectional design does not allow us to make any conclusions on causality. Yet, this survey provides unique opportunities for future analyses of potential causes and consequences of job satisfaction and well-being among GPs.

Comparison with the literature

The number of Danish GPs who face complete burnout has increased twofold since 2012 and fourfold since 2004; this is mainly due to increased emotional exhaustion and depersonalisation [41, 42]. During the same period, a decrease in job satisfaction has been seen; we found a mean WCW sum score in this study at 48 compared with 55 in 2012 and 57 in 2004 [43]. This development is in accordance with the previously reported reciprocal relationship between burnout and job satisfaction among GPs [7, 44]. Earlier studies included GPs in only one region of Denmark. However, this is not expected to impair the comparability since job satisfaction and burnout did not vary significantly across regions in the current study. Compared with the general population, participating GPs had lower levels of general well-being, and more GPs perceived high levels of stress, especially in comparison with subpopulations with similar length of education [38, 45]. This is notable as we expect GPs in general to be more aware of the importance of mental health compared to professionals outside the healthcare system.

Burnout is considered a consequence of long-term job-related stress, and the emotional exhaustion component of burnout has been described as an individual stress experience. Thus, the finding that GPs more often report high emotional exhaustion than high levels of perceived stress might appear contradictory. However, the measures are intended to measure different concepts; the emotional exhaustion subscale of the MBI aims to measure job-related exhaustion (depletion of emotional resources), whereas the PSS-10 is constructed to measure perceived stress in life in general. Moreover, both scales measure symptom degree as a continuum, and the somewhat arbitrary cut-off points have been established differently. Hence, the two measures were expected to overlap, but only to some extent. Moreover, burnout and stress were expected to overlap with poor general well-being, and similar overlap between positive

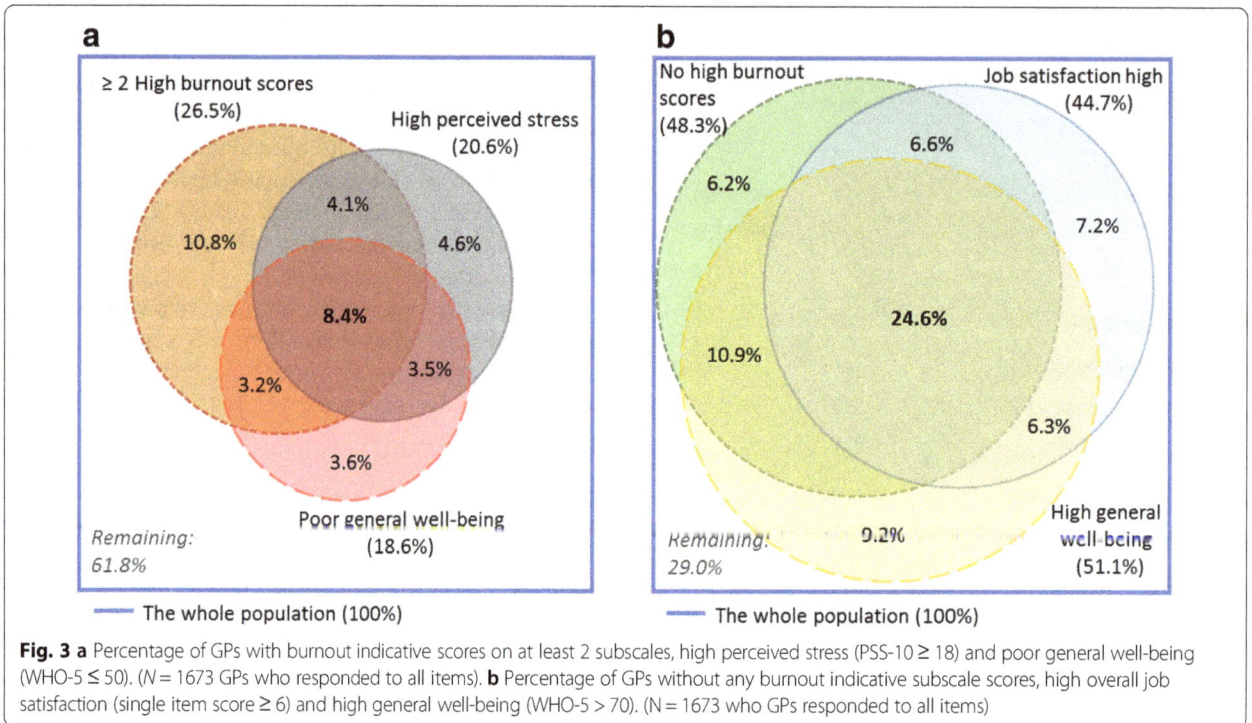

Fig. 3 a Percentage of GPs with burnout indicative scores on at least 2 subscales, high perceived stress (PSS-10 ≥ 18) and poor general well-being (WHO-5 ≤ 50). (N = 1673 GPs who responded to all items). **b** Percentage of GPs without any burnout indicative subscale scores, high overall job satisfaction (single item score ≥ 6) and high general well-being (WHO-5 > 70). (N = 1673 who GPs responded to all items)

outcomes was also expected [27, 46]. The wide span in mental health and job satisfaction among GPs may relate to differences in self-care strategies, personality traits and other factors unrelated to work. However, differences in working conditions are likely to contribute as well. The changes in working conditions that we have witnessed in recent years may weigh heavier on GPs practicing in areas characterised by deprivation, many elderly patients and/or workforce shortage [25, 47].

The increasing prevalence of mental distress and job dissatisfaction among Danish GPs mirrors the findings from physician studies in other countries [3–6]. However, the reported prevalence of distress and dissatisfaction varies substantially across countries [10].

Few other studies have measured GP burnout using the MBI-HSS. Despite marked increases in high EE (30.6%) and high DP (21.0%) among Danish GPs, most recent GP studies from elsewhere in Europe and North America have reported even higher prevalence with high EE ranging from 46% (UK) to 53% (Ireland) and high DP ranging from 32% (Ireland) to 46% (Canada) [48–50]. Still, lower prevalence of high EE (25%) and high DP (16%) was reported in one Portuguese study [51]. Additional categorisation of burnout status based on MBI subscale scores has been approached in multiple ways, but consensus on the diagnostic criteria is lacking [26]. Only few GP studies report prevalence of GPs with high burnout scores on all MBI-HSS subscales (complete burnout syndrome). In a recent Irish study, the prevalence of GPs with complete burnout was 6.6% [48]. In

earlier studies, the prevalence ranged from 3.5% in a Swiss study from 2002 to 12% (with wide inter-country variation) in a GP survey across 12 European countries from 2000 [7, 51, 52].

Low overall job satisfaction was less common in our sample (22%) than in a study among GPs in the UK from 2015 (32%) using the WCW-JSS single item [5]. In contrast, studies from Switzerland in 2009 and Norway in 2008 reported higher levels of GP job satisfaction [53, 54]. However, to our knowledge, no recent publications explore whether the job satisfaction among GPs has declined in these countries, as has been the case in Denmark.

The pronounced inter-country variation in the reported GP distress and discontentment may relate to sociodemographic and cultural differences and to different research methods and response rates [2]. However, different working conditions may also contribute substantially as the contextual factors associated with working in general practice (e.g. working hours, time per patient and type of employment) vary substantially across countries [55]. Job-related factors that are consistently reported to influence the levels of distress and dissatisfaction among GPs include lack of recognition, dissatisfaction with income, increased number of administrative tasks, long working hours, workload intensity and time pressure [13, 19]. Working conditions that undermine the GPs' experience of providing high-quality patient care may reduce the professional fulfilment, which has been described as the satisfying inner experience of being useful and making progress and has been

Table 3 Associations between GP-reported well-being and job satisfaction and gender, age and type of practice. Odds ratios with 95% confidence intervals adjusted for GP gender, age and type of practice

| | Male | 46–59 years | ≥ 60 years | Group practice |
	(female as ref.)	(≤ 45 years as ref.)		(solo practice as ref.)
Negative aspects				
EE high	1.00 (0.81–1.24)	1.15 (0.90–1.46)	**0.70 (0.51–0.94)**	0.84 (0.65–1.07)
DP high	**1.56 (1.23–1.99)**	0.96 (0.73–1.26)	**0.50 (0.35–0.71)**	0.92 (0.70–1.22)
PA low	1.11 (0.91–1.37)	1.15 (0.91–1.46)	0.96 (0.72–1.28)	0.85 (0.68–1.07)
Job satisfaction low[a]	**1.55 (1.23–1.95)**	**1.44 (1.10–1.90)**	1.32 (0.96–1.86)	0.93 (0.72–1.20)
Perceived stress high	0.83 (0.65–1.08)	1.06 (0.81–1.40)	**0.49 (0.34–0.71)**	0.88 (0.66–1.17)
General well-being poor	1.08 (0.84–1.40)	1.03 (0.77–1.40)	**0.46 (0.31–0.68)**	0.77 (0.58–1.03)
Self-rated health poor or fair	1.00 (0.69–1.45)	**1.55 (1.00–2.40)**	1.06 (0.62–1.82)	0.81 (0.54–1.21)
Work-life balance poor	0.87 (0.66–1.15)	0.91 (0.68–1.23)	**0.52 (0.35–0.77)**	**0.72 (0.53–0.97)**
Strains in private life (some/a lot)	0.87 (0.67–1.13)	1.17 (0.87–1.58)	0.85 (0.59–1.24)	0.94 (0.70–1.26)
Combinations of measures				
Complete burnout syndrome (EE high, DP high and PA low) (Fig. 2)	**1.50 (1.08–2.07)**	**1.45 (1.01–2.08)**	0.66 (0.40–1.09)	0.91 (0.64–1.30)
Poor overall mental health (≥ 2 burnout symptoms, high perceived stress and poor general well-being) (Fig. 3a)	**1.65 (1.16–2.36)**	1.24 (0.83–1.83)	**0.39 (0.22–0.70)**	0.80 (0.53–1.20)
Positive aspects				
EE low	**1.23 (1.01–1.51)**	0.95 (0.75–1.20)	**1.56 (1.19–2.06)**	0.89 (0.76–1.12)
DP low	**0.73 (0.60–0.89)**	1.02 (0.81–1.29)	**1.77 (1.35–2.34)**	0.87 (0.69–1.09)
PA high	0.92 (0.70–1.21)	1.09 (0.80–1.50)	1.29 (0.90–1.88)	0.89 (0.66–1.20)
Job satisfaction high[b]	**0.77 (0.61–0.98)**	**0.65 (0.50–0.84)**	0.87 (0.64–1.19)	0.88 (0.67–1.15)
General well-being high	1.15 (0.94–1.41)	**1.47 (1.16–1.85)**	**2.57 (1.93–3.40)**	1.09 (0.87–1.37)
Work-life balance good	**1.31 (1.07–1.62)**	1.23 (0.97–1.57)	**2.11 (1.58–2.79)**	1.23 (0.97–1.56)
Combinations of measures				
Engagement (EE low, DP low and PA high)	1.01 (0.72–1.43)	1.26 (0.83–1.91)	**1.70 (1.07–2.70)**	0.92 (0.64–1.34)
No burnout symptoms, high general well-being and high overall job satisfaction (Fig. 3b)	0.96 (0.76–1.21)	0.93 (0.70–1.21)	1.28 (0.94–1.74)	0.86 (0.67–1.12)

[a]Low: 1st quartile (WCW-JSS score ≤ 41)
[b]High: 4th quartile (WCW-JSS score ≥ 59)
EE Emotional exhaustion, *DP* Depersonalisation, *PA* Personal accomplishment
Bold indicates statistically significant results ($p \leq 0.05$)

identified as a key motivator for physicians' engagement in clinical work and healthcare development [56].

The finding that male GPs more often reported negative mental health and low job satisfaction is in accordance with previous research [48, 53]. Barriers to help-seeking and the propensity among physicians to ignore indicators of distress may be more pronounced in men [57]. This may contribute to increased risk of severe negative mental health among male GPs. The finding that male GPs more often reported low EE is consistent with previous research [7].

Superior mental health among GPs in the oldest age band echoes previous research [48]. This may be due to early retirement among GPs who experience low job satisfaction, workload pressure and poor health, whereas delayed retirement is seen among GPs who thrive in the job [58]. Other explanatory factors may include a cohort effect and age-related obligations unrelated to work (e.g. children living at home). This is supported by the finding that GPs of higher age reported better work-life balance. Furthermore, work-related strains may seem less intruding when retirement is approaching and you have many years of clinical experience. The high job satisfaction among the youngest GPs and the high prevalence of severe burnout symptoms among GPs in mid-career is in line with previous research [7, 52]. This increased burnout risk in middle-aged GPs compared with younger colleagues may reflect gradual development of burnout over time due to gradual depletion of resources [26].

Implications

The high prevalence of severe mental distress implicates a need for enhanced support to the affected GPs. Special attention should be paid to subgroups at high risk (e.g. male GPs and GPs in mid-career). The variation in GP responses concerning external factors calls for future research to examine the significance of differences in size and composition of patient populations.

The substantial increase in GP distress and discontentment signifies an urgent need to address the working conditions in general practice in order to maintain a sustainable GP workforce. Further exploration of the personal and environmental factors that are related to (positive and negative) well-being and satisfaction among GPs is suggested. Initiatives aiming to enhance GP well-being, career satisfaction and engagement are recommended to strengthen primary care and support the provision of high-quality patient care in a health care sector characterised by increasing workloads and looming workforce shortage.

Conclusion

This study documents a high and increasing level of mental distress and discontentment among GPs in Denmark. More than one in five reported low overall job satisfaction, one in three reported emotional exhaustion, and one in ten experienced complete burnout (emotional exhaustion, depersonalisation and sense of inefficacy). Furthermore, one in five perceived high levels of stress and poor general well-being. Nearly one in ten of the GPs experienced a combination of at least two burnout symptoms, high stress and poor general well-being. The risk of negative mental health and dissatisfaction was generally high for both genders and across age band and practice type, but it was particularly high among GPs in mid-career and male GPs. In contrast to the substantial minority of distressed GPs, a larger group expressed positive mental health and high job satisfaction. This indicates that GPs constitute a heterogeneous population. Targeted interventions are needed to addresses GP mental health and job satisfaction.

Abbreviations

CI: Confidence interval; DP: Depersonalisation; EE: Emotional exhaustion; GP: General practitioner; MBI-HSS: Maslach Burnout Inventory - Human Services Survey; OR: Odds ratio; PA: Personal accomplishment; PLO: Organisation of General Practitioners in Denmark; PSS-10: Cohen's Perceived Stress Scale, 10-item Danish version; SD: Standard deviation; WCW-JSS: Warr, Cook and Wall Job Satisfaction Scale; WHO-5: The World Health Organisation Well-Being Index

Acknowledgements

The authors would like to thank the PLO and all the GPs who took part in this study.

Funding

This project was supported by the Danish National Research Foundation for Primary Care and by the Health Foundation.

Authors' contributions

All authors contributed substantially to the design of the study. KBN performed the statistical analyses in consultation with PV. KBN wrote the first draft of the article. AFP, FB and PV assisted in writing and revising the manuscript. All authors read and approved the final manuscript.

Ethics approval and consent to participate

The project was approved by the Danish Data Protection Agency (J.no. 2016-41-4648). According to Danish law, approval by the Danish National Committee on Health Research Ethics was not required as no biomedical intervention was performed.
Respondents gave their content to participate by responding to the questionnaire. Personally identifiable information on GPs and patients were re-coded and anonymised at Statistics Denmark prior to data analysis.

Competing interests

The authors declare that they have no competing interests. The Organisation of General Practitioners in Denmark (PLO) had no access to the data or any influence on the analyses or conclusions.

Author details

[1]Research Unit for General Practice, Department of Public Health, Aarhus University, Bartholins Allé 2, 8000 Aarhus C, Denmark. [2]Research Unit for General Practice & Department of Clinical Medicine, Aarhus University, Aarhus, Denmark.

References

1. Imo UO. Burnout and psychiatric morbidity among doctors in the UK: a systematic literature review of prevalence and associated factors. BJPsych Bull. 2017;41(4):197–204.
2. Hayes B, Prihodova L, Walsh G, Doyle F, Doherty S. What's up doc? A national cross-sectional study of psychological wellbeing of hospital doctors in Ireland. BMJ Open. 2017;7(10):e018023. -2017-018023
3. Shanafelt TD, Hasan O, Dyrbye LN, Sinsky C, Satele D, Sloan J, West CP. Changes in burnout and satisfaction with work-life balance in physicians and the general US working population between 2011 and 2014. Mayo Clin Proc. 2015;90(12):1600–13.
4. Rothenberger DA. Physician burnout and well-being: a systematic review and framework for action. Dis Colon Rectum. 2017;60(6):567–76.
5. Gibson J, Checkland K, Coleman A, Hann M, McCall R, Spooner S: Eighth National GP Worklife Survey, 2015. http://research.bmh.manchester.ac.uk/healtheconomics/research/Reports/EighthNationalGPWorklifeSurveyreport/, (asssessed 25 Feb 2018).
6. Arigoni F, Bovier PA, Sappino AP. Trend of burnout among Swiss doctors. Swiss Med Wkly. 2010;140:w13070.
7. Soler JK, Yaman H, Esteva M, Dobbs F, Asenova RS, Katic M, Ozvacic Z, Desgranges JP, Moreau A, Lionis C, Kotanyi P, Carelli F, Nowak PR, de Aguiar

Sa Azeredo Z, Marklund E, Churchill D, Ungan M. European general practice research network burnout study group: burnout in European family doctors: the EGPRN study. Fam Pract. 2008;25(4):245–65.

8. Wallace JE, Lemaire JB, Ghali WA. Physician wellness: a missing quality indicator. Lancet. 2009;374(9702):1714–21.

9. Scheepers RA, Boerebach BC, Arah OA, Heineman MJ, Lombarts KM. A systematic review of the impact of Physicians' occupational well-being on the quality of patient care. Int J Behav Med. 2015;22(6):683–98.

10. Kumar S. Burnout and doctors: prevalence, prevention and intervention. Healthcare (Basel). 2016;4(3) https://doi.org/10.3390/healthcare4030037.

11. Osborn R, Moulds D, Schneider EC, Doty MM, Squires D, Sarnak DO. Primary care physicians in ten countries report challenges caring for patients with complex health needs. Health Aff (Millwood). 2015;34(12):2104–12.

12. Baird B, Charles A, Honeyman M, Maguire D, Das P: Understanding the pressures in general practice. Kings Fund, 2016 https://wwwkingsfundorguk/publications/pressures-in-general-practice, (assessed 26 May 2018).

13. Marchand C, Peckham S. Addressing the crisis of GP recruitment and retention: a systematic review. Br J Gen Pract. 2017;67(657):e227–37.

14. Landon BE, Reschovsky J, Blumenthal D. Changes in career satisfaction among primary care and specialist physicians, 1997-2001. JAMA. 2003;289(4):442–9.

15. Whitebird RR, Solberg LI, Crain AL, Rossom RC, Beck A, Neely C, Dreskin M, Coleman KJ. Clinician burnout and satisfaction with resources in caring for complex patients. Gen Hosp Psychiatry. 2017;44:91–5.

16. Leiter MP, Frank E, Matheson TJ. Demands, values, and burnout: relevance for physicians. Can Fam Physician. 2009;55(12):1224–5. 1225.e1–6

17. Agana DF, Porter M, Hatch R, Rubin D, Carek P. Job satisfaction among academic family physicians. Fam Med. 2017;49(8):622–5.

18. Dale J, Potter R, Owen K, Parsons N, Realpe A, Leach J. Retaining the general practitioner workforce in England: what matters to GPs? A cross-sectional study. BMC Fam Pract. 2015;16:140–015. 0363-1.

19. Van Ham I, Verhoeven AA, Groenier KH, Groothoff JW, De Haan J. Job satisfaction among general practitioners: a systematic literature review. Eur J Gen Pract. 2006;12(4):174–80.

20. Hobbs FD, Bankhead C, Mukhtar T, Stevens S, Perera-Salazar R, Holt T, Salisbury C. National Institute for Health Research School for Primary Care Research: Clinical workload in UK primary care: a retrospective analysis of 100 million consultations in England, 2007-14. Lancet. 2016;387(10035):2323–30.

21. Organisation of General Practitioners (PLO), Denmark: Fact sheet on Danish General Practice 2017., https://www.laeger.dk/sites/default/files/plo_faktaark_2017.pdf, (assessed 6 Dec 2017).

22. Loeb DF, Bayliss EA, Candrian C, deGruy FV, Binswanger IA. Primary care providers' experiences caring for complex patients in primary care: a qualitative study. BMC Fam Pract. 2016;17:34.

23. Moth G, Vestergaard M, Vedsted P. Chronic care management in Danish general practice–a cross-sectional study of workload and multimorbidity. BMC Fam Pract. 2012;13:52–2296. 13-52

24. Adams WL, McIlvain HE, Lacy NL, Magsi H. Ea: Primary care for elderly people: Why do doctors find it so hard? Gerontologist. 2002;42(6):835–42.

25. Pedersen AF, Vedsted P. Understanding the inverse care law: a register and survey-based study of patient deprivation and burnout in general practice. Int J Equity Health. 2014;13(1):121.

26. Schaufeli WB, Leiter MP, Maslach C. Burnout: 35 years of research and practice. Career Development International. 2009;14(3):204–20.

27. Maslach C, Leiter MP. Understanding the burnout experience: recent research and its implications for psychiatry. World Psychiatry. 2016;15(2):103–11.

28. Pavlic DR, Sever M, Klemenc-Ketis Z, Svab I, Vainieri M, Seghieri C, Maksuti A. Strength of primary care service delivery: a comparative study of European countries, Australia, New Zealand, and Canada. Prim Health Care Res Dev. 2018:1–11.

29. Vedsted P, Sokolowski I, Olesen F. Open access to general practice was associated with burnout among general practitioners. Int J Family Med. 2013;2013:383602.

30. Andersen CM: The association between attachment and delay in the diagnosis of cancer in primary care. *Ph.D dissertation*. Aarhus University, Health; 2016.

31. Pedersen CD. The Danish civil registration system. Scand J Public Health. 2011;39(7 Suppl):22–5.

32. Sundararajan V, Quan H, Halfon P, Fushimi K, Luthi JC, Burnand B, Ghali WA. International methodology consortium for coded health information (IMECCHI): cross-national comparative performance of three versions of the ICD-10 Charlson index. Med Care. 2007;45(12):1210–5.

33. Thygesen SK, Christiansen CF, Christensen S, Lash TL, Sorensen HT: The predictive value of ICD-10 diagnostic coding used to assess Charlson comorbidity index conditions in the population-based Danish National Registry of patients. BMC Med Res Methodol 2011, 11:83–2288–11-83.

34. Maslach C, Jackson E, Leiter MP. Maslach burnout inventory manual, 3rd edition. USA: Consulting Pshychologists Press, Pao Alto, Calif; 1996.

35. Warr P, Cook J, Wall T. Scales for the measurement of some work attitudes and aspects of psychological well-being. J Ocupp Psychol. 1979;52:129.

36. Cohen S, Kamarck T, Mermelstein R. A global measure of perceived stress. J Helath Soc Behav. 1983;24(4):385.

37. Cohen S, Williamson G. Perceived stress in a probability sample in the United States. In: Spacapan S, Oskamp S, editors. The Social Psychology of Health: The Claremont Symposium on Apllied Soc Psychol SAGE publications inc; 1988. p. 31.

38. Prior A, Fenger-Gron M, Larsen KK, Larsen FB, Robinson KM, Nielsen MG, Christensen KS, Mercer SW, Vestergaard M. The association between perceived stress and mortality among people with multimorbidity: a prospective population-based cohort study. Am J Epidemiol. 2016;184(3):199–210.

39. Ware J, Jr KM, Keller SD. A 12-item short-form health survey: construction of scales and preliminary tests of reliability and validity. Med Care. 1996;34(3):220–33.

40. Barclay S, Todd C, Finlay I, Grande G, Wyatt P. Not another questionnaire! Maximizing the response rate, predicting non-response and assessing non-response bias in postal questionnaire studies of GPs. Fam Pract. 2002;19(1):105–11.

41. Pedersen AF, Andersen CM, Olesen F, Vedsted P. Risk of burnout in Danish GPs and exploration of factors associated with development of burnout: a two-wave panel study. Int J Family Med. 2013;2013:603713.

42. Pedersen AF, Andersen CM, Olesen F, Vedsted P. Stress and burnout increase among general practitioners in Denmark. Ugeskr Laeger. 2014;176(2):135.

43. Brøndt A, Vedsted P, Olesen F. General practitioners' job satisfaction. Ugeskr Laeger. 2007;169(26):2521.

44. Bovier PA, Arigoni F, Schneider M, Gallacchi MB. Relationships between work satisfaction, emotional exhaustion and mental health among Swiss primary care physicians. The European Journal of Public Health. 2009;19(6):611–7.

45. Topp CW, Ostergaard SD, Sondergaard S, Bech P. The WHO-5 well-being index: a systematic review of the literature. Psychother Psychosom. 2015;84(3):167–76.

46. Vicentic S, Gasic MJ, Milovanovic A, Tosevski DL, Nenadovic M, Damjanovic A, Kostic BD, Jovanovic AA. Burnout, quality of life and emotional profile in general practitioners and psychiatrists. Work (Reading, Mass). 2013;45(1):129.

47. Hoffmann K, Wojczewski S, George A, Schäfer WLA, Maier M. Stressed and overworked? A cross-sectional study of the working situation of urban and rural general practitioners in Austria in the framework of the QUALICOPC project. Croat Med J. 2015;56(4):366–74.

48. O'Dea B, O'Connor P, Lydon S, Murphy AW. Prevalence of burnout among Irish general practitioners: a cross-sectional study. Irish J Med Sci. 2017;186(2):447–53.

49. Orton P, Orton C, Pereira Gray D. Depersonalised doctors: a cross-sectional study of 564 doctors, 760 consultations and 1876 patient reports in UK general practice. BMJ Open. 2012, 2:e000274–2011. 000274. Print 2012

50. Lee FJ, Stewart M, Brown JB. Stress, burnout, and strategies for reducing them: what's the situation among Canadian family physicians? Can Fam Physician. 2008;54(2):234–5.

51. Marcelino G, Cerveira JM, Carvalho I, Costa JA, Lopes M, Calado NE, Marques-Vidal P. Burnout levels among Portuguese family doctors: a nationwide survey. BMJ Open. 2012;2(3):e001050.

52. Goehring C, Bouvier Gallacchi M, Kunzi B, Bovier P. Psychosocial and professional characteristics of burnout in Swiss primary care practitioners: a cross-sectional survey. Swiss Med Wkly. 2005;135(7–8):101–8.

53. Goetz K, Jossen M, Szecsenyi J, Rosemann T, Hahn K, Hess S. Job satisfaction of primary care physicians in Switzerland: an observational study. Fam Pract. 2016;33(5):498–503.

54. Nylenna M, Aasland OG. Job satisfaction among Norwegian doctors. Tidsskr Nor Laegeforen. 2010;130(10):1028–31.

55. Masseria C, Irwin R, Thomson S, Gemmill M, Mossialos E. Primary Care in Europe, policy brief. London, UK: London School of Economics and Political Science; 2009.

56. Lindgren A, Baathe F, Dellve L. Why risk professional fulfilment: a grounded theory of physician engagement in healthcare development. Int J Health Plann Manag. 2013;28(2):e138–57.

57. Spiers J, Buszewicz M, Chew-Graham CA, Gerada C, Kessler D, Leggett N, Manning C, Taylor AK, Thornton G, Riley R. Barriers, facilitators, and survival strategies for GPs seeking treatment for distress: a qualitative study. Br J Gen Pract. 2017;67(663):e700–8.

58. Silver MP, Hamilton AD, Biswas A, Warrick NI. A systematic review of physician retirement planning. Hum Resour Health. 2016;14(1)

6

The effectiveness of shared decision-making followed by positive reinforcement on physical disability in the long-term follow-up of patients with nonspecific low back pain in primary care

Ariëtte R. J. Sanders[1]* (iD), Jozien M. Bensing[2,3], Tessa Magnée[2], Peter Verhaak[2] and Niek J. de Wit[1]

Abstract

Background: Although the recovery of patients suffering from low back pain is highly context dependent, patient preferences about treatment options are seldom incorporated into the therapeutic plan. Shared decision-making (SDM) offers a tool to overcome this deficiency. The reinforcement by the general practitioner (GP) of a 'shared' chosen therapy might increase patients' expectations of favourable outcomes and thus contribute to recovery.

Methods: In the Netherlands, a clustered randomised controlled trial was performed to assess the effectiveness of shared decision-making followed by positive reinforcement of the chosen therapy (SDM&PR) on patient-related clinical outcomes. Overall, 68 GPs included 226 patients visiting their GP for a new episode of non-chronic low back pain. GPs in the intervention group were trained in implementing SDM&PR using a structured training programme with a focus on patient preferences in reaching treatment decisions. GPs in the control group provided care as usual. The primary outcome was the change in physical disability measured with the Roland-Morris disability questionnaire (RMD) during the six-month follow-up after the first consultation. Physical disability (RMD), pain, adequate relief, absenteeism and healthcare consumption at 2, 6, 12 and 26 weeks were secondary outcomes. A multivariate analysis with a mixed model was used to estimate the differences in outcomes.

Results: Of the patients in the intervention and the control groups, 66 and 62%, respectively, completed the follow-up. Most patients (77%) recovered to no functional restrictions due to back pain within 26 weeks. No significant differences in the mean scores for any outcome were observed between intervention patients and controls during the follow-up, and in multivariate analysis, there was no significant difference in the main outcome during the six-month follow-up. Patients in the intervention group reported more involvement in decision-making.

(Continued on next page)

* Correspondence: alennep@umcutrecht.nl
[1]Julius Centre for Health Sciences and Primary Care, University Medical Centre Utrecht, PO Box 85500 3508, GA, Utrecht, the Netherlands
Full list of author information is available at the end of the article

(Continued from previous page)

Conclusion: This study did not detect any improvement in clinical outcome or in health care consumption of patients with non-chronic low back pain after the training of GPs in SDM&PR. The implementation of SDM merely introduces task-oriented communication. The training of the GPs may have been more effective if it had focused more on patient-oriented communication techniques and on stressing the expectation of favourable outcomes.

Keywords: Low back pain, General practice, Patient-oriented outcome, Shared decision-making, Randomised controlled trial

Background

Nonspecific low back pain is defined as back pain localised below the costal margin and the inferior gluteal folds, with or without referred leg pain, and without a specific somatic origin [1, 2].

Low back pain can be divided into acute, with a duration of complaints < 6 weeks, subacute, with a duration of complaints between 6 and 12 weeks, and chronic, with complaints lasting longer than 3 months [1–3].

Low back pain has a lifetime prevalence of 60–85% [4]. Most episodes of low back pain resolve after two weeks, but the recurrence rate is high; three-quarters of patients have a second episode within one year [4]. Because of related health costs, absenteeism and disability, low back pain is a substantial economic burden to society [2, 5].

The therapeutic guidelines on low back pain focus on the continuation of physical activity, as the effectiveness of most therapeutic interventions does not exceed the placebo effect [1]. In addition, the guidelines recommend considering patient preferences in the choice of the therapeutic regimen because contextual factors determine the speed of recovery [1, 6]. Contextual factors include the patient, the physician, and their relationship [6].

The illness perceptions of a patient, such as avoidance beliefs and fear of the duration of the illness, predict the patient's recovery and their return to work [7–9]. In medical decision-making, little attention is paid to the patient perspective, and even if considered, it is often misinterpreted [9–11]. However, the patient perspective is generally considered essential for medical decision-making, as stated in the Salzburger Statement on shared decision-making (SDM) [12].

SDM is defined as follows: A situation in which the professional and patient share their perspective and jointly decide on a treatment plan. SDM provides the possibility of incorporating patient preferences into clinical decision-making [13]. The philosophy of this concept is that patients will have more autonomy in decisions about their personal health if the doctor-patient relationship shifts from paternalistic to a more equal relationship [14]. Glyn Elwyn operationalised this concept into a three-talk model of shared decision-making. Team talk places an emphasis on the need to provide support to patients when they are made aware of choices, and Option talk refers to the task of comparing alternatives by using risk communication principles. Decision talk refers to the task of arriving at decisions that reflect the informed preferences of patients, guided by the experience and expertise of health professionals. In this broadly accepted model, patients are informed about the decision process and the pros and cons of treatment options [15].

Since the introduction of SDM in clinical care, research has focused on the process of SDM implementation and its effect on clinical outcomes [16]. At present, the findings related to clinical outcomes are scarce and unconvincing [16].

For patients with low back pain, SDM could improve the prognosis if patients were more adherent to treatment, as the expectation of a favourable outcome is incorporated into the treatment decisions [17].

It has been empirically proven that the positive outcome expectations of the patient benefit the health status of the patient, and the reinforcement of these treatment expectations could endorse these effects [18, 19].

Although widely advocated in guidelines, the effectiveness of SDM in the management of low back pain has not been evaluated in general practice [20].

Therefore, we conducted a large randomised controlled trial among primary care patients with non-chronic low back pain in the Netherlands and report the effectiveness of SDM followed by positive reinforcement of the therapeutic choice (SDM&PR) on recovery and healthcare consumption.

Methods

Aim

The aim is to assess the effectiveness of shared decision-making followed by a positive reinforcement of the chosen therapy (SDM&PR) on patient-related clinical outcomes in patients with non-chronic low back pain in general practice.

Design and setting

A cluster-randomised controlled trial was performed in the practices of 68 general practitioners (GPs) in the academic primary care network around Utrecht in the Netherlands.

Participants

GPs were recruited between August 2009 and May 2011. Each participating GP was requested to include ten patients with non-chronic nonspecific low back pain.

The inclusion criteria were as follows:

1. between 18 and 65 years of age, and
2. in consultation for a new episode of non-chronic nonspecific low back pain (as defined by the guidelines of the Dutch College of General Practitioners and the Cochrane Collaboration) [2, 21].

The exclusion criteria were as follows:

1. duration of low back pain longer than three months,
2. any previous episode of low back pain within the three months prior to the onset of the present episode,
3. pregnancy, and
4. insufficient mastery of the Dutch language.

Because the causes and pathophysiology of low back pain might be different in patients younger than 18 or older than 65 years, those who are pregnant or in those with a longer disease duration, we excluded these patients [1, 21].

Randomisation, data collection and blinding

GPs were randomly assigned to the usual care (UC) group or the intervention (IV) group immediately after consenting to participate in the trial. Randomisation was done by research staff members who were not otherwise in the research project. Allocation was blinded using allocation cards in sealed envelopes in an initial block of 40 followed by blocks of ten envelopes. GPs in the control group were kept unaware of the communicative techniques that were trained. Auxiliary staff members recruited the patients. Patients and auxiliary practice staff members were not informed about the allocation of the GP or about the communicative techniques in the training programme. Auxiliary practice staff members collected questionnaires from the patients after inclusion. A follow-up questionnaire with a pre-paid envelope was given to each patient with instructions on when to complete it and send it to the research team. Patients were reminded to send the questionnaires two, six, twelve and twenty-six weeks after the consultation by

email or phone just before the correct time and, if necessary, again two weeks later.

Intervention

GPs in the intervention group were trained to perform SDM&PR during their consultations with the included patients. SDM followed the following process steps: inform the patient about therapeutic options, discuss the patient's preferences, concerns and expectations, confirm the patient's understanding, assess the patient's preferred level of involvement in decision-making and finally make a joint decision about the optimal therapeutic regimen. GPs were trained to positively reinforce treatment outcomes after SDM.

Training

GPs in the intervention group received two training sessions of two and a half hours. Training sessions were held in small groups of approximately three to five participants and were given by a peer GP with expertise in training SDM skills (AS).

The training was based on the learning principles of Kolb and the behavioural process elements of Elwyn [22]. To support SDM performance during consultations, the participating GPs received a desktop card summarising all consecutive process elements for SDM and a decision aid specifically developed for this trial according to the International Patient Decision Aids Standards (IPDAS)-guidelines (Additional file 1 Appendix 1) [23, 24]. Finally, they received individual feedback on their SDM performance based on observation by the trainer (AS) of videotapes of the consultation of each included patient. Details of the training are reported elsewhere [23]. The fidelity of the intervention was checked by measuring behavioural changes and consultation duration differences between the intervention and the control group using the OPTION instrument on videotaped consultations [23].

Control group

In the control group, the GPs provided the usual standard of care. Although routine management was not predefined in the instructions for the study, GPs in the Netherlands are reported to follow the professional guidelines on low back pain in 70% of patients [25]. Discussion of the favourable prognosis of low back pain is part of the suggested management in the guideline, but SDM is not [2].

Outcome

The primary outcome was the difference between the intervention and the control group in the course of functional disability during the six-month follow-up. Functional disability was measured daily during the first two weeks and at two, six, twelve and twenty-six weeks after the first consultation.

As secondary outcomes, we assessed the difference in functional disability at the time of each of the separate measurements (2, 6, 12 and 26 weeks), the difference in severity of back pain and the percentage of patients with adequate relief on separate measurement dates and at the end of the study.

As indicators of economic effect, we evaluated the differences in absenteeism and health care consumption between groups over the complete study period and on the separate measurement dates.

To be able to test for potential confounding, we measured illness perceptions at the baseline. To check the fidelity of the intervention, we questioned patients after the consultation about the level of involvement in decision-making.

Measurements and instruments

Functional disability was assessed by the Dutch version of the Roland-Morris disability questionnaire (RMD). This validated questionnaire contains 24 closed questions about restrictions in daily activities during the previous day. The score is the total number of positive answers [26]. Pain severity was quantified by the validated continuous visual analogue scale (VAS), in which the patients indicate the level of pain during the past week on a continuous line that ranges from zero (no pain) to ten cm (the most terrible pain I can imagine), with outcomes measured in mm. [27]. Adequate relief (AR) of pain was assessed with one closed question referring to the recovery experienced since the previous questionnaire and was expressed as the percentage of patients with AR in each group.

Absenteeism was measured by the response to a question referring to the time before the baseline or since the previous questionnaire: 'Because of my back pain, I refrained from work (absenteeism),' yes/no/not applicable (expressed as a percentage of patients), followed by an inquiry about the number of days of sick leave.

Healthcare consumption data were derived from patient questionnaires by counting follow-up contacts, via telephone or at the practice, and expressed as the mean number of contacts per patient since the previous questionnaire.

Illness perceptions were assessed by the Dutch version of the abbreviated illness perception questionnaire (IPQ) [28]. This instrument measures eight separate dimensions of perceptions about low back pain using a scale rating from zero to ten. This instrument has been proven to be valid [29].

The actual level of shared decision-making, as experienced by the patient, was evaluated by their response to one simple question immediately after the consultation: 'Were you involved in decision-making?' Mean scores were calculated from a range of one to four points corresponding to the answers 'no,' 'mostly no,' mostly yes' or 'yes'.

The observed effects of the training were reported in a separate article on the evaluation of the training [23].

The primary outcome (RMD) and the VAS was assessed daily during the first 14 days by a diary and at two, six, twelve and twenty-six weeks after consultation by questionnaires. All other secondary outcomes were assessed at two, six, twelve and twenty-six weeks (Fig. 1). Baseline measurements, potential confounders and the manipulation check were assessed through questionnaires completed by all patients before and immediately after the consultation.

Sample size

To reach a minimum standardised difference of 0.3 in the primary outcome between the intervention and control groups, which is more than 1 point on RMD scores with a standard deviation of 5, using a beta of 0.80 and an alpha of 0.05, 352 patients would be required [26]. As we randomised at the level of the GP but measured patient outcomes, we controlled for clustering effects. Based on clustering effects reported in earlier trials, we applied an intra-class correlation of 0.03 [30]. Presuming a 10% dropout rate, we calculated that 426 patients should be included by 60 GPs.

Statistical analysis

Differences in baseline characteristics between dropouts and patients who completed the follow-up were tested for significance using a t-test for continuous variables and a X^2-test for dichotomous and categorical variables.

The effect of the intervention on the separate measurement dates at two, six, twelve and twenty-six weeks was tested univariately. In multivariate analysis, differences in primary and secondary outcomes were estimated with a mixed model corrected for potential confounders: age, sex, educational level and the corresponding baseline value of the outcome. A random intercept was included for clustering at the level of the GP, and a random intercept and a random effect for time at the patient level were included to incorporate the effect over time. All analysis was performed on an intention-to-treat basis.

The potential confounding effect of each of the illness perception dimensions was assessed with mixed models, with restrictions at 12 weeks as the outcome variable and correction for all confounders.

Mixed models are robust for individual patients with missing follow-up measurements. In the analysis, we originally included the baseline measurement of the corresponding outcome as a covariate. Consequently, any measurement of any patient with a missing baseline measurement would be excluded from the analysis, thus

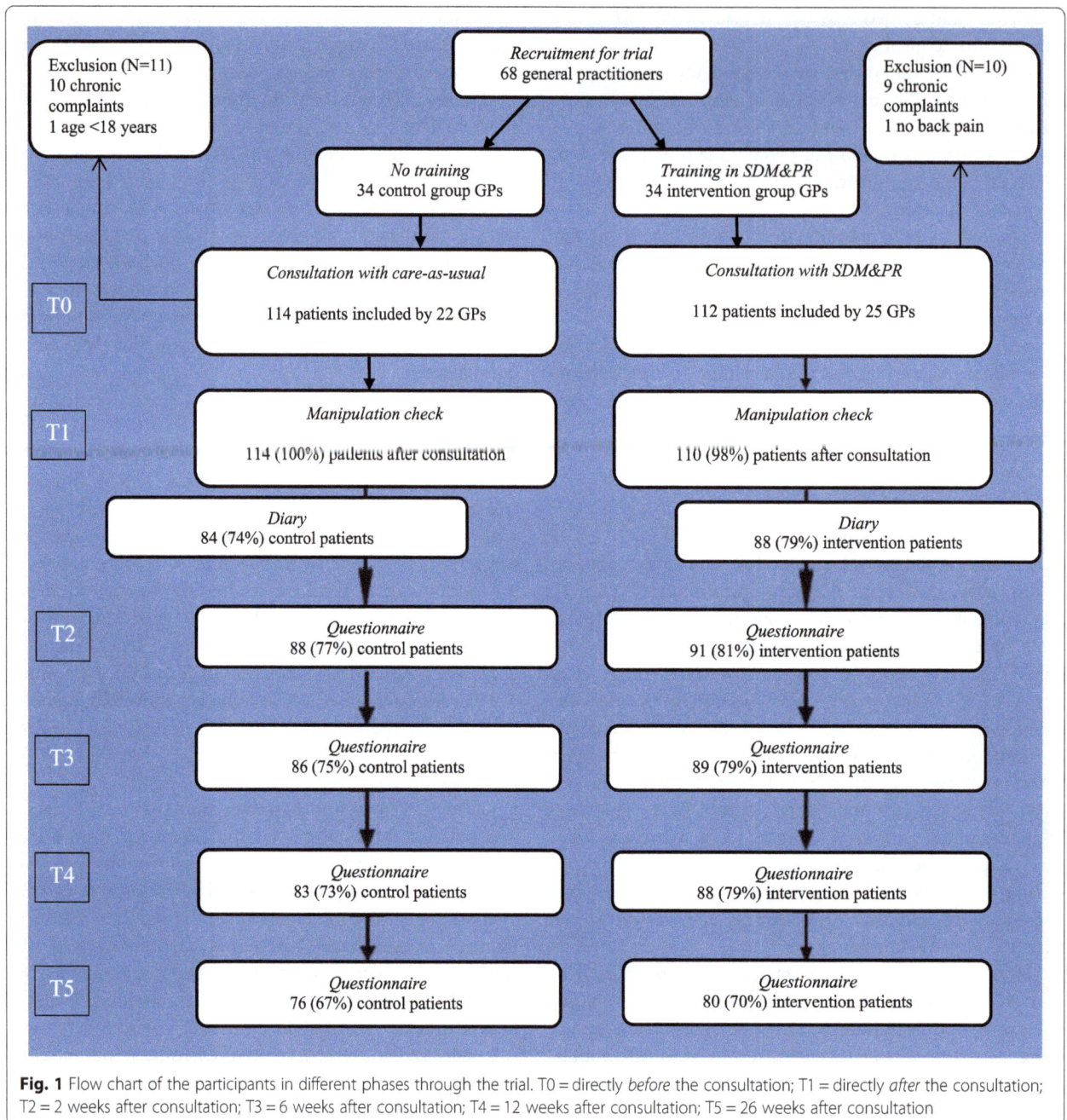

Fig. 1 Flow chart of the participants in different phases through the trial. T0 = directly *before* the consultation; T1 = directly *after* the consultation; T2 = 2 weeks after consultation; T3 = 6 weeks after consultation; T4 = 12 weeks after consultation; T5 = 26 weeks after consultation

reducing power and potentially introducing bias. We therefore decided to use multiple imputation to impute baseline variables and missing confounders measured at the baseline [31, 32].

Age, sex, educational level, absenteeism, all illness perceptions, the treatment allocation and all baseline measurements of primary and secondary outcomes were included in the multiple imputation. The numbers of imputed missing variables per baseline variable are described in Table 1. Five imputed datasets were created. Univariate and multivariate analyses were performed on

each imputation; the results reported here were combined with Rubin's rule [33].

Results

Participants

Sixty-eight GPs agreed to participate and were randomised to the intervention (*n* = 34) or the control group (*n* = 34). GPs in the intervention group did not differ from control GPs with regard to sex, age, professional age, number of included patients or percentage of GP trainers per group.

Table 1 Baseline demographic and clinical characteristics of patients *in the complete* dataset. Continuous variable values are represented as means (standard deviation). Dichotomous variable values are represented as numbers (percentages)

	intervention group	control group
Patient characteristics	(*n* = 112)	(*n* = 114)
mean age (years)	45.4 (13.2)	44.3 (14.4)
male†	52 (47%)	55 (49%)
Dutch origin‡	97 (91%)	103 (93%)
educational level‡		
primary only	15 (14%)	19 (17%)
secondary	56 (52%)	53 (48%)
college, university	36 (34%)	39 (35%)
employed§	73 (70%)	71 (70%)
Baseline clinical characteristics		
functional disability score (RMD 0–24) (primary measure)¶	10.7 (5.0)	10.3 (5.2)
pain severity at baseline (VAS 0–100 mm)‖	48.6 (16.0)	46.7 (16.7)
absenteeism (yes/no)‖	39 (35%)	19 (20%)
illness perception dimensions (IPQ)(0–10)§		
consequences	6.3 (2.3)	6.1 (2.5)
timeline	4.2 (2.8)	3.5 (2.4)
personal control	5.0 (2.2)	5.4 (2.1)
treatment control	6.6 (1.9)	6.9 (1.9)
identity	6.9 (1.6)	7.2 (1.6)
concerns	4.5 (2.5)	4.8 (2.6)
illness comprehensibility	6.0 (2.3)	6.1 (2.3)
emotional response	5.0 (2.5)	5.2 (2.6)

RMD = Roland-Morris disability questionnaire (a higher score indicates a more favourable outcome). VAS = visual analogue scale combined score of low back pain, leg pain and both (a lower score indicates a more favourable outcome). IPQ = Illness Perception Questionnaire. ¶ *n* = 3 missing. ‖ *n* = 34 missing. † *n* = 4 missing. ‡ *n* = 8 missing. § *n* = 19 missing

Between January 2010 and January 2012, forty-seven GPs included 247 patients (range 0–10). Twenty-one of these patients did not meet the inclusion criteria because they did not align with the definition of non-chronic low back pain (*n* = 19), did not have back complaints (*n* = 1) or were younger than 18 years old (*n* = 1). Ultimately, 114 patients in the control group and 112 in the intervention group were included in the analysis (Fig. 1).

Patients in the intervention and control groups were comparable across most baseline measurements (Table 1 and Additional file 2 Appendix 2 for the imputed dataset). Patients in the intervention group reported more absenteeism from work due to their low back pain, and they more frequently expected their pain to last longer than did the controls.

During the follow-up, 76 (67%) of the control patients and 80 (70%) of the intervention patients completed all questionnaires. Overall, 71 (62%) patients in the control group and 75 (66%) patients in the intervention group completed the diary and all questionnaires (Fig. 1). Patients who did not complete the follow-up were more frequently of non-Dutch origin (15% non-Dutch natives in dropouts versus 5% non-Dutch natives in the analysed group; *p* = 0.017) and were younger (a mean age of 39.2 years for dropouts versus 47.4 years for the analysed group; *p* = 0.000). They did not differ significantly in other baseline measurements.

Intervention effect

The mean disability score among the patients in the intervention and the control groups declined to 4.1 (SDM&PR group) and 4.3 (control group) after 2 weeks (difference 0.2; *p*-value 0.789), 2.1 (SDM&PR) and 2.3 (controls) after 12 weeks (difference 0.2; *p*-value 0.720) and 2.0 for both groups after 26 weeks (difference 0.0; p-value 0.949) (Table 2 and Fig. 2).

The mean pain score in the two groups was 18.9 (SDM&PR) and 20.3 (controls) after 2 weeks (difference 1.4; *p*-value 0.675), 14.2 (SDM&PR) and 12.4 (controls) after 12 weeks (difference 1.8; p-value 0.577) and 13.6 (SDM&PR) and 16.3 (controls) after 26 weeks (difference 2.7; p-value 0.385). The percentage of patients with adequate relief was 70% (SDM&PR) and 62% (controls) after 2 weeks (p-value 0.888), 49% in both groups after 6 weeks, 69% (SDM&PR) and 62% (controls) after 12 weeks, and 66% (SDM&PR) and 64% (controls) after 26 weeks. The mean number of days of absenteeism and mean health care consumption at 2, 6, 12 and 26 weeks did not differ between the two groups (Table 2).

In the multilevel, multivariate analysis, correcting for baseline differences, patient characteristics and the clustering effect, the mean difference in disability scores between the intervention and control groups during the six-month follow-up was – 0.259 (*p*-value 0.582) (Table 3). The mean difference in pain score between the two groups in the six-month follow-up was – 2.269 (p-value 0.306). During the follow-up, the two groups did not differ in the percentage of patients with adequate relief, the number of days of absenteeism or in healthcare consumption (Table 3).

Of the 8 dimensions of illness perception, only consequences (β = 1.24 confidence interval (CI) 0.14–2.35), timeline (β = 1.38 CI 0.27–2.48) and concern (β = 1.45 CI 0.34–2.56) were significantly associated with disability at 12 weeks. However, when the interaction term of each of these three items with the intervention was added to the multivariate model, no significant effect of illness perception on disability at 12 weeks was found.

Table 2 Univariate mean score per group in primary and secondary outcomes in the imputed dataset without correction for clustering

	MEAN SCORE AT 2 WEEKS			Mean score at 12 weeks			mean score at 26 weeks		
	IV	CO	p-value	IV	CO	p-value	IV	CO	p-value
Clinical parameters									
Disability (RMD) (0–24)	4.1 (5.3)	4.3 (4.8)	0.789	2.1 (4.0)	2.3 (3.7)	0.720	2.0 (3.7)	2.0 (3.6)	0.949
Pain (VAS) (0–100 mm)	18.9 (21.7)	20.3 (20.9)	0.675	14.2 (22.6)	12.4 (17.5)	0.577	13.6 (17.3)	16.3 (21.2)	0.385
Adequate relief (yes/no)†	70 (81%)	62 (81%)	0.888	45 (69%)	38 (62%)	0.416	35 (66%)	32 (64%)	0.830
Societal impact									
Absenteeism (days)	1.47 (3.35)	2.05 (4.03)	0.359	0.93 (5.65)	0.800 (3.63)	0.888			*
Absenteeism (yes/no)‡	18 (28%)	20 (27%)	0.924	3 (5%)	4 (8%)	0.552	7 (11%)	6 (14%)	0.650
healthcare consumption									
Telephone consultations (per patient)	0.35 (0.71)	0.29 (0.60)	0.556	1.18 (0.50)	1.18 (0.51)	0.672			*
Practice consultations (per patient)	0.21 (0.51)	0.11 (0.39)	0.134	1.12 (0.43)	1.15 (0.52)	0.965	1.11 (0.45)	1.10 (0.38)	0.914

RMD = Roland-Morris disability questionnaire (a higher score indicates a more favourable outcome). VAS = visual analogue scale (a lower score indicates a more favourable outcome). Mean score of low back pain, leg pain and both. IPQ = illness perception questionnaire. CO = control group. IV = intervention group. *Cannot be computed because the group is zero

In both groups, patients reported a substantial degree of involvement in decision-making. However, the patients in the intervention group reported a significantly higher level of patient involvement (2.92 standard deviation (SD) 1.21; range 1–4) than the controls (2.44 SD 1.23) (difference 0.48; *p*-value 0.005).

When studying the fidelity of the intervention, we measured significant differences in the SDM behaviour in favour of the intervention group and a mean duration of the consultation of 16 min for the intervention group versus 13 min for the control group [23].

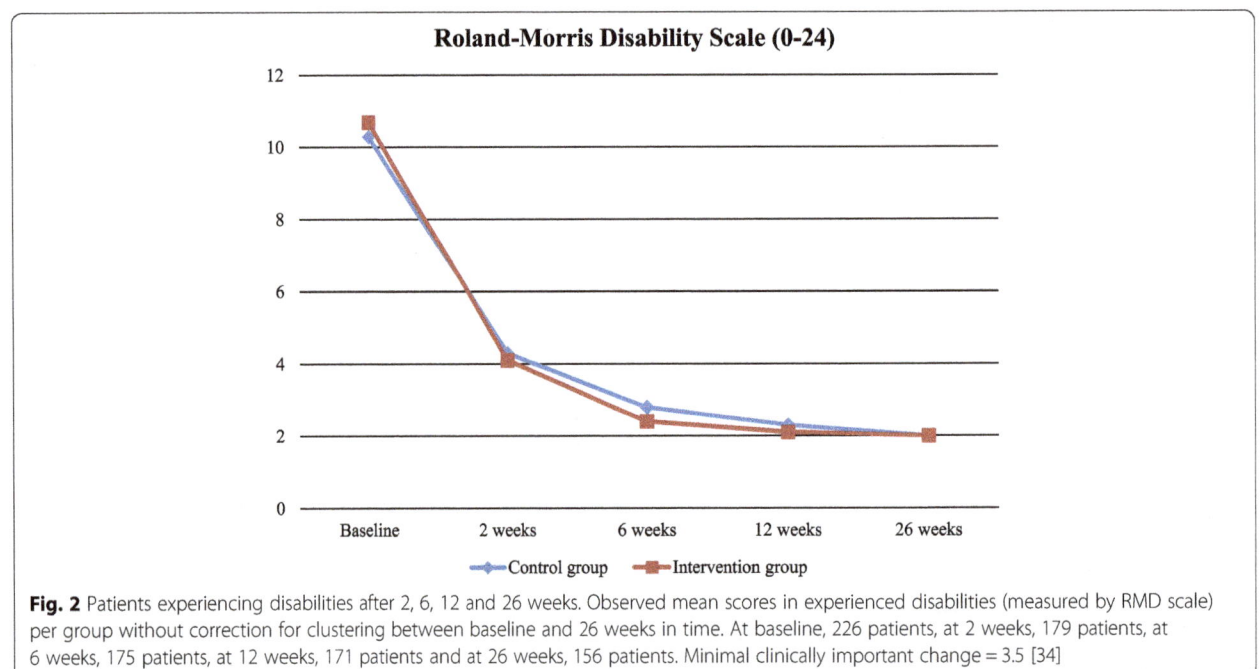

Fig. 2 Patients experiencing disabilities after 2, 6, 12 and 26 weeks. Observed mean scores in experienced disabilities (measured by RMD scale) per group without correction for clustering between baseline and 26 weeks in time. At baseline, 226 patients, at 2 weeks, 179 patients, at 6 weeks, 175 patients, at 12 weeks, 171 patients and at 26 weeks, 156 patients. Minimal clinically important change = 3.5 [34]

Table 3 Difference in mean scores between the control and intervention groups *in the imputed dataset* during the six-month follow-up

	UNIVARIATE ANALYSIS*			multivariate analysis	
	mean difference/ rate ratio	CI	p-value	mean difference/ rate ratio	p-value
ENDPOINT					
Disability (RMD) (scale 0–24) ¶	−0.233	−1.258 to 0.791	0.655	−0.259	0.582
Secondary outcomes					
Pain (VAS) (scale 0–100 mm) ¶	−1.120	−6.133 to 3.893	0.662	−2.269	0.306
Adequate relief (yes/no) †	1.118	0.510–1.567	0.696	1.119	0.730
Absenteeism (in days) ‡	1.032	0.927–1.338	0.249	0.332	0.506
Healthcare consumption					
Telephone consultations (number per patient) §	1.0142	1.001–1.018	0.845	1.020	0.789
Practice consultations (number per patient) §	1.0143	0.880–1.169	0.845	1.067	0.245

RMD = Roland-Morris disability questionnaire (a higher score indicates a more favourable outcome). VAS = visual analogue scale (a lower score indicates a more favourable outcome). Mean score of low back pain, leg pain and both. *Corrected for clustering effect. ¶ Mean difference between control and intervention groups over 26 weeks. † Odds ratio without baseline correction. ‡ Rate ratio in the multilevel model corrected for dichotomous baseline value. § Rate ratio without baseline correction

Discussion

This training of general practitioners in SDM&PR did not improve the symptom recovery of patients with non-chronic low back pain in primary care, even though the GPs effectively involved patients in the choice of treatment after the training. At no point in the follow-up did the mean disability or pain score of the patients whose GP was trained in SDM&PR differ from those patients whose GP provided the usual standard of care (Fig. 2). Patients in both groups reported that pain and physical limitations gradually declined and returned to a normal population level at 26 weeks [34].

The comparable clinical discourse in the two groups was also reflected in pain-related absenteeism from work and in health care consumption during the follow-up.

Patients who attributed much importance to the consequences of their back pain, those who expected the pain to last long and those who had many concerns about the pain had a poorer prognosis for symptom recovery. However, the prognosis was independent of the performance of SDM&PR by the GPs.

Strengths of the study

Most research on SDM thus far has focused on process outcomes and not on patient-related clinical outcomes [20].

We performed a randomised controlled trial among patients with low back pain recruited in daily primary care and evaluated the effectiveness of SDM on relevant clinical outcomes. Based on current knowledge, we constructed a multifaceted intervention and training programme that was grounded in a theoretical concept of SDM, involving both participants in the decision process [20].

Participating GPs were well trained, and the positive SDM performance during consultations after the training was acknowledged by the patients [23]. We used a mixed model analysis because these are robust for individual patients with missing follow-up measurements under the assumption of missing values completely at random or missing values at random dependent on another variable included in the mixed model. As in most studies, the correctness of this assumption of 'random missing' cannot be proven in our study. In our view, however, it is very unlikely that a treatment effect was not observed due to the multiple imputation procedure because the complete case analyses confirmed the lack of a treatment effect (Additional file 3 Appendix 3).

Limitations of the study

The patient recruitment met only half (53%) of the pre-set sample size. Participating GPs experienced problems that hampered recruitment, possibly due to unforeseen changes in the healthcare system, such as the introduction of direct access physiotherapy. However, the fact that the results of the patients in the intervention and control groups did not differ in any of the outcome measures at any moment in time demonstrates in our view the consistency of the results, and even if differences were demonstrated at the pre-set sample size, these differences would have been small and of questionable clinical relevance.

Dropout rates of GPs and patients are similar in the intervention and control groups and are in line with other studies on patients suffering from nonspecific low back pain in primary care in the Netherlands [35]. We cannot think of any reason why the intervention should have influenced the dropout rate of patients, but we estimate that dropout is not related to the intervention but is rather related to the complex disease course of nonspecific low back pain and the mismatch between patient expectations and the professional's management.

Although we have observed significant differences in the perception of SDM between the experimental groups, we believe that the difference should be evaluated in the context of treatment fidelity. In a recent publication evaluating the intervention from an observational perspective, we found significant differences in the use of physical examination and in the consultation duration between groups [23]. Moreover, we question whether the patient perspective was sufficiently considered to incorporate the patient's positive expectations into the actual decision despite significant differences in the SDM behaviour of GPs between the groups.

Unfortunately, as with many other studies on the effects of SDM on health outcomes, the effects are too small to allow conclusions about the impact of the separate communicative techniques, SDM and positive reinforcement of treatment expectations. Theoretically, we expected a positive interaction between the two techniques. The consistent pattern of very small potential positive treatment effects of the combined intervention above the usual standard of care could be explained by a stronger positive effect of one technique counteracted by the effect of the other (Fig. 2). For instance, in a study by a physiotherapist on the effects of SDM on the prognosis of low back pain, even negative expectations of patients were suggested to be responsible for poorer health outcomes after SDM than the usual standard of care [36]. Conversely, in a study evaluating the placebo effect on chronic low back pain, positive treatment expectations and a supportive environment were considered responsible for short-term relief from complaints [16, 23].

Studies on the effects of learned communicative strategies frequently face problems with blinding. We downsized the risk of non-blinding by sorting patients per GP, by recruiting patients via auxiliary staff members unaware of the allocation, and by not providing details of the trained communicative strategy to control GPs, auxiliary staff members and patients.

We did not perform a full health economic assessment but restricted the economic impact analysis to measuring the absenteeism of workers. However, in a detailed cost-effectiveness analysis, the reported 20% difference in the duration of the consultation time should be considered [23].

Possible explanations

As in other studies on interventions for non-chronic low back pain, we did not find substantial or significant effects [37].

This finding could be attributed to different factors. Such as an excessively diverse study population in the duration of the complaints or in patient characteristics [36–38].

Although we think that the risk of contamination was limited, GPs in the control group may have incorporated SDM in their consultations as well. This might be reflected in the fact that the mean score for the question of whether patients felt involved in the decision-making was between 'mostly yes' and 'mostly no'. The difference in the results of the intervention group, where the mean score was 'mostly yes', was significant but limited. However, the observational study demonstrates low levels of SDM in both groups despite the significant effect of training in SDM behaviour [11, 23, 39, 40].

Because most patients quickly recover from their back pain, the intervention simply might not have had sufficient discriminative content above the spontaneous course. In their review of psychosocial interventions for non-chronic low back pain in primary care, Ramond et al. [38] advise the integration of several psychosocial factors with multicomponent interventions to overcome this problem.

Contextual factors play an important role in the symptom perception, prognosis and recovery of low back pain [1, 4]. We identified three subgroups of patients with a poorer prognosis for symptom recovery in the analysis of the effect of each of the illness perception dimensions on the restrictions at twelve weeks. Patients with more negative illness perceptions or with a longer duration of complaints before they contact their GP might be better helped by more positive treatment expectations, but unfortunately, our dataset did not allow subgroup analysis on the effect of the intervention for particular patient characteristics [38]. Differences between the contextual factors of patients in the intervention and control groups may have influenced the results. Although the patients were not randomised, we have no indication that the recruitment to the intervention and control groups resulted in selection bias [18, 28, 41, 42].

Although the GPs were extensively trained before participating in the intervention group and the patients recognised SDM during the actual consultations, we question, based on the results of the evaluation of the training, whether the training did result in adequate SDM performance [40, 43].

Trained GPs became more aware of the need to better inform patients about treatment options and to incorporate patients' expectations during the intake phase of the consultation, but they persisted in providing a paternalistic, guideline-oriented choice.

In a review on the effects of the implementation of SDM in clinical encounters measured by an external observer, Couët et al. [40] reported similar training effects and noticed that only incidentally is clinical management adjusted to patient preferences. In the evaluation of the training, we confirm this observation and conclude that patient preferences were insufficiently considered in the actual decision-making to incorporate the patient's positive treatment expectations into the treatment choice [23]. When patient preferences are not reflected in treatment choices, the impact of positive reinforcement of the therapeutic plan on patient recovery will diminish.

So far, task-oriented issues, such as performing process steps and information exchange, are emphasised in the implementation of SDM [20]. However, the effects of knowledge transfer on proportional understanding are questionable, and the effects on recovery are unclear [20, 43].

Future research on the involvement of patients in treatment decisions should therefore focus more on professional attitude and equality in the patient professional relationship as a condition for successful SDM.

Conclusion

Training of GPs in the application of SDM&PR during consultations with patients with non-chronic low back pain did not significantly improve clinical recovery. Although it may have improved the 'knowledge and rationalise expectations' of the patients, this did not lead to less functional impairment, shorter pain duration or less absenteeism from work than routine practice. Most patients recovered from their low back-pain within 12 weeks, and this positive effect was persistent at the 26-week follow-up, which confirms the benign natural course of low back-pain as reported in the literature. A potential small positive effect of either SDM or positive reinforcement of treatment expectations cannot be excluded. As the prognosis of low back pain is predominantly determined by psychosocial factors, we suggest that further research on the positive health effects of communicative techniques should focus on a more patient-oriented approach, combined with the reinforcement of positive recovery expectations, than on task-oriented techniques such as SDM.

Abbreviations

AR: Adequate relief; AS: Ariëtte Sanders; CI: Confidence interval; GP: General practitioner; IPDAS: International Patient Decision Aids Standards; IPQ: Illness perception questionnaire; IV: Intervention; NTR: The Netherlands National Trial Register; RMD: Roland-Morris disability questionnaire; SD: Standard deviation; SDM: Shared decision-making; SDM&PR: Shared decision-making followed by a positive reinforcement of the chosen therapy; UC: Usual care; VAS: Visual analogue scale

Acknowledgements

The authors wish to thank all patients and GPs who voluntarily participated in the trial, William Verheul for developing the concept, Peter Zuithoff and Peter Spreeuwenberg for statistical support and Emily van Dedem-Fick and all students who supported the sample acquisition and sequence data processing.

Authors' contributions

All authors were involved in critical review of the manuscript and have seen and approved the final version. Specific contributions are as follows: study conception and design: JB and AS; analysis of epidemiological and sequence data: PV, TM, AS; drafting the manuscript: NW, JB, PV and AS. All authors had full access to all the study data and take responsibility for the integrity of the data and the accuracy of the data analysis. All authors read and approved the final version of the manuscript.

Ethics approval and consent to participate

The study protocol for the trial was assessed by the Ethics Committee of the University Medical Centre of Utrecht and exempted from full assessment because participants are not subject to medical proceedings or behavioural changes as referred to in the definition of medical scientific research in the Medical Research Involving Human Subjects Act (article 1b). Patients with back pain were individually informed by the medical staff about the trial and the consequences of participation, including the videotaping. They signed a written informed consent form in the waiting room. Before the recording started, the GP checked the permission together with the patient.
The manuscript has been drafted according to the CONSORT guidelines.

Competing interests

The authors declare that they have no competing interests to disclose.

Author details

¹Julius Centre for Health Sciences and Primary Care, University Medical Centre Utrecht, PO Box 85500 3508, GA, Utrecht, the Netherlands. ²NIVEL (Netherlands Institute for Health Services Research), PO Box 1568 3500, BN, Utrecht, the Netherlands. ³Faculty of Social and Behavioural Science, Utrecht University, Utrecht, the Netherlands.

References

1. van Tulder M, Becker A, Bekkering T, Breen A, del Real MT, Hutchinson A, et al. Chapter 3. European guidelines for the management of acute nonspecific low back pain in primary care. Eur Spine J. 2006;15(Suppl 2): S169–91.
2. Bons SCS, Borg MAJP, Van den Donk M, et al. NHG-Standaard Aspecifieke lagerugpijn (Tweede herziening). In: Richtlijnen en praktijk. Het Nederlands Huisartsen Genootschap. 2017. https://www.nhg.org/standaarden/volledig/nhg-standaard-aspecifieke-lagerugpijn. Accessed 20 June 2018.
3. Dionne CE, Dunn KM, Croft PR, Nachemson AL, Buchbinder R, Walker BF, et al. A consensus approach toward the standardization of back pain definitions for use in prevalence studies. Spine. 2008;33:95–103.
4. Krismer M, van Tulder M. Strategies for prevention and management of musculoskeletal conditions. Low back pain (non-specific). Best Pract Res Clin Rheumatol. 2007;21:77–91.
5. Dagenais S, Caro J, Haldeman S. A systematic review of low back pain cost of illness studies in the United States and internationally. Spine J. 2008;8:8–20.
6. Di Blasi Z, Harkness E, Ernst E, Georgiou A, Kleijnen J. Influence of context effects on health outcomes: a systematic review. Lancet. 2001;357:757–62.
7. Iles RA, Davidson M, Taylor NF. Psychosocial predictors of failure to return to work in non-chronic non-specific low back pain: a systematic review. Occup Environ Med. 2008;65:507–17.
8. Iles RA, Davidson M, Taylor NF, O'Halloran P. Systematic review of the ability of recovery expectations to predict outcomes in non-chronic non-specific low back pain. J Occup Rehabil. 2009;19:25–40.
9. van Tol-Geerdink JJ, Stalmeier PF, van Lin EN, Schimmel EC, Huizenga H, van Daal WA, et al. Do patients with localized prostate cancer treatment really want more aggressive treatment? J Clin Oncol. 2006;24:4581–6.
10. Bensing J. Bridging the gap. The separate worlds of evidence-based medicine and patient-centered medicine. Patient Educ Couns. 2000;39:17–25.
11. Stalmeier PFM, van Tol-Geerdink JJ, van Lin ENJT, Schimmel E. Huizenga H, van Daal WA, et al. [the patient chooses for feasibility and effectiveness]. NedTijdschrGeneeskd. 2009;153:600–6.

12. Salzburg Global Seminar. Salzburg statement on shared decision making. BMJ. 2011;342:d1745.

13. Edwards A, Elwyn G. Inside the black box of shared decision making: distinguishing between the process of involvement and who makes the decision. Health Expect. 2006;9:307–20.

14. Stiggelbout AM, Van der Weijden T, De Wit MP, et al. Shared decision making: really putting patients at the Centre of healthcare. BMJ. 2012;344:e256.

15. Elwyn G, Durand MA, Song J, et al. A three-talk model for shared decision making: multistage consultation process. BMJ. 2017;359:j4891.

16. Légaré F, Stacey D, Turcotte S, Cossi MJ, Kryworuchko J, Graham ID, et al. Interventions for improving the adoption of shared decision making by healthcare professionals. Cochrane Database Syst Rev. 2014;9:CD006732.

17. Stacey D, Légaré F, Lewis K, Barry MJ, Bennett CL, Eden KB, et al. Decision aids for people facing health treatment or screening decisions. Cochrane Database Syst Rev. 2011;10:CD001431.

18. Benedetti F, Amanzio M. Mechanisms of the placebo response. Pulm Pharmacol Ther. 2013;26:520–3.

19. Thomas KB. General practice consultations: is there any point in being positive? Br Med J (Clin Res Ed). 1987;294:1200–2.

20. Légaré F, Ratté S, Stacey D, Kryworuchko J, Gravel K, Graham ID. Interventions for improving the adoption of shared decision making by healthcare professionals. Cochrane Database Syst Rev. 2010;5:CD006732.

21. Saragiotto BT, Machado GC, Ferreira ML, Pinheiro MB, Abdel Shaheed C, Maher CG. Paracetamol for low back pain. Cochrane Database Syst Rev. 2016;6:CD012230.

22. Elwyn G, Hutchings H, Edwards A, Rapport F, Wensing M, Cheung WY, Grol R. The OPTION scale: measuring the extent that clinicians involve patients in decision-making tasks. Health Expect. 2005;8:34–42.

23. Sanders AR, Bensing JM, Essed MA, Magnée T, de Wit NJ, Verhaak PF. Does training general practitioners result in more shared decision making during consultations? Patient Educ Couns. 2017;100:563–74.

24. Elwyn G, O'Connor AM, Bennett C, Newcombe RG, Politi M, Durand MA, et al. Assessing the quality of decision support technologies using the international patient decision aid standards instrument (IPDASi). PLoS One. 2009;4:e4705.

25. Schers H, Wensing M, Huijsmans Z, van Tulder M, Grol R. Implementation barriers for general practice guidelines on low back pain a qualitative study. Spine (Phila Pa 1976). 2001;26:E348–53.

26. Brouwer S, Kuijer W, Dijkstra PU, Göeken LN, Groothoff JW, Geertzen JH. Reliability and stability of the Roland Morris disability questionnaire: intra class correlation and limits of agreement. Disabil Rehabil. 2004;26:162–5.

27. Ostelo RW, de Vet HC. Clinically important outcomes in low back pain. Best Pract Res Clin Rheumatol. 2005;19:593–607.

28. Foster NE, Bishop A, Thomas E, Main C, Horne R, Weinman J, et al. Illness perceptions of low back pain patients in primary care: what are they, do they change and are they associated with outcome? Pain. 2008;136:177–87.

29. Broadbent E, Petrie KJ, Main J, Weinman J. The brief illness perception questionnaire. J Psychosom Res. 2006;60:631–7.

30. Jellema P, van der Windt DA, van der Horst HE, Blankenstein AH, Bouter LM, Stalman WA. Why is a treatment aimed at psychosocial factors not effective in patients with (sub)acute low back pain? Pain. 2005;118:350–9.

31. Donders AR, van der Heijden GJ, Stijnen T, Moons KG. A gentle introduction to imputation of missing values. J Clin Epidemiol. 2006;59:1087–91.

32. Sterne JA, White IR, Carlin JB, Spratt M, Royston P, Kenward MG, et al. Multiple imputation for missing data in epidemiological and clinical research: potential and pitfalls. BMJ. 2009;338:b2393.

33. Rubin LH, Witkiewitz K, Andre JS, Reilly S. Methods for handling missing data in the behavioral neurosciences: don't throw the baby rat out with the bath water. J Undergrad Neurosci Educ. 2007;5:A71–7.

34. Kovacs FM, Abraira V, Royuela A, Corcoll J, Alegre L, Cano A, et al. Minimal clinically important change for pain intensity and disability in patients with nonspecific low back pain. Spine (Phila Pa 1976). 2007;32:2915–20.

35. Jellema P, van der Windt DA, van der Horst HE, Twisk JW, Stalman WA, Bouter LM. Should treatment of (sub)acute low back pain be aimed at psychosocial prognostic factors? Cluster randomised clinical trial in general practice. BMJ. 2005;331:84.

36. Gysels M, Richardson A, Higginson IJ. Communication training for health professionals who care for patients with cancer: a systematic review of effectiveness. Support Care Cancer. 2004;12:692–700.

37. Pengel HM, Maher CG, Refshauge KM. Systematic review of conservative interventions for subacute low back pain. Clin Rehabil. 2002;16:811–20.

38. Ramond-Roquin A, Bouton C, Gobin-Tempereau AS, Airagnes G, Richard I, Roquelaure Y, et al. Interventions focusing on psychosocial risk factors for patients with non-chronic low back pain in primary care–a systematic review. Fam Pract. 2014;31:379–88.

39. Schers H, Braspenning J, Drijver R, Wensing M, Grol R. Low back pain in general practice: reported management and reasons for not adhering to the guidelines in the Netherlands. Br J Gen Pract. 2000;50:640–4.

40. Couët N, Desroches S, Robitaille H, Vaillancourt H, Leblanc A, Turcotte S, et al. Assessments of the extent to which health-care providers involve patients in decision making: a systematic review of studies using the OPTION instrument. Health Expect. 2015;18:542–61.

41. Benedetti F, Lanotte M, Lopiano L, Colloca L. When words are painful: unraveling the mechanisms of the nocebo effect. Neuroscience. 2007; 147:260–71.

42. Patel S, Ngunjiri A, Hee SW, Yang Y, Brown S, Friede T, et al. Primum non nocere: shared informed decision making in low back pain–a pilot cluster randomised trial. BMC Musculoskelet Disord. 2014;15:282.

43. Braddock CH 3rd. The emerging importance and relevance of shared decision making to clinical practice. Med Decis Mak. 2010;30:5S–7S.

7

Job satisfaction and career intentions of registered nurses in primary health care: an integrative review

Elizabeth Halcomb* ⓘ, Elizabeth Smyth and Susan McInnes

Abstract

Background: There has been a significant growth of the international primary health care (PHC) nursing workforce in recent decades in response to health system reform. However, there has been limited attention paid to strategic workforce growth and evaluation of workforce issues in this setting. Understanding issues like job satisfaction and career intentions are essential to building capacity and skill mix within the workforce. This review sought to explore the literature around job satisfaction and career intentions of registered nurses working in PHC.

Methods: An integrative review was conducted. Electronic databases including: CINAHL, MEDLINE, Scopus and Web of Science, and reference lists of journal publications were searched for peer-reviewed literature published between 2000 and 2016 related to registered nurse job satisfaction and career intentions. Study quality was appraised, before thematic analysis was undertaken to synthesise the findings.

Results: Twenty papers were included in this review. Levels of job satisfaction reported were variable between studies. A range of factors impacted on job satisfaction. Whilst there was agreement on the impact of some factors, there was a lack of consistency between studies on other factors. Four of the six studies which reported career intentions identified that nearly half of their participants intended to leave their current position.

Conclusion: This review identifies gaps in our understanding of job satisfaction and career intentions in PHC nurses. With the growth of the PHC nursing workforce internationally, there is a need for robust, longitudinal workforce research to ensure that employment in this setting is satisfying and that skilled nurses are retained.

Keywords: Primary health care, Nursing, Workforce, Job satisfaction, Retention, Career intention

Background

The recruitment and retention of nurses is problematic worldwide. There is a maldistribution of human resources for health, a shortage in the overall number of qualified nurses and an aging nursing workforce [1]. Job satisfaction has been cited as an important factor contributing to the turnover of nurses and as an antecedent to nursing retention [2–4]. Therefore, understanding factors that impact on job satisfaction is important to inform recruitment and retention strategies.

The concept of job satisfaction is multifaceted and complex. Job satisfaction has been the focus of much research around organisational behaviour. Lu, et al. [5]

define job satisfaction as not only how an individual feels about their job but also the nature of the job and the individuals' expectation of what their job should provide. To this end, job satisfaction is comprised of various components, including; job conditions, communication, the nature of the work, organisational policies and procedures, remuneration and conditions, promotion / advancement opportunities, recognition / appreciation, security and supervision / relationships [5]. Whilst levels of job satisfaction vary, several common factors emerge across studies [6, 7]. These include working conditions and the organisational environment, levels of stress, role conflict and ambiguity, role perceptions and content and organisational and professional commitment [5–8]. Given these factors it becomes clear that research about job satisfaction cannot be undertaken across the nursing

* Correspondence: ehalcomb@uow.edu.au
School of Nursing, University of Wollongong, Northfields Ave, Wollongong, NSW 2522, Australia

profession as a whole, but rather needs to consider various settings and organisational environments to understand the issues facing different nursing groups.

Career intentions can be described as the intention to leave ones' job voluntarily [9]. This process may start with a psychological response to negative situations in the workplace or undesirable aspects of the job. Subsequently, a cognitive decision is made to leave the position and withdrawal behaviours occur as the person moves out of the workplace [10]. Like job satisfaction, a number of common determinants for career intention have been identified. These include organisational factors, management style, workload and stress, role perceptions, empowerment, remuneration and employment conditions and opportunities for advancement [10]. In several studies, job satisfaction has been shown to impact on career intentions [11, 12].

Despite the common themes in this workforce literature, much of the research around job satisfaction and career intentions reported to date has focussed on acute care nurses [2, 5, 6, 10, 11, 13, 14]. Given the impact of organisational factors, roles and employment conditions it is important to consider different groups of nurses, such as those employed in PHC, who are employed in settings unlike those of their acute care colleagues. PHC nurses practice in a range of settings, including general practices, schools, refugee health services, correctional settings, non-government organisations and community health centres [15]. As such, their employment conditions and work environments are unlike those of acute care nurses who are employed by large health providers or government funded health services (17). The small business nature of primary care in many countries and the predominance of charities and non-government health providers makes employment in the PHC setting unique [16–18]. Lorenz and De Brito Guirardello [19] describe the PHC work environment as "not always favourable to the professional practice of nurses"(p. 927), citing lack of equipment, inappropriate physical environment and occupational risks as key contributors to dissatisfaction. Additionally, there are significant difference between the roles, responsibilities and work environments of acute and PHC nurses [20]. These differences and the impact of such factors on job satisfaction and career intentions mean that acute care nursing workforce research cannot be simply generalised to the PHC setting. With the growth in the PHC nursing workforce and the need for a strong nursing workforce in this setting it is timely to explore the job satisfaction and career intentions of PHC nurses. Therefore, this review sought to critically synthesise the literature around the job satisfaction and career intentions of registered nurses working in PHC.

The underlying research questions are:

- What was known about the main outcomes of studies regarding PHC registered nurses job satisfaction?
- What was known about the career intentions of PHC registered nurses?

Registered nurses are the focus of the review as they are the largest nursing workforce in PHC [21].

Methods
Design
This integrative literature review is informed by Whittemore and Knafls [22] framework. It provides a thorough examination of the existing literature following the five stages of review: problem identification, literature search, data evaluation, data analysis and presentation [22].

Search strategy
A systematic search strategy was designed to guide the search of electronic databases: CINAHL, MEDLINE, Scopus and Web of Science. Key search terms included; nurs*, primary health care, community care and job satisfaction or career intention. The search was confined to English language peer reviewed papers of original research. Given the significant changes in PHC systems internationally, only papers published between January 2000 and 2016 were considered. The reference lists of publications were also reviewed to identify further literature.

Inclusion criteria
Table 1 details the inclusion and exclusion criteria. Papers were excluded if they focussed on a particular nursing specialty (e.g. community mental health nurses) or were based in residential care settings (e.g. nursing homes), as the issues with this workforce are somewhat different to other PHC settings. Studies that focussed on nurse practitioners and/or advanced practice nurses (e.g. [23]), or specifically on nurse managers were excluded as these nurses may have different perceptions and experiences to registered nurses. Remoteness itself was not considered to constitute PHC nursing, therefore, papers focussed on rural or remote nurses without being specifically PHC focussed were excluded. Research articles were also excluded if the findings did not isolate PHC nurses from acute care nurses or other health professionals.

Study selection
After removal of duplicates, 477 citations were yielded from the search. These citations were exported to Endnote X8™ for review of their titles, followed by closer evaluation of the abstract. This process identified that 346 papers did not meet the inclusion criteria, leaving

Table 1 Inclusion / Exclusion Criteria

Inclusion Criteria	Exclusion Criteria
• Published between 2000 and 2016. • Written in English language. • Peer-reviewed original research. • Explores issues related to job satisfaction and the retention of registered nurses employed in PHC settings.	• Literature reviews, discussion papers, dissertations and theses. • Papers focussed on advanced practice nurses / Nurse Practitioners. • Papers focussed on nursing speciality areas. • Data about nurses aggregated with other nursing specialties and health professionals. • Nurses employed in residential settings.

131 papers where the full-text was retrieved. Of these papers, 111 did not meet the inclusion criteria, and so were excluded. This left 20 papers for inclusion in the review. (Fig. 1).

Appraisal of methodological quality

Determining the methodological quality of the included studies was difficult due to the broad sampling frame and various research designs [22]. As identified by Whittemore and Knafl [22], there is no gold standard for evaluating quality in research reviews. In this review we conducted quality appraisal using the tool provided by the Center for Evidence Based Management [25]. The major areas of concern were around the quality of reporting of the instrument development and validity / reliability measures in some papers [26–31]. Given the relatively small number of included papers and the minor nature of the limitations identified none of the

studies were excluded based on their methodological quality.

Data abstraction and synthesis

Once the included papers were identified all data was abstracted into a summary table. The main characteristics that were extracted included;

- Citation
- Country
- Study design
- Sample
- Study aim
- Methods
- Main outcomes related to job satisfaction or career intention

The nature of the included papers, in terms of the heterogeneity of the measures used, meant that thematic analysis was the most appropriate technique for aggregating the findings. Therefore, data is presented in a narrative form around the key themes that emerged from the literature.

Results

Of the 20 included papers (Table 2), 15 (75%) described quantitative studies, 4 (20%) papers described qualitative projects, and the remaining paper (5%) employed a mixed-method approach. Most of the included papers reported research undertaken in Canada ($n = 8$, 40%), with other studies coming out of the United Kingdom ($n = 4$, 20%), the United States of America ($n = 5$, 25%),

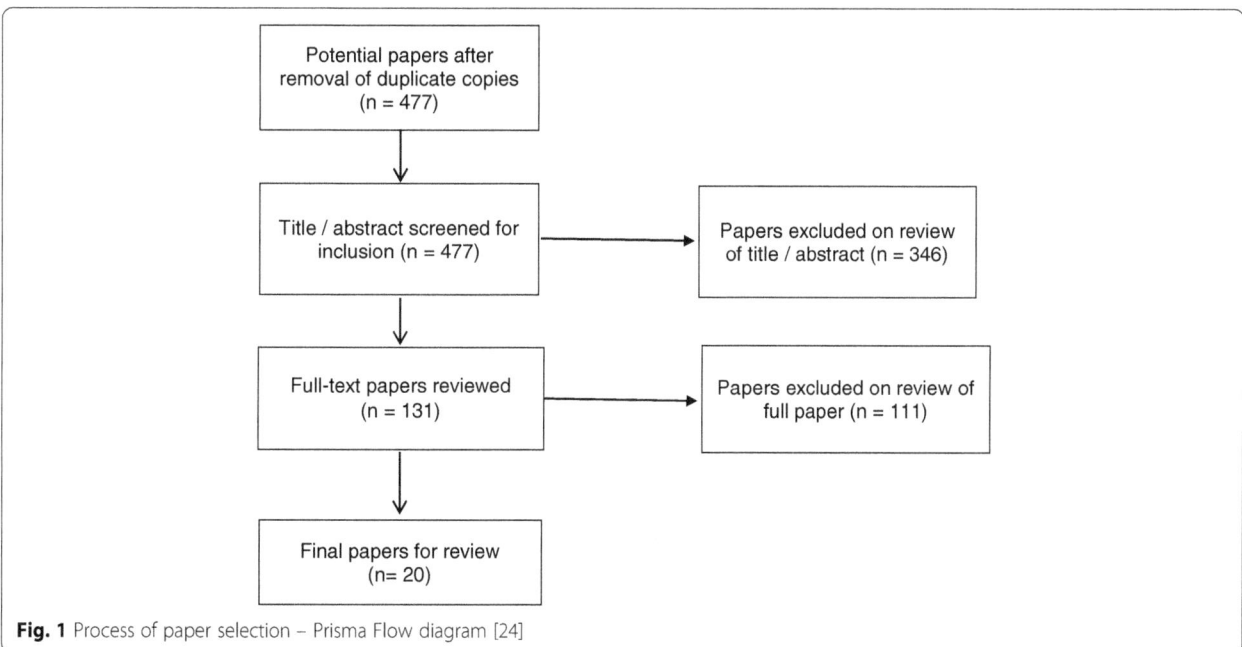

Fig. 1 Process of paper selection – Prisma Flow diagram [24]

Table 2 Summary table

Reference	Aim	Country	Sample	Methods	Findings
Almalki et al. [42]	Examine the relationship between quality of work life (QWL) and turnover intention	Saudi Arabia	508 PHC nurses (87% response)	Survey Brooks Quality of Nursing Work Life Anticipated Turnover Scale	• 67.3% female. 44% aged between 20 and 29 years. • Mean time in current PHC organisation 6.6 years and mean 6.1 years in current position. • Brooks' scale can range from 42 to 252. Participants scored from 45 to 218 (mean 139.45), indicating they were dissatisfied with work life. • 40% respondents indicated a desire to leave their current PHC workplace. • Turnover was significantly related to quality of work life, explaining 26% of variance ($p < 0.001$). • Quality of work life and demographics explained 32.1% of variance ($p < 0.001$). • In the final model, work context ($p < 0.001$), duration in positional ($p < 0.05$), payment per month ($p < 0.05$), and gender ($p < 0.05$) were statistically significant.
Armstrong-Stassen [26]	Compare work-related concerns, job satisfaction, and factors influencing retention	Canada	1044 PHC nurses (52% response)	Survey	• 98% female. Mean age 44 years • Employed in the position and agency for a mean of 8 years. • 4/5 highest ranked concerns were the same across the 3 settings, namely; inadequate staffing, increasingly complex needs of clients, working with vulnerable families with many problems, and dealing with difficult clients. • There were significant differences for 15 of the 17 work-related concerns between nurses from the 3 settings ($p < 0.001$). • Community Care Access Centre nurses expressed greatest concern about the emotional effects of the job. HCNs reported significantly greater concern over working conditions and safety issues. PHNs reported significantly greater concern about poor facilities. • There was a significant difference between the three groups for 6 of the 7 job satisfaction items ($p < 0.001$). • 3 /5 highest ranked retention items were identical across the three settings, although the ranking order varied.
Best and Thurston [33]	Test standardised job satisfaction tool	Canada	PHC Nurses Pre: $n = 44$ (60% response). Post: $n = 43$ (49% response)	Survey Index of Worklife Satisfaction (IWS)	• Most important components of job satisfaction were autonomy then pay. • Participants most satisfied with professional status. • Satisfaction with professional status and interaction significantly increased over the study ($p < 0.01$). • Aspects of work life giving the most satisfaction were quality client care / making a difference. Other factors identified included; autonomy/independence, colleague relationships, and opportunities for health teaching, respect/recognition, and client appreciation. • An open-ended question asking about what respondents would change identified administrative concerns, the need for more educational opportunities, more time for client care, more respect/recognition, and more opportunity for independence/autonomy.
Betkus and MacLeod [43]	Examine job and community satisfaction; how these relate to retention	Canada	124 PHC nurses in rural and small urban communities (76% response)	Survey Piedmonte's Work Satisfaction Index (WSI)	• 99% female. Mean age 43 years, 67% aged over 40 years. • 60% were first licensed ≥20 years ago. 50% had worked 5 years or longer in PHC nursing, and 49% were in PPT positions • Overall, most were satisfied. Most satisfied with professional status, professional interactions, and autonomy. Least satisfied with salary. • PHC nurses had varied perceptions of the organisational environment. • Nil correlation between age and job satisfaction ($p > 0.05$). • 52% indicated intent to stay in position for 5 years or more; • No correlation between job satisfaction and retention. • 52% intended to stay in their job for ≥5 years. 28% planned to leave within 2 years – this was 43% of those aged ≤35 yrs.

Table 2 Summary table *(Continued)*

Reference	Aim	Country	Sample	Methods	Findings
Campbell, et al. [34]	Impact of organisational structure on job satisfaction	USA	192 PHC nurses (55% response)	Survey Alexander Structure Instrument (ASI) McCloskey / Mueller Satisfaction Survey (MMSS)	• Factors impacting on decisions to stay were age, retirement, family circumstances and the economy. • Job satisfaction and community satisfaction were correlated ($p < 0.001$). • 96.9% female. 40.5% aged between 41 and 50 years. • 85.9% worked full-time, 48% had worked in nursing ≥20 years, and 40% had been employed in their department < 5 years. • The more that supervisors and subordinates work together concerning tasks and decisions and the more that individuals are involved in decision making and task definition, the higher job satisfaction. • Increased vertical participation and horizontal decision-making opportunities equate to higher job satisfaction. • Full-time staff reported higher levels of vertical participation compared to part-time staff ($p < 0.002$). • 'Formalization' (i.e. standardised policy, practices and position responsibilities) was not significantly related to job satisfaction. • Significant differences found between position classifications for total ASI score ($p = 0.000$), and vertical and horizontal participation subscales ($p = 0.000$). • Global job satisfaction scores ranged from 75 to 144 (Mean 113.04; SD = 6.32). As 94 is the lowest score that indicates satisfaction, most participants were satisfied. • No significant differences for job satisfaction were associated with current position or primary work assignment. • Educational preparation made a difference to job satisfaction with MSN prepared nurses (8.5%) scoring highest on MMSS. • To make the job more satisfying 27% indicated "better pay", 19% wanted increased management feedback and staff recognition, 15% indicated a desire to have more input and decision-making opportunity in their jobs, and 4% sought to increase role clarity. • 98% of participants planned to remain working in their health department. • Enjoyment of what they do, autonomy, flexibility, scheduling, benefits, and low stress were reported as intention to remain working.
Cameron, et al. [35]	Nurse satisfaction and retention in hospital and community settings	Canada	644 Community nurses (54% response)	Survey	• Most participants female (97.5%), Mean age of 45.07 years and 60% work full-time • Community nurses were significantly more likely than hospital nurses to report greater cohesiveness in the work place and a higher degree of support from supervisors related to feedback and recognition. • Community nurses were significantly more likely than hospital nurses to report higher autonomy and greater satisfaction with work demands. • Hospital nurses were significantly more likely than community nurses to be satisfied with remuneration.
Curtis & Glacken [37]	Level of and factors affecting job satisfaction	Ireland	351 PHC nurses (35.1% response)	Survey (IWS)	• 35% aged 36–45 years. 34.5% practiced as PHN 1-to-5 years • 53.3% hadn't worked as part of a primary care team previously. • IWS score of 12.62 (range 0.5–39.7) suggests a low level of job satisfaction. • Variables considered most important to their job satisfaction were: autonomy, interaction and pay. Task requirements were rated as least important to their job satisfaction. • Statistically significant differences in IWS scores noted for 3 age groups ($p < 0.05$): < 35 years, 35–45 years, and 45 years ($p = 0.000$). • The > 45 years age group were significantly more satisfied than younger colleagues. • There was no significant difference in job satisfaction between the < 35 years

Table 2 Summary table (Continued)

Reference	Aim	Country	Sample	Methods	Findings
					group and the 35–45 years group ($p = 0.574$). • Those employed as PHNs for > 10 years had a significantly higher job satisfaction compared to those with < 5 years ($p = 0.001$) and 6–10 years experience ($p = 0.006$). There was no significant difference between participants with < 5 years and 6–10 years experience ($p = 0.995$). • There was no statistically significant difference between job satisfaction and educational background ($p = 0.478$), rurality of practice ($p = 0.137$) or if participants were members of a constituted primary care team ($p = 0.16$).
Cole, et al. [36]	Difference in job satisfaction between nurse managers and nurses	Canada	88 PHC nurses (20 managers and 68 staff nurses) (56% response)	Survey Stember's model of job satisfaction	• 94% female, 75% worked full-time and 75% had flexibility in work schedules. • Job experience: Managers 20–42 yrs. (mean 29.7 yrs); Staff nurses 1–50 yrs. (mean 21.6 yrs). • Both managers and staff reported high job satisfaction – a mean > 3 for each subscale. • There was no significant differences between managers and staff nurses on the total job satisfaction scores ($p = 0.530$). • Managers were significantly less satisfied than staff nurses in both the 'influence' (participation in decision making) ($p = 0.026$) and 'interpersonal relationship' ($p = 0.008$) subscales. • The comparison of education levels and job satisfaction was inconclusive.
Delobelle et al. [2]	Examine the relationship between job satisfaction, turnover intent and demographic variables	South Africa	143 Rural PHC nurses (82% response)	Mixed-methods Survey & focus group	• 87% female, 58% were aged > 40 yrs. • 83% had been working in the unit for 10 years or less. • 51% of participants considered turnover within 2 years. • Job satisfaction was reportedly moderate (Mean = 3.2; SD 0.5). • Higher mean scores were attained for work itself and co-workers, and lower scores for pay and work conditions. • There was a significant difference in job satisfaction amongst professional ranks - NA and ENs were more satisfied than RNs ($p < 0.001$) • Job satisfaction negatively correlated with unit tenure ($p < 0.05$), professional rank ($p < 0.01$) and turnover intent ($p < 0.01$). • There was no significant difference between job satisfaction and age, education or years of nursing. • Turnover intent was statistically significantly explained by job satisfaction, age and education ($p < 0.001$) • Younger and more highly educated nurses are more likely to show turnover intent. • Nurses who reported more satisfaction with supervision were nearly 40% less likely to consider a job change. • The most satisfying aspects of job were the nature of work itself, staff and patient relationships, adequate staffing and resources. • The least satisfying aspects of the job were; work conditions (including lack of space), adequate staffing, lack of equipment and supplies, inadequate security, high workload, and the time spent doing non-nursing activities. Participants were also dissatisfied with their pay and benefits, lack of training and promotion, and lack of recognition and support from supervisors. • When asked what factors would help in their work respondents identified work conditions and equipment (88%), improved pay (69%), additional training (60%) and more staffing (49%).
Doran et al. [38]	Relationship between employment, job	Canada	700 HCNs (479 RNs, 211 RPNs, and 9	Survey Nursing Job	• 98% female, mean age 45 years, mean 8.2 years of community experience, 30% full-time.

Table 2 Summary table (Continued)

Reference	Aim	Country	Sample	Methods	Findings
	satisfaction and perceived job security		APNs) (49.0% response)	Satisfaction Scale	• A mean score of 3.84 (SD = 0.54) demonstrated that participants were moderately satisfied with work enjoyment. • Of the items measuring work enjoyment, participants were least satisfied with the conditions of the job (1.69) and balance between work and leisure (2.14). A mean score of 2.62 (SD = 1.28) indicated a low level of satisfaction with job security. • There were significant differences in nurses' work enjoyment between agencies (p < 0.05). • Older nurses rated work enjoyment higher than younger nurses. • There were significant differences in participants' satisfaction with time for care among agencies (p < 0.05). • Participants who had been employed by the same agency for a longer period were less satisfied with time for care than those who had been employed by the same agency for a shorter period. • Participants paid on an hourly basis were more satisfied with their time for care than those paid on a per-visit basis. • Participants who were employed on a casual basis perceived less job security than those employed full-time.
Flynn and Deatrick [27]	Identify attributes important to professional practice and job satisfaction	USA	58 HCNs	Focus groups	• 91% female, Mean age 44.7 years, and had worked in HC 7 years or longer (50%). • Continuing education opportunities were identified by all to enhance retention. • There were 6 major categories and 8 sub-categories identified to positively influence job satisfaction and retention if present or working towards; – 'An extensive, preceptor-based orientation' – 'An organised and supportive office environment' including; Real-time phone support, Interdisciplinary coordination and follow-up and Adequate and efficient clerical assistance – 'Reasonable working conditions' including Realistic workload, Adequate staffing and Scheduled days off – 'Accessible field security' – 'Competent and supportive management', including; Competent nursing supervisors and Supportive administrative practices – 'Patient-centred mission and values'
Graham et al. [39]	Examine relationship between autonomy, control-over-practice, workload and job satisfaction	Canada	271 PHC nurses (79.7% response)	Survey	• Mean age 42.5 years, 52% permanent full-time, 50% worked in PHC for < 7 years. • 53.5% reported being very satisfied with their jobs. • Control-over practice (p = 0.01) and workload (p < 0.01) were reliable predictors for job satisfaction. • As workload increased job satisfaction decreased. • Increases in control over practice scores were related to increased job satisfaction. • Interaction between autonomy and workload was a significant predictor for job satisfaction (p < 0.01). • The interaction between age and workload was a significant predictor for job satisfaction (p < 0.01).
Junious, et al. [28]	Explore job satisfaction and changes needed to boost levels of job satisfaction	USA	71 School Nurses (78.9% response)	Focus Groups	• All female, 55% worked in an elementary school, 84% had ≥3 years' experience. • 83% of participants reported being satisfied with their job. • 17% were dissatisfied with their job, primarily related to poor remuneration and lack of trust / support from administration. • Four major themes arose: (a) benefits, (b) resources, (c) autonomy, and (d) coping • Theme 1 Benefits. Issues related to job satisfaction included things such as creativity, freedom, growth, power, work standards, and ethics. Participants were very satisfied with job flexibility and paid holidays.

Table 2 Summary table (*Continued*)

Reference	Aim	Country	Sample	Methods	Findings
					• Theme 2 Resources. Resources, such as salary and supplies, were areas where participants were least satisfied with their jobs. Participants also wanted to be appreciated, valued, and compensated fairly for job performance. • Theme 3 Autonomy. Autonomy was considered the ability to act independently within one's scope of professional practice. When autonomy was not expressed, "isolation" emerged as the divergent theme. Over half of the participants stated that working with outside agencies increased satisfaction (53%). • Strategies that could be implemented to increase satisfaction included; career or pay scale differentiating qualifications (52%), increased professional development (32%), supervision by another nurse rather than nonnurse (24%), and a designated budget / supplies (17%). • Factors that negatively impacted on job satisfaction were; uncooperative staff and parents (61%), constant interruptions (48%), and the expectation that they would use their personal vehicle for work (13%).
Lorenz & Guiradello [19]	Relationship between burnout, satisfaction at work, quality of work and the intention to quit	Brazil	168 PHC nurses (58.5% response)	Survey Nursing Work Index-Revised Maslach Burnout Inventory	• 88.4% female, Mean age 36.3 years, 6.6 years' experience in primary care; employed 4.9 years at current job. • Satisfaction measure on Likert scale. 62.6% considered that they were satisfied at work. 34.9% were dissatisfied. • Satisfaction at work was significantly related to organisational support ($p < 0.01$) and control over the practice environment ($p < 0.01$). • The intention to quit their job was significantly related to autonomy ($p < 0.01$)
O'Donnell, et al. [41]	Degree of professional support felt by PHC nurses and their career intentions	Scotland	200 PHC nurses (61% response)	Survey	• All female, 49% aged 40–49 years and 29% were aged > 50 years. Employed as PHC nurse for a mean of 10 years (Range 0.5–24.0 years). • 15.5% intended to leave general practice in the next 5 years. • There was a significant association between age and intention to leave employment ($p = 0.001$), with 60% of those intending to leave aged ≥50 years, although 40% were aged under 50 years. • Isolated nurses are less likely to intend staying in practice nursing ($p = 0.009$). • 52.3% felt isolated at least sometimes, 43.7% reported feeling isolated sometimes, and 31% of nurses worked alone. • 77.3% of isolated nurses intended to continue working for the coming 5 years compared to 91.4% of non-isolated nurses. • Factors contributing to feelings isolation are generally located in the work environment. • Training and qualifications being used to the full and a productive appraisal both significantly reduce feelings of isolation, as did the intention to continue working in the future.
Royer [32]	Perceptions of work and workplace to identify factors affecting tenure intent	USA	478 C/PHC nurses (76% response)	Survey TCM Work Commitment Survey	• 73% clinical nurses, 11.6% were in management/administrative positions and 22% supervisors • 70.5% of respondents were middle aged or nearing or at retirement age • 1/3 were either thinking about leaving, looking into leaving, or planning to leave the job in 1 year • Of the 70% of respondents aged > 45 years, 1/3 were planning to leave within 1 year. • 46% of those aged 35–45 years were looking into leaving, and almost 40% of those aged 56–65 were thinking about leaving. • Respondents aged 35–45 years are 4.3 times more likely to be looking into leaving compared with those nurses who are older. • Respondents who have the least tenure (1–36 months) are 0.35 times less likely to

Table 2 Summary table (Continued)

Reference	Aim	Country	Sample	Methods	Findings
					be planning to leave < 1 year than those with greater tenure.
					• Respondents who have increasing attachment (affective commitment) to the job are also 1.7 times more likely to be looking into leaving and three times more likely to be planning to leave within 1 year than those who are committed in other ways.
					• Respondents who hold obligatory or loyalty commitment (normative) to the job are 1.4 times more likely to be planning to leave within 1 year than those who are committed by attachment or cost.
Storey et al. [29]	Impact of age on retention	England	485 PHC nurses (61% response)	Survey	• 78% respondents were aged between 40 and 59 years. 47% worked full-time.
					• 178 district nurses, 114 health visitors, 56 school nurses, and 137 practice nurses
					• 61% indicated that their role lived up to expectations. There was no significant difference across professional groups.
					• Older nurses are more likely to report that their role lived up to expectations opposed to younger ones (p = 0.001).
					• There was no difference in happiness in their current role between those aged under and over 50 years.
					• Older nurses were more likely to report being happy working in nursing than those < 50 years (p = 0.006).
					• Stress and job satisfaction were identified as key factors contributing to respondents views of working as a nurse.
					• School nurses were significantly less happy than other groups in their current role (p = 0.006).
					• Sources of unhappiness were identified as excessive workload, low morale, disillusionment, high administrative workload, perceived lack of support and staff shortages.
					• In terms of job satisfaction, 'relationships with other people at work' (62%), 'the actual job itself' (60%),' the level of job security in your present job' (55%) were highest scored.
					• There was a statistically significant difference between those aged under and over 50 years on nine items related to job satisfaction.
					• There was a statistically significant difference between those aged under and over 50 years on nine items related to factors encouraging them to stay.
					• Highest scored scales of dissatisfaction related to salary relative to experience (27%), change management' (21%), and organisational communications (18%).
					• Enhanced pay is a factor encouraging retention (p = 0.044) for those with degree-level qualifications.
					• Significant potential causes of nurses leaving were high administrative workloads, problems in combining work and family commitments (p > 0.001), and lack of workplace support (p = 0.029).
Stuart et al. [30]	Workload management, job satisfaction and challenges	Scotland	31 district nurses	Focus groups & interviews	• Most job satisfaction is derived from the 'hands-on nature' of patient care using clinical knowledge and skills.
					• Nurses liked the 'personal nature' of caring for patients in this setting and the formation of ongoing and sometimes intergenerational relationships.
					• Job dissatisfaction arises with overwhelming workloads, increased time pressure and policy change that negatively affects patient care and feeling devalued.
					• Nurses are dissatisfied as administrative tasks are taking them away from patient care.

Table 2 Summary table (Continued)

Reference	Aim	Country	Sample	Methods	Findings
Tourangeau [31]	Factors affecting intention to remain employed	Canada	50 PHC nurses	Focus groups	• 6 categories were found to influence nurse intention to remain employed: I. Job characteristics: variation in clientele and wide use of nursing skills, autonomous nature of work, decision authority; II. Work structures: continuity of care, appropriateness of client expectations, and flexibility in scheduling work hours, workload and use of technology. III. Relationships and communication: clients and families, physicians nursing colleagues, supervisors, CCAC case managers; IV. Work environment: professional practice environment: orientation, education and training; physical work environment: travel demands, access to resources and personal safety; V. Nurse responses to work: work-life balance, meaningfulness of work. VI. Employment conditions: employment status, union status, pay and benefits, unpaid work, work-related expenses, and income stability; • Job satisfaction was not a reported concept affecting intention to remain employed.
Tullai-McGuinness [40]	Predictors of job satisfaction	USA	201 PHC nurses (42.5% response)	Survey Nurse Work Index-Revised Global Appraisal of Autonomous Practice	• Mean age 45 years. Mean experience 17.8 years, with a mean of 8.3 years HC experience. 75% employed fulltime. • Almost 77% of HC nurses were satisfied (ratings > 60). • Diploma nurses had lower satisfaction (69.25%), compared to baccalaureate (74.43%) and associate degree (75.21%) nurses ($p > 0.05$). • There was an inverse relationship between years worked as a home healthcare nurse and satisfaction ($p < 0.01$). • Controlling for years of experience significant predictors of satisfaction were control over practice decisions and practice setting decisions.

one paper each from Saudi Arabia, South Africa, and Brazil.

The sample sizes of included studies varied from 31 [30] to 1044 participants [26]. Participants spanned the scope of PHC and included community nurses, primary health nurses, general practice nurses, school nurses, and district nurses. In some studies the data from various primary care nursing groups was reported in an aggregated form [32], whilst in other papers there was an attempt to tease out the differences between groups [26, 29].

Eleven (55%) papers focussed on job satisfaction only [27, 28, 30, 33–40], and three (15%) papers reported only data on career intention or turnover [31, 32, 41]. A further six (30%) papers combined measures of job satisfaction and career intention within the same study [2, 19, 26, 29, 42, 43].

The key features and predominant findings of papers are summarised in Table 2. Five overarching themes emerged, namely; levels of job satisfaction, factors that enhanced job satisfaction, factors that reduced levels of job satisfaction, career intentions, and, factors that impacted on career intentions.

Levels of job satisfaction

The variation in measurement of job satisfaction across studies and the differences in respondent characteristics makes comparison difficult. Most tools measured job satisfaction quantitatively using a Likert scale (agree to disagree) [2, 19, 26, 37–39], whilst one study used qualitative data collected from focus groups and interviews [28]. Studies measured different aspects of job satisfaction including; overall satisfaction (enjoyment, pride), specific aspects of the job (pay, rewards, resources, task requirements, work conditions, training, quality of care, time) and supervision (authority, autonomy, feedback, appreciation, organisational policies, interaction).

In some studies just over half of the respondents were reported to be satisfied with their job [19, 39], whilst in other studies a greater majority indicated that they were satisfied [28]. A small number of studies reported moderate [2, 38] to low levels of satisfaction [37, 42]. Those studies which reported lower levels of satisfaction used more items to measure satisfaction (42 items and 80 items respectively) [37, 42], compared to studies reporting high levels of satisfaction which used only 4 items [19, 39].

Factors influencing job satisfaction

The ten studies which explored the relationship between job satisfaction and demographics / professional variables demonstrated significant variation [2, 19, 29, 34, 36–40, 43].

Whilst two studies found that age had no significant impact on job satisfaction [2, 43], three others demonstrated that older nurses were more satisfied than their younger colleagues [29, 37, 38]. Similarly, there were variable findings related to the impact of education, with three papers finding no relationship with job satisfaction or inconclusive findings [2, 36, 37], and two papers demonstrating that nurses with higher educational qualifications had reported higher work satisfaction [34, 40]. In contrast, Delobelle et al. [2] found that Nursing Assistants and Enrolled Nurses were more satisfied than Registered Nurses.

Curtis and Glacken [37] reported that those employed for over 10 years had a significantly higher level of job satisfaction than other nurses. However, other studies reported an inverse relationship between years worked in PHC and satisfaction [40] and no significant differences between satisfaction and years of nursing [2].

Other factors that positively contributed to satisfaction included control over clinical practice and decision-making [19, 34, 39, 40], community satisfaction [43], organisational support [19], remuneration [38], and workload [39].

There was significant agreement between studies in terms of the factors that contributed positively to job satisfaction. These included the professional role, respect and recognition from clients and managers, workplace relationships, autonomy, access to resources and the flexibility of the role [2, 27–31, 33, 34, 37, 43].

Factors negatively impacting job satisfaction

There was a high level of agreement amongst included studies about factors that negatively impacted respondents' levels of satisfaction. Seven studies identified concerns about adequate remuneration [2, 28, 29, 34, 35, 37, 43]. When comparing hospital and community nurses, Campbell, et al. [34] identified that hospital nurses were significantly more likely than community nurses to be satisfied with their pay.

Another key factor identified in several studies related to the time pressures and high administrative workloads that impact on patient care [2, 26, 30, 33, 37]. Other factors identified to negatively impact job satisfaction included; a lack of recognition [2, 28, 33, 34], poor role clarity [30, 34, 37] and poor organisational communication [29, 34].

Career intentions

The included studies present an important picture around career intentions. However, caution needs to be applied in the interpretation of these data, as most studies comprise of an ageing workforce who will naturally retire in the near future. Six studies sought to explore the factors impacting on retention [2, 32, 34, 41–43] The highest reported career intentions was reported by Delobelle, et al. [2] with half of all nurse participants (*n*

= 69; 51.1%) considering leaving PHC in the next 2 years. Both Betkus and MacLeod [43] and Almalki, et al. [42] also reported that nearly half (48 and 40%) intended to leave their current PHC job in the next year. Royer [32] similarly identified that some 46% of participants aged 35–45 years were considering leaving, and almost 40% of those aged 56–65 were thinking about leaving. The remaining two studies reported that few participants intended to leave their current position [34, 41].

The findings of the three studies which explored job satisfaction and quality of worklife [2, 42, 43], lacked consistency. Almalki, et al. [42] demonstrated that quality of worklife was significantly related to turnover intent ($p < 0.001$), however, this only explained 26% of the variance and was not included in the final model. Whilst Betkus and MacLeod [43] reported no correlation between job satisfaction and retention, Delobelle, et al. [2] found that turnover intent was significantly explained by job satisfaction, age and education ($p < 0.001$). Other factors that were identified as having an impact on career intentions included gender [42], work environment [42], remuneration [42], education [2, 41, 42], satisfaction with supervision [2], feelings of isolation [41], length of time in position / years of experience [32, 42].

Discussion

This review provides the first synthesis of the literature around job satisfaction and career intentions of registered nurses working in PHC. Given the differences in organisational context, employment conditions and practice environment that likely impact job satisfaction and career intention [17–19] it is important that this group are explored beyond the context of the broader nursing workforce. Considering the imperatives to grow the workforce in PHC settings, to meet community demand, understanding this literature is important to inform both practice and policy. Dissatisfaction with nursing employment is reported in the broader nursing workforce literature. In their survey of 33,659 medical–surgical nurses across 12 European countries, Aiken, et al. [44] concluded that more than one in five nurses were dissatisfied with their employment. The variation in job satisfaction identified in this review highlights the need for further large well-designed longitudinal investigations of the PHC nurse workforce to monitor workforce issues, such as satisfaction and career intentions, over time. Given the links between nurse satisfaction and both retention and patient outcomes [44], this issue should be prioritised.

Our review demonstrated agreement between studies in terms of the positive impact of a professional role, respect, recognition, workplace relationships and autonomy upon job satisfaction. This is consistent with the acute care nursing literature where modifiable factors within the workplace have been demonstrated to influence both job and career satisfaction [45]. In their study, Nantsupawat, et al. [46] demonstrated that job dissatisfaction and intention to leave were significantly lower in nurses who worked in a better work environment. Similarly, in their systematic review, Cicolini, et al. [14] found a significant link between nurses empowerment and satisfaction. The significant role of such modifiable factors highlights an opportunity for managers, employers and policy makers to implement strategies which can improve the workplace and, subsequently, enhance satisfaction.

A key finding of this review was the negative impact of poor remuneration on job satisfaction. Whilst concerns about pay have been previously identified in the acute sector [44, 47], the challenge of lower rates of pay in PHC compared to the acute sector has long been reported [17, 48]. This review adds to the evidence-base around the impact of this disparity on the PHC nursing workforce and highlights the significant implications of not addressing this issue.

Our review also revealed that in many studies large numbers of nurses were intending to leave PHC employment in the near future [2, 42, 43]. This clearly has significant implications for the workforce and service delivery. However, measures of the factors affecting career intentions were variable across included studies as were findings. The difficulties in synthesising such disparate data have been previously identified in the acute care literature [13]. Despite this, there were clear similarities between our review and the broader literature around nurse turnover and intention to leave. In their systematic review of nurses intention to leave their employment, Chan, et al. [13] identified that intention to leave was impacted by a complex combination of organisational and individual factors. Organisational factors included the work environment, culture, commitment, work demands and social support. In contrast, individual factors related to job satisfaction, burnout and demographic factors. The complex interplay of multiple factors that underlie retention is probably the reason that retention is the highest when interventions such as mentoring and in-depth orientations are used to support staff [49].

In their study of acute care nurses Galletta, et al. [50] conclude that the quality of relationships among staff is an important factor in nurses' decisions to leave. Interprofessional relationships in PHC have long been identified as presenting unique challenges [48, 51]. The complex environment of PHC, whereby services are funded by small businesses or non-government agencies [52], combines with the relatively rapid shift towards interdisciplinary care to create challenges for staff in developing positive relationships [53]. The importance of positive relationships, respect of roles and recognition of value between co-workers demonstrated in our review highlights the value of further work to enhance interprofessional collaboration.

Limitations

Whilst this review synthesised the available literature, the variation in measurement instruments and sample sizes made comparison difficult. Since not all papers reported the reliability or validity of the instruments they used it is possible that these instruments had issues in their validity. The data presented, however, represents the best available evidence to address the research question.

A further limitation is the variation between PHC settings and international PHC systems that makes comparison difficult. Whilst this review has included all papers written about PHC nurses internationally, local variations mean that care needs to be taken when generalising findings to other contexts, even within PHC.

Conclusion

This review has identified some key factors that impact on both job satisfaction and career intentions amongst PHC nurses. The importance of the work environment and workplace relationships highlights the need to implement strategies that enhance modifiable workplace factors. The numbers of nurses across studies indicating an intention to leave is a significant concern at a time when we need to build the PHC workforce internationally. Findings from this review highlight the need for action by managers, educators, employers and policy makers to enhance support for nurses in PHC.

Implications for practice and research

There is urgent need to build capacity within the PHC nursing workforce internationally to meet service demands. This review has highlighted a number of issues around job satisfaction and career intention that impact on the retention of nurses in PHC. Exploring strategies to address the modifiable antecedents to nurse job dissatisfaction has the potential to improve retention. Maintaining happy and skilled nurses in the workforce has the potential to build workforce capacity and enhance patient outcomes.

This review has demonstrated that gaps remain in our knowledge around job satisfaction and career intention among PHC registered nurses. Further well-designed longitudinal research is required to explore the trajectory of careers in PHC. Additionally, mixed methods approaches are likely required to explore not only quantitative job satisfaction, but also to reveal how the aspects of satisfaction impact on PHC nurses.

Abbreviation
PHC: Primary Health Care

Funding
No funding was received for this study.

Authors' contributions
EH conceived the study, conducted the initial search and participated in the data analysis and drafting of the paper. ES confirmed the initial search and participated in the data analysis and drafting of the paper. SM participated in the data analysis and drafting of the paper. All authors read and approved the final manuscript.

Competing interests
Professor Elizabeth Halcomb is an Associate Editor of BMC Family Practice. Nil other competing interests.

References
1. Buchan J, Twigg D, Dussault G, Duffield C, Stone PW. Policies to sustain the nursing workforce: an international perspective. Int Nurs Rev. 2015;62(2):162–70.
2. Delobelle P, Rawlinson JL, Ntuli S, Malatsi I, Decock R, Depoorter AM. Job satisfaction and turnover intent of primary healthcare nurses in rural South Africa: a questionnaire survey. J Adv Nurs. 2011;67(2):371–83.
3. AbuAlRub R, El-Jardali F, Jamal D, Al-Rub NA. Exploring the relationship between work environment, job satisfaction, and intent to stay of Jordanian nurses in underserved areas. ANR. 2016;31:19–23.
4. Spence Laschinger HK, Zhu J, Read E. New nurses' perceptions of professional practice behaviours, quality of care, job satisfaction and career retention. J Nurs Manag. 2016;24(5):656–65.
5. Lu H, Barriball KL, Zhang X, While AE. Job satisfaction among hospital nurses revisited: a systematic review. Int J Nurs Stud. 2012;49(8):1017–38.
6. Hayes B, Bonner A, Pryor J. Factors contributing to nurse job satisfaction in the acute hospital setting: a review of recent literature. J Nurs Manag. 2010; 18(7):804–14.
7. Atefi N, Abdullah K, Wong L, Mazlom R. Factors influencing registered nurses perception of their overall job satisfaction: a qualitative study. Int Nurs Rev. 2014;61(3):352–60.
8. Khamisa N, Oldenburg B, Peltzer K, Ilic D. Work related stress, burnout, job satisfaction and general health of nurses. Int J Environ Res Public Health. 2015;12(1):652–66.
9. Takase M, Yamashita N, Oba K. Nurses' leaving intentions: antecedents and mediating factors. J Adv Nurs. 2008;62(3):295–306.
10. Hayes LJ, O'Brien-Pallas L, Duffield C, Shamian J, Buchan J, Hughes F, Laschinger HKS, North N. Nurse turnover: a literature review – an update. Int J Nurs Stud. 2012;49(7):887–905.
11. Kim J-K, Kim M-J. A review of research on hospital nurses' turnover intention. J Korean Acad Nurs. 2011;17(4):538–50.
12. Liu Y. Job satisfaction in nursing: a concept analysis study job satisfaction in nursing. Int Nurs Rev. 2016;63(1):84–91.
13. Chan ZC, Tam WS, Lung MK, Wong WY, Chau CW. A systematic literature review of nurse shortage and the intention to leave. J Nurs Manag. 2013; 21(4):605–13.
14. Cicolini G, Comparcini D, Simonetti V. Workplace empowerment and nurses' job satisfaction: a systematic literature review. J Nurs Manag. 2014;22(7):855–71.

15. Australian Institute of Health and Welfare: Australian Nursing and Midwifery Workforce Data and additional information. Canberra, Australia; 2014.

16. Freund T, Everett C, Griffiths P, Hudon C, Naccarella L, Laurant M. Skill mix, roles and remuneration in the primary care workforce: who are the healthcare professionals in the primary care teams across the world? Int J Nurs Stud. 2015;52(3):727–43.

17. Halcomb E, Ashley C, James S, Smythe E. Employment conditions of Australian PHC nurses. Collegian. 2018;25(1):65–71.

18. Halcomb EJ, Ashley C. Australian primary health care nurses most and least satisfying aspects of work. J Clin Nurs. 2017;36(3–4):535–45.

19. Lorenz VR, De Brito Guirardello E. The environment of professional practice and burnout in nurses in primary healthcare. Rev Lat Am Enfermagem. 2014;22(6):926–33.

20. Poghosyan L, Liu J, Shang J, D'Aunno T. Practice environments and job satisfaction and turnover intentions of nurse practitioners: implications for primary care workforce capacity. Health Care Manag Rev. 2015;

21. Health Workforce Australia: Health Workforce 2025 - Doctors, Nurses and Midwives. Adelaide; 2012.

22. Whittemore R, Knafl K. The integrative review: updated methodology. J Adv Nurs. 2005;52(5):546–53.

23. Desborough J, Parker R, Forrest L. Nurse satisfaction with working in a nurse led primary care walk in Centre: an Australian experience. Aust J Adv Nurs. 2013;31(1):11–9.

24. Moher D, Liberati A, Tetzlaff J, Altman DG. Preferred reporting items for systematic reviews and meta-analyses: the PRISMA statement. Int J Surg. 2010;8(5):336–41.

25. Center for Evidence Based Management. Critical Appraisal Checklist for Cross-Sectional Study. 2014. https://www.cebma.org/wp-content/uploads/Critical-Appraisal-Questions-for-a-Cross-Sectional-Study-july-2014.pdf. Accessed May 22 2017.

26. Armstrong-Stassen M, Cameron SJ. Concerns, satisfaction, and retention of Canadian community health nurses. J Community Health Nurs. 2005;22(4):181–94.

27. Flynn L, Deatrick JA. Home care Nurses' descriptions of important agency attributes. J Nurs Scholarsh. 2003;35(4):385–90.

28. Junious DL, Johnson RJ, Peters RJ Jr, Markham CM, Kelder SH, Yacoubian GS Jr. A study of school nurse job satisfaction. Journal of School Nursing (Allen Press Publishing Services Inc). 2004;20(2):88–93.

29. Storey C, Cheater F, Ford J, Leese B. Retaining older nurses in primary care and the community. J Adv Nurs. 2009;65(7):1400–11.

30. Stuart EH, Jarvis A, Daniel K. A ward without walls? District nurses' perceptions of their workload management priorities and job satisfaction. J Clin Nurs. 2008;17(22):3012–20.

31. Tourangeau A, Patterson E, Rowe A, Saari M, Thomson H, MacDonald G, Cranley L, Squires M. Factors influencing home care nurse intention to remain employed. J Nurs Manag. 2014;22(8):1015–26.

32. Royer L. Empowerment and commitment perceptions of community/public health nurses and their tenure intention. Public Health Nurs. 2011;28(6):523–32.

33. Best MF, Thurston NE. Canadian public health nurses' job satisfaction. Public Health Nurs. 2006;23(3):250–5.

34. Campbell SL, Fowles ER, Weber BJ. Organizational structure and job satisfaction in public health nursing. Public Health Nurs. 2004;21(6):564–71.

35. Cameron S, Armstrong-Stassen M, Bergeron S, Out J. Recruitment and retention of nurses: challenges facing hospital and community employers. Can J Nurs Leadersh. 2004;17(3):79–92.

36. Cole S, Ouzts K, Stepans MB. Job satisfaction in rural public health nurses. J Public Health Manag Pract. 2010;16(4):E1–6.

37. Curtis EA, Glacken M. Job satisfaction among public health nurses: a national survey. J Nurs Manag. 2014;22(5):653–63.

38. Doran D, Pickard J, Harris J, Coyte PC, MacRae AR, Laschinger HS, Darlington G, Carryer J. The relationship between managed competition in home care nursing services and nurse outcomes. Can J Nurs Res. 2007;39(3):151–65.

39. Graham KR, Davies BL, Woodend AK, Simpson J, Mantha SL. Impacting Canadian public health nurses' job satisfaction. Can J Public Health. 2011;102(6):427–31.

40. Tullai-McGuinness S. Home healthcare practice environment: predictors of RN satisfaction. Res Nurs Health. 2008;31(3):252–60.

41. O'Donnell C, Jabareen H, Watt G. Practice nurses' workload, career intentions and the impact of professional isolation: a cross-sectional survey. BMC Nurs. 2010;9(1):2.

42. Almalki MJ, Fitzgerald G, Clark M. The relationship between quality of work life and turnover intention of primary health care nurses in Saudi Arabia. BMC Health Serv Res. 2012;12:314.

43. Betkus MH, MacLeod MLP. Retaining public health nurses in rural British Columbia: the influence of job and community satisfaction. Can J Public Health. 2004;95(1):54–8.

44. Aiken LH, Sloane DM, Bruyneel L, Van den Heede K, Sermeus W. Nurses' reports of working conditions and hospital quality of care in 12 countries in Europe. Int J Nurs Stud. 2013;50(2):143–53.

45. Laschinger HKS. Job and career satisfaction and turnover intentions of newly graduated nurses. J Nurs Manag. 2012;20(4):472–84.

46. Nantsupawat A, Kunaviktikul W, Nantsupawat R, Wichaikhum OA, Thienthong H, Poghosyan L. Effects of nurse work environment on job dissatisfaction, burnout, intention to leave. Int Nurs Rev. 2017;64(1):91–8.

47. Al-Dossary R, Vail J, Macfarlane F. Job satisfaction of nurses in a Saudi Arabian university teaching hospital: a cross-sectional study. Int Nurs Rev. 2012;59(3):424–30.

48. Halcomb EJ, Davidson PM, Griffiths R, Daly J. Cardiovascular disease management: time to advance the practice nurse role? Aust Health Rev. 2008;32(1):44–55.

49. Lartey S, Cummings G, Profetto-McGrath J. Interventions that promote retention of experienced registered nurses in health care settings: a systematic review. J Nurs Manag. 2014;22(8):1027–41.

50. Galletta M, Portoghese I, Battistelli A, Leiter MP. The roles of unit leadership and nurse–physician collaboration on nursing turnover intention. J Adv Nurs. 2013;69(8):1771–84.

51. McInnes S, Peters K, Bonney A, Halcomb E. An integrative review of facilitators and barriers influencing collaboration and teamwork between general practitioners and nurses working in general practice. J Adv Nurs. 2015;71(9):1973–85.

52. McInnes S, Peters K, Bonney A, Halcomb E. The influence of funding models on collaboration in Australian general practice. Aust J Prim Health. 2017;23(1):31–6.

53. Williams A, Sibbald B. Changing roles and identities in primary health care: exploring a culture of uncertainty. J Adv Nurs. 1999;29(3):737–45.

8

How well do public sector primary care providers function as medical generalists in Cape Town: a descriptive survey

Renaldo Christoffels and Bob Mash[*]

Abstract

Background: Effective primary health care requires a workforce of competent medical generalists. In South Africa nurses are the main primary care providers, supported by doctors. Medical generalists should practice person-centred care for patients of all ages, with a wide variety of undifferentiated conditions and should support continuity and co-ordination of care. The aim of this study was to assess the ability of primary care providers to function as medical generalists in the Tygerberg sub-district of the Cape Town Metropole.

Methods: A randomly selected adult consultation was audio-recorded from each primary care provider in the sub-district. A validated local assessment tool based on the Calgary-Cambridge guide was used to score 16 skills from each consultation. Consultations were also coded for reasons for encounter, diagnoses and complexity. The coders inter- and intra-rater reliability was evaluated. Analysis described the consultation skills and compared doctors with nurses.

Results: 45 practitioners participated (response rate 85%) with 20 nurses and 25 doctors. Nurses were older and more experienced than the doctors. Doctors saw more complicated patients. Good inter- and intra-rater reliability was shown for the coder with an intra-class correlation coefficient of 0.84 (95% CI 0.045–0.996) and 0.99 (95% CI 0. 984–0.998) respectively. The overall median consultation score was 25.0% (IQR 18.8–34.4). The median consultation score for nurses was 21.6% (95% CL 16.7–28.1) and for doctors was 26.7% (95% CL 23.3–34.4) ($p = 0.17$). There was no difference in score with the complexity of the consultation. Ten of the 16 skills were not performed in more than half of the consultations. Six of the 16 skills were partly or fully performed in more than half of the consultations and these included the more biomedical skills.

Conclusion: Practitioners did not demonstrate a person-centred approach to the consultation and lacked many of the skills required of a medical generalist. Doctors and nurses were not significantly different. Improving medical generalism may require attention to how access to care is organised as well as to training programmes.

Keywords: Primary care, Primary health care, Nurse practitioners, General practitioners, Consultation, Communication, Person centredness, Medical generalism, South Africa

* Correspondence: rm@sun.ac.za
Division of Family Medicine and Primary Care, Stellenbosch University, Box
241, Cape Town 8000, South Africa

Background

Effective primary health care is an essential part of any successful health system and strengthening primary health care is a priority in South Africa especially with the huge burden of disease [1, 2]. South Africa's vision of universal health coverage and national health insurance requires strong primary health care as a prerequisite [3]. According to the World Health Organization (WHO) one of the key reforms required of primary health care is to become more people-centred and to move away from a focus on selected diseases and vertical programmes [4]. Putting people first requires a primary care workforce that focuses on people's health needs, is based on enduring personal relationships, is characterised by comprehensive, continuous and person-centred care, and is orientated towards tackling the underlying determinants of ill-health in a collaborative manner [5, 6].

In South Africa clinical nurse practitioners (CNPs) became the main primary care providers (PCPs) because of the shortage of doctors [7] and in order to reduce healthcare costs [8]. The adoption of nurses as the main PCP also necessitated a change in their scope of practice to be able to diagnose and prescribe. Primary care facilities include community health centres and clinics. Community health centres are larger facilities in metropolitan areas or towns and have a broader range of services offered by a multidisciplinary team that includes CNPs and doctors. Clinics are smaller facilities where services are offered by CNPs, sometimes with support from visiting doctors [9]. Pressure is placed on primary care to be comprehensive and to decrease referrals to the referral hospitals. In South Africa therefore the main medical generalist is a nurse supported by doctors.

The Royal College of General Practitioners defines medical generalism as an approach to the delivery of health care, be it to individuals, families, groups or communities, which is characterised by "whole person medicine" [10]. This broadly implies seeing a patient as a whole in the context of his or her family and community, being able to deal with undifferentiated symptoms and illness, providing a platform for continuity and coordination of care and the ability to form a collaborative relationship with both the patient and other health care providers to foster comprehensive management [11–13]. Effective communication skills are at the heart of effective generalism and the generalist must have the skills to manage these often complex consultations [14]. Direct links exist between effective communication and better health outcomes, symptom relief, reduced psychological distress, improved adherence to medication, increased patient satisfaction and less litigation [15, 16]. The principles of information sharing and concordant decision making between practitioner and patient also leads to a more effective consultation, further strengthens the therapeutic environment, and assists in providing continuity of care [13, 14]. Any health care worker that wants to function as a medical generalist, therefore, must possess and practice these capabilities [17].

Many low and middle income countries rely on nurses or mid-level doctors to provide primary care and the question therefore arises as to whether they are adequately prepared as medical generalists. Most of the evidence available is from high income countries, is qualitative and does not distinguish between CNPs working independently versus as an adjunct to the doctor. The evidence, however, suggests that patients may prefer to see a doctor if given a choice and nurses may be less prepared to offer a patient centred approach [18]. However, both doctors and nurses may provide technically competent clinical care in terms of exploring symptoms, giving acceptable advice and providing ample explanation of tests and medical terms [18]. Outcomes of care as measured by physical function, general health and vitality, social function, mental health and emotional welfare may also be similar regardless of whether care is received from a CNP or doctor [19]. In some instances CNPs had longer consultations, requested more special investigations and were less capable of providing chronic care, but had better record keeping than doctors and scored higher on amount of advice given [20, 21].

This study will add to the evidence base from a middle income country in an African setting and investigate the extent to which PCPs in public sector primary care display the attributes of a medical generalist. The findings should provide insight into the training and continuing professional development of CNPs and medical officers (MOs) functioning within a primary care team. The aim of the study was to assess the ability of PCPs to function as medical generalists in the Tygerberg sub-district of the Cape Town Metropole.

Methods

Study design

The study was a descriptive survey of PCPs using indirect observation of the consultation and an assessment tool.

Setting

Cape Town has a population of 4 million people and approximately 80% are dependent on the public health services. The city is divided into eight sub-districts and this study was based in the Tygerberg sub-district, which has 10 community health centres. Two of these facilities provide 24 h emergency care whilst the others are only functioning during office hours. Three facilities also have a midwife obstetric unit providing uncomplicated obstetric care. All facilities provide emergency care, chronic care for non-communicable diseases, HIV and TB, antenatal care and integrated management of childhood illnesses.

Three facilities have a family physician (specialist in family medicine) and other specialities provide outreach via their registrars. Nursing staff consist of general registered nurses, advanced midwives, CNPs, advanced psychiatric nurses, and nurses trained in initiating antiretroviral treatment. Medical staff include established medical officers, community service medical officers and interns. The reception or triage staff allocate patients to doctors or CNPs according to prior appointments or the complexity of the problem, as doctors are meant to see more complicated patients. Patients may also be referred by the CNPs to the doctors if they need help or the guidelines require a doctor's involvement in the management.

Study population
The study intended to include all 53 PCPs that were consulting adults in the sub-district's health centres and required a participation rate of at least 70% to be representative. As all PCPs in the sub-district were invited to participate there was no need to sample or select.

Data collection
A single audio recording was made of a consultation from each PCP who gave consent. Each patient, aged 18 years and above, was randomly selected from the pool of patients waiting to see the specific PCP using a random number generator smartphone application. If consent was granted by the selected patient, then the consultation with the PCP was recorded. If the selected patient declined participation in the study, another patient was chosen with the same randomisation process. The randomisation process ensured that a range of typical patients were selected. Patients could consult in either English or Afrikaans the predominate languages in the communities served.

The Stellenbosch University Observation Tool was used for assessing the consultation. This tool is based on the Calgary-Cambridge guide to the consultation, which summarises the international evidence base for consultation skills required by medical generalists [22, 23]. Its content and construct have been validated previously by experts within the Division of Family Medicine and Primary Care. The tool has been published and is used nationally for the assessment of registrars in family medicine in all nine training programmes [24–26]. The Calgary-Cambridge guide has been shown to have reasonable score distribution with no points in the extremes, a good test-retest reliability and low inter-rater variability due to its check point system [11, 27].

The tool evaluated 16 different consultation skills (Table 1) as "not done" (score = 0), "partially done" (score = 1) or "fully done" (score = 2). Each item could also be assessed as "not applicable" to the specific consultation.

The assessment tool was adapted by the addition of two items to assess continuity and co-ordination of care

Table 1 Skills assessed in the observation tool

1. Makes appropriate greeting / introduction and demonstrates interest and respect

2. Identifies and confirms the patient's problem list or issues

3. Encourages patient's contribution / story

4. Makes an attempt to understand the patient's perspective

5. Thinks family, and obtains relevant family, social and occupational information

6. Obtains sufficient information to ensure no serious condition is likely to be missed

7. Appears to make a clinically appropriate working diagnosis

8. There is a clear explanation of the diagnosis and management plan

9. Gives patient an opportunity to ask for other information and / or seeks to confirm patient's understanding

10. The explanation takes account of and relates to the patient's perspective

11. Involves the patient where appropriate in decision making

12. Chooses an appropriate management plan

13. Show a commitment to co-ordination of care

14. Shows a commitment to continuity of care

15. Closes consultation successfully

16. Provides appropriate safety netting for the patient

as these were part of the definition of medical generalism. The definition of these concepts were also informed by the Primary Care Assessment Tool [28], which is another validated tool for assessing core dimensions of primary care (although not in a recorded consultation). Any statement that the healthcare worker made that indicated a commitment to informational continuity received a "partially done" score, while any statement that demonstrated a commitment to relational continuity received a "fully done" score. Any statement that the healthcare worker made which attempted to co-ordinate care between people in the facility received a "partially done" score, while any statement that indicated a commitment to co-ordinate care between external agencies in the community or the next level of care (e.g. advocating for the patient by telephone to the referral centre or local non-government organisation) received a "fully done" score. If continuity or co-ordination of care was not required, then this item was scored as "not applicable".

Items 6, 7 and 12 were guided by the Practical Approach to Care Kit guidelines for consultation with adults in primary care, which is an evidence-based and integrated guideline for the management of common symptoms and chronic conditions in the Western Cape [29–31]. Scores were awarded on how completely the algorithm was followed; 2 was given if 75% or more of the content in the assessment or management algorithms were followed, 1 if between 50 and 74% of the content was followed and 0 if it was less than 50%.

The reasons for encounter and the diagnoses made in each consultation were coded using the International Classification of Primary Care [32]. Consultations were grouped in classes of different complexities based on the number of reason for encounter and the number of diagnoses involved in the consultation with low complexity being 1 to 2 reasons for encounter or with 1 diagnosis involved, moderate complexity 3 to 4 reasons for encounters or 2 diagnoses and high complexity having 5 or more reasons for encounter or 3 or more diagnoses [33, 34].

Data analysis

All data was captured in Microsoft Excel and checked for errors. Data was analysed with the help of a biostatistician from Stellenbosch University's Faculty of Medicine and Health Sciences, Biostatistics Unit, using the Statistical Package for Social Sciences software, version 24 (IBM Corp. Released 2015. IBM SPSS Statistics for Windows, Version 24.0. Armonk, NY: IBM Corp.).

Three randomly selected recordings were graded by three assessors (the researcher, an academic CNP and a family physician who were all familiar with the tool) to ensure that the primary rater had an acceptable level of reliability. For this, the Kappa value of each variable and total was calculated using Fleiss-Kappa [35, 36]. An Intra-class Correlation Coefficient was calculated to determine the level of reliability with a ratio of < 0.40 seen as poor, 0.60 to 0.74 as good and 0.75 to 1.00 as excellent [37]. The primary rater alone then re-assessed 15 randomly selected consultations four weeks after the initial assessment to determine intra-rater reliability. The Cohen-Kappa values were calculated for each individual variable and an Intra-class Correlation Coefficient was calculated to determine intra-rater reliability.

Descriptive statistics used means and standard deviations or medians and interquartile ranges for continuous data, depending on its distribution, or frequencies and percentages for categorical data.

Inferential statistics were used to compare the CNPs and MOs. The Pearson's Chi-Square test was used to compare categorical variables between independent groups and the Mann Whitney U-test to compare median scores between practitioners (binary categories) and the Kruskal-Wallis test to compare median scores between different levels of complexity in the consultation (multiple categories). A 0.05 level of statistical significance was used.

Results

Profile of participants

Altogether 45 health workers were included, which gave a response rate of 45/53 (85%). Of these participants 20 were CNPs (19 females, 1 male) and 25 were MOs (19 females, 7 male). Table 2 presents their characteristics and

shows that the medical officers were significantly younger and less experienced.

Rater reliability

Good inter-rater reliability was shown with an intra-class correlation coefficient for the overall assessment score of 0.84 (95% CI 0.045–0.996). High intra-rater reliability was also shown with an intra-class correlation coefficient of 0.99 (95% CI 0.984–0.998).

Types of consultations

Table 3 shows the complexity of the cases seen by the CNPs and MOs. As expected MOs saw more complex cases than the CNPs, although overall there was a good spread of complexity across the sample. The mean consultation time was 14 min with the shortest consultation being 3 min and the longest 46 min. Table 4 shows the top 10 reasons for encounter and diagnoses involved in consultations by the PCPs.

Evaluation of consultation skills

Figure 1 shows the distribution of total scores as a percentage (out of maximum possible score of 32). The median score was 8.0 (IQR 6.0–11.0) and median percentage was 25.0% (IQR 18.8–34.4). The median percentage score for CNPs was 21.6% (95% CL 16.7–28.1) and for MOs was 26.7% (95% CL 23.3–34.4) ($p = 0.17$). The median percentage scores obtained for different levels of complexity in the consultation were 28.1% (95% CL 18.8–40.0) for high complexity, 23.3% (95% CL 15.6–34.4) for moderate complexity and 23.3% (95% CL 20.0–28.1) for low complexity ($p = 0.609$).

Table 5 shows how all participants performed for each skill. Ten of the 16 skills were not performed in more than half of the consultations. These missing skills were across the whole consultation and were the more patient-centred skills of building rapport, attending to the person's perspective and context, ensuring they understood what was said and enabling shared decision making. There was little commitment to continuity of care and to safety netting for the patient. Six of the 16 skills were partly or fully performed in more than half of the consultations and these included the more practitioner-centred and biomedical skills such as collecting sufficient medical information, making an appropriate diagnosis (no diagnosis was needed in 15 consultations) or management plan and communicating these to the patients. There was some commitment to co-ordinating care.

CNPs and MOs did not differ significantly in the percentage of skills that were fully done apart from for "obtaining sufficient information to ensure no serious condition was missed", where the MOs performed better than the CNPs (CNPs 10% vs MOs 40%, $p = 0.009$).

Table 2 Profile of participants

Characteristics	Clinical nurse practitioners Mean (SD)	Medical officers Mean (SD)
Age (years)	45.7 (8.5)	34.7 (10.1)
Years since qualifying as professional nurse or doctor	20.6 (8.7)	10.5 (9.3)
Years in primary care as a CNP or MO	11.8 (6.2)	5.1 (4.9)

Discussion
Summary of key findings
PCPs did not function well as medical generalists in the consultation and were particularly poor at being patient-centred. Nurses also struggled to obtain sufficient medical information to ensure no serious conditions were missed and this was an area where doctors performed significantly better. Nurses and doctors did not differ in any of the other consultation skills, although doctors were seeing more complex patients. Most consultations appeared to make an appropriate diagnosis and management plan. There was some commitment to co-ordinating care for patients, but little commitment to continuity of care. The findings suggest that despite person-centeredness being a key goal of the health system in the Western Cape [38, 39] there is a huge gap between aspiration and reality.

Discussion of key findings
This gap in effective communication and lack of patient-centredness is likely to be one of the factors behind poor adherence to treatment [20, 21, 40], poor control of chronic diseases [18, 41] and less than ideal health outcomes in terms of quality of life and mortality [19, 42, 43]. It may also relate to increased litigation and reduced satisfaction with medical care [44]. The primary care system itself may be one of the modifiable factors behind the capacity of health workers to consult effectively. If one assumes that PCPs are capable of more holistic and effective consultations, they may be limited in their ability to perform by a high workload that necessitates large numbers of brief consultations on a daily basis. Many primary care facilities measure practitioners in terms of the number of patients seen and not the quality of the interaction or the outcomes. Many practitioners working under these stressful conditions

Table 3 Complexity of consultations

Complexity	All N = 45 n (%)	CNPs N = 20 n (%)	MOs N = 25 n (%)
High	17 (37.8)	4 (20.0)	13 (52.0)
Moderate	13 (28.9)	8 (40.0)	5 (20.0)
Low	15 (33.3)	8 (40.0)	7 (28.0)

CNP Clinical nurse practitioners, MO Medical officers

suffer from burnout and depression [45] and this may also limit their ability to offer care [46].

There may, however, be a more fundamental gap in the capability of PCPs to communicate effectively as medical generalists. The training of clinical nurse practitioners (1-year Diploma) may not focus sufficiently on patient-centred consultation skills and may lack the opportunity to practice these skills and receive feedback [47]. The training of doctors (6-years Degree) may not consistently reinforce effective patient-centred communication skills and they may not see these skills modelled by other doctors in practice [48]. These skills are often developed further by postgraduate training in family medicine and primary care, yet few PCPs engage with such training and it is not compulsory or incentivised. The new national Diploma in Family Medicine aimed at primary care doctors does make consultation skills a core competency in the programme [49]. The training of family physicians also makes patient-centred communication a core competency (at Stellenbosch University the assessment tool used in this study was standardised at a pass mark of 60% for their exit examination, which is much higher than the median of 25% scored in actual primary care practice).

Continuity of care requires a longitudinal interaction with the same team of PCPs so that you develop a trusting and knowledgeable relationship [50–52]. This improves the efficiency and accuracy of care as ongoing management is based on a foundation of prior understanding and knowledge of the person [53]. A commitment to continuity of care was not found in this study and may reflect a lack of a systematic approach to enabling it. A lack of relational continuity is normative in these health centres [54]. These large urban community health centres do not register or link patients to specific practitioners and do not create practice teams with a sense of ongoing responsibility for a specific group of patients.

Doctors performed better than nurses in terms of gathering sufficient medical information and making an appropriate diagnosis, while also seeing more complex patients. Studies from other countries suggest that nurses can manage minor injuries in an emergency department, [8, 55] decreasing the overall workload and improving cost-effectiveness [56]. In primary care they have been shown to improve satisfaction of care, decrease the numbers referred to emergency departments, improve biomedical markers

Table 4 Top 10 reasons for encounter and diagnoses

	Reason for encounter (N = 102)	n (%)		Diagnosis (N = 93)	n (%)
1	Follow up appointment	14 (13.7)	1	Hypertension	14 (15.1)
2	Cough	8 (7.8)	2	Osteoarthritis	9 (9.7)
3	Back pain	7 (6.9)	3	Respiratory infection	8 (8.6)
4	Abdominal pain	6 (5.9)	4	HIV	8 (8.6)
5	Headache	6 (5.9)	5	Diabetes	6 (6.6)
6	Chest pain	5 (4.9)	6	Soft tissue injury	5 (5.4)
7	Dyspnoea	5 (4.9)	7	Urinary tract infection	4 (4.3)
8	Fatigue	4 (3.9)	8	Dyslipidaemia	4 (4.3)
9	Rash	4 (3.9)	9	Cardiac failure	3 (3.2)
10	Peripheral oedema	3 (2.9)	10	Epilepsy	3 (3.2)
11	Seizures	3 (2.9)	11	Eczema	3 (3.2)

and health outcomes [57]. Nurses, however, in these more highly resourced settings may have had more relevant training and work more in collaboration with doctors rather than as replacements for them.

Methodological issues and limitations
The behaviour of practitioners may have been affected by the presence of the audio-recorder. Such a Hawthorne effect, however, might be expected to lead to an extra effort to perform well, which would imply the scores might be lower in actual practice. If the practitioner was unduly anxious about being recorded this could also lead to a reduced performance. The audio-recorder was small and unobtrusive and may well have been forgotten as the consultation progressed. Non-verbal communication and medical record keeping were not observed. The assessment of some of the consultation skills, such as making an appropriate management plan or informational continuity of care, could have been enhanced by this collateral data.

The medical officer pool included three people with post graduate training in Family Medicine (one family physician and 2 registrars) who scored much better than their peers and this would have influenced the results. Eight practitioners refused informed consent, although it is unlikely that the overall results would have been significantly different if they were included. The PCPs included in the study are typical of such practitioners in the Western Cape, although one cannot claim they are representative of PCPs throughout South Africa.

Recommendations
Although not measured directly in this study it is clear that enabling patient-centred primary care may require managers to consider the availability of sufficient human and other resources as well as the way access is organised (e.g. appointment systems, opening times, patient flow) to ensure a reasonable consultative workload on each practitioner and the potential to offer more holistic care [58].

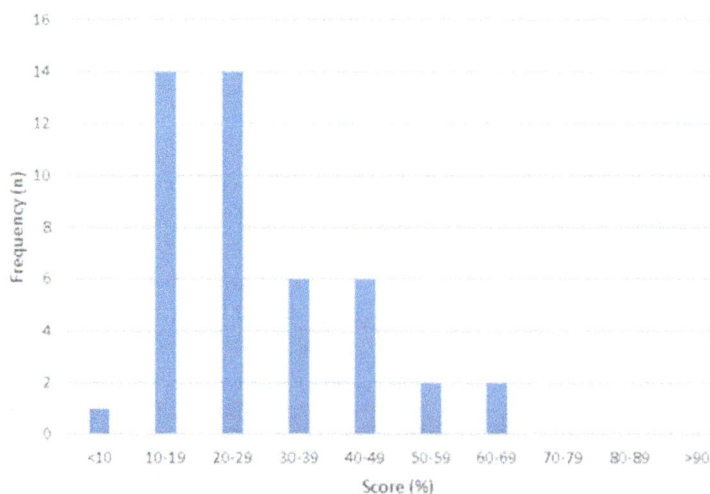

Fig. 1 Distribution of consultation scores (N = 45)

Table 5 Summary of performance for each skill

Consultation skill	Not done n (%)	Partially done n (%)	Fully done n (%)
1. Makes appropriate greeting / introduction and demonstrates interest and respect	29 (64.4)	7 (15.6)	9 (20.0)
2. Identifies and confirms the patient's problem list or issues	38 (84.4)	4 (8.9)	3 (6.7)
3. Encourages patient's contribution / story	26 (57.8)	13 (28.9)	6 (13.3)
4. Makes an attempt to understand the patient's perspective	40 (88.9)	3 (6.7)	2 (4.4)
5. Thinks family, and obtains relevant family, social and occupational information	36 (80.0)	8 (17.8)	1 (2.2)
6. Obtains sufficient information to ensure no serious condition is likely to be missed	13 (28.9)	20 (44.4)	12 (26.7)
7. Appears to make a clinically appropriate working diagnosis	9 (20.0)	11 (24.4)	10 (22.2)
8. There is a clear explanation of the diagnosis and management plan	13 (30.2)	20 (46.5)	10 (23.3)
9. Gives patient an opportunity to ask for other information and / or seeks to confirm patient's understanding	34 (75.6)	7 (15.6)	4 (8.9)
10. The explanation takes account of and relates to the patient's perspective	42 (93.3)	1 (2.2)	2 (4.4)
11. Involves the patient where appropriate in decision making	37 (82.2)	7 (15.6)	1 (2.2)
12. Chooses an appropriate management plan	7 (15.6)	18 (40.0)	20 (44.4)
13. Show a commitment to co-ordination of care	18 (40.0)	17 (37.8)	8 (17.8)
14. Shows a commitment to continuity of care	25 (55.6)	16 (35.6)	4 (8.9)
15. Closes consultation successfully	7 (15.6)	25 (55.6)	13 (28.9)
16. Provides appropriate safety netting for the patient	34 (75.6)	5 (11.1)	6 (13.3)

Pre-service training programmes for CNPs and MOs may need to give more attention to the development of patient-centred communication skills. Training needs to include theory, modelling and simulated practice, to be formally assessed and reinforced through the curriculum [47]. Thought should also be given to in-service training for existing CNPs and MOs in the form of short courses or post graduate Diplomas.

Clinical governance activities should also prioritise the acquisition of these skills and support training opportunities, quality improvement cycles and routine indicators that support the development of patient-centred communication skills.

The primary care system needs to support the development of a commitment to continuity of care by creating practice teams that take responsibility for a defined group of patients. Such an approach may dovetail with recent interest in community orientated primary care that links specific groups of households to community health workers and through them to specific health facilities and PCPs.

Comparative research could be done in rural areas, other provinces or in private general practice.

Conclusions

PCPs did not demonstrate a person-centred approach to the consultation and lacked many of the skills required of a medical generalist. Primary care doctors, mostly without postgraduate training, and clinical nurse practitioners were not significantly different, although doctors did collect more essential medical information and saw more complex patients. Most consultations appeared to make an appropriate diagnosis and management plan. There was little commitment to continuity of care and moderate commitment to co-ordination of care. Improving person-centredness and medical generalism may require attention to how access to care is organised as well as to pre-service, postgraduate and in-service training programmes.

Abbreviations
CNP: Clinical nurse practitioner; HIV: Human immunodeficiency virus; MO: Medical officer; PCP: Primary care provider; TB: Tuberculosis; WHO: World Health Organization

Acknowledgements
A consultant (Ms T Esterhuizen) at the Biostatistics Unit within the Centre for Evidence Based Health Care (CEHBC), Stellenbosch University assisted with the analysis of this study through support from the Faculty of Medicine and Health Science's dean's fund. The authors also acknowledge Sister Hilary Rhode who assisted with the reliability testing and Mr. Jayson Sefela who helped to collect the data.

Authors' contributions
RC performed this research for the Master of Medicine degree under the supervision of RM. RC conceptualised the research, collected and analysed the data, and wrote the final report. RM supervised each step of the research process and prepared the manuscript for publication. Both authors approved the final version.

Competing interests
The authors declare that they have no competing interests.

References

1. Pillay-van Wyk V, Msemburi W, Laubscher R, Dorrington RE, Groenewald P, Glass T, et al. Mortality trends and differentials in South Africa from 1997 to 2012: second National Burden of Disease Study. Lancet Glob Heal. 2012;4(9): e642–53. https://doi.org/10.1016/S2214-109X(16)30113-9.
2. Strandberg EL, Ovhed I, Borgquist L, Wilhelmsson S. The perceived meaning of a (w)holistic view among general practitioners and district nurses in Swedish primary care: a qualitative study. BMC Fam Pract. 2007;8(8):1–8.
3. South African Department of Health. National Health Insurance for South Africa: Towards Universal Health Coverage. Pretoria; 2015. Available from: https://www.health-e.org.za/wp-content/uploads/2015/12/National-Health-Insurance-for-South-Africa-White-Paper.pdf. Accessed 25 June 2013.
4. World Health Organization. The world health report: primary health care. Geneva: World Health Organization; 2008.
5. West N. National Health Insurance: the first 18 months. SAMJ. 2014;103(3):156–8.
6. Howarth G. National Health Insurance: a lofty ideal in need of cautious, planned implementation. South Afr J Bioeth Law. 2012;5(1):4–10.
7. Breier M. The shortage of medical doctors in South Africa: a multiple source identification and verification of scarce and critical skills in the South African labour market. 2008. [cited 2007 Nov 27]. Available from: www.labour.gov.za/research. Accessed 25 June 2013.
8. Marten R, Mcintyre D, Travassos C, Shishkin S, Longde W, Reddy S, et al. An assessment of progress towards universal health coverage in Brazil, Russia, India, China, and South Africa (BRICS). Lancet. 2014;384(9960):2164–71. https://doi.org/10.1016/S0140-6736(14)60075-1.
9. South African Department of Health. Department of Health Annual Report 2014/2015. Pretoria; 2015 [cited 2015 Sep 21]. Available from: https://www.health-e.org.za/2015/10/20/report-department-of-health-annual-report-201415/. Accessed 21 Sept 2015.
10. Royal College of General Practitioners. Medical Generalism: impact report. 2013. p. 1–8. Available from: http://www.rcgp.org.uk/policy/rcgp-policy-areas/~/media/Files/Policy/A-Z-policy/Medical-Generalism-Impact-Report-March-2013.ashx. Accessed 21 Sept 2015.
11. Howe A. What's special about medical generalism? The RCGP's response to the independent commission on Generalism. Br J Gen Pract. 2012;62(600):342–3.
12. Royal College of General Practitioners. Guiding patients through complexity: Modern Medical Generalism. 2011 [cited 2011 Oct 7]. p. 38. Available from: www.health.org.uk/publication/guiding-patients-through-complexity-modern-medical-generalism. Accessed 7 Oct 2011.
13. Schirmer JM, Mauksch L, Lang F, Marvel MK, Zoppi K, Epstein RM, et al. Assessing communication Competence : a review of current tools. Fam Med. 2005;37(3):184–92.
14. Robinson J, Walley T, Pearson M, Taylor D, Barton S. Measuring consultation skills in primary care in England: evaluation and development of content of the MAAS scale. Br J Gen Pract. 2002;52(484):889–93.
15. Burt J, Abel G, Elmore N, Campbell J, Roland M, Benson J, et al. Assessing communication quality of consultations in primary care: initial reliability of the global consultation rating scale, based on the Calgary-Cambridge guide to the medical interview. Br Med J. 2014;4:1–8.
16. Silverman J, Draper J, Kurtz SM. Skills for communicating with patients. Second edi. Oxford: Radcliffe Medical Press; 2006.
17. Enzer I, Robinson J, Pearson M, Barton S, Walley T. A reliability study of an instrument for measuring general practitioner consultation skills: the LIV-MAAS scale. Int J Qual Heal Care. 2003;15(5):407–12.
18. Klemenc-Ketis Z, Kravos A, Poplas-Susic T, Svab I, Kersnik J. New tool for patient evaluation of nurse practitioner in primary care settings. J Clin Nurs. 2013;23:1323–31.
19. Mundinger MO, Kane RL, Lenz ER, Totten AM, Cleary PD, Friedewald WT, et al. Primary care outcomes in patients treated by nurse practitioners or physicians. JAMA. 2000;283(1):59–68.
20. Poulton BC. Use of the consultation satisfaction questionnaire to examine patients' satisfaction with general practitioners and community nurses: reliability, replicability and discriminant validity. Br J Gen Pract. 1996;46(402):26–31.
21. Martínez-González NA, Djalali S, Tandjung R, Huber-Geismann F, Markun S, Wensing M, et al. Substitution of physicians by nurses in primary care: a systematic review and meta-analysis. BMC Health Serv Res 2014; Vol. 14. [cited 2013 Jun 25]. Available from: http://www.biomedcentral.com/1472-6963/14/214. Accessed 25 June 2013.
22. Kurtz S, Silverman J, Benson J, Draper J. Marrying content and process in clinical method teaching: enhancing the Calgary–Cambridge guides. Acad Med. 2003;78(8):802–9.
23. Kurtz S, Silverman J, Draper J. Teaching and learning communication skills in medicine. Oxford: Radcliffe Medical Press; 1998.
24. De Villiers M, Van Heusden M. A comparison of clinical communication skills between two groups of final-year medical students with different levels of communication skills training. South African Fam Pract. 2007;49(7):16.
25. Cooper V, Hassell A. Teaching consultation skills in higher specialist training: experience of a workshop for specialist registrars in rheumatology. Rheumatology. 2002;41:1168–71.
26. The Colleges of Medicine of South Africa: Fellowship of the College of Family Physicians of South Africa. 2017 [cited 2005 May 20]. Available from: https://www.cmsa.co.za/view_college.aspx?collegeid=6. Accessed 20 May 2005.
27. Kurtz S, Silverman J. The Calgary-Cambridge referenced observation guides: an aid to defining the curriculum and organizing the teaching in communication training programmes. Med Educ. 1996;30(2):83–9.
28. Sayed A, Bresick G, Bhagwan S, Manga C. Adaptation and cross-cultural validation of the United States primary care assessment tool (expanded version) for use in South Africa. African J Prim Heal Care Fam Med. 2015;7(1):1–11.
29. Practical Approach to Care Kit. BMJ. 2017 [cited 2015 May 5]. Available from: http://pack.bmj.com/. Accessed 5 May 2015.
30. Practical Approach to Care Kit. Knowledge Translation Unit, Univerity of Cape Lung Institute. 2017 [cited 2016 Jun 14]. Available from: http://knowledgetranslation.co.za/programmes/pack-adult-wc-sa/. Accessed 14 June 2016.
31. Fairall L, Bateman E, Cornick R, Faris G, Timmerman V, Folb N, et al. Innovating to improve primary care in less developed countries: towards a global model. BMJ Innov. 2015;1:196–203.
32. WONCA International Classification Committee. International classification of primary care (ICPC-2). Oxford: Oxford University Press; 1998.
33. Soler JK, Okkes I. Reasons for encounter and symptom diagnoses: a superior description of patients' problems in contrast to medically unexplained symptoms (MUS). Fam Pract. 2012;29:272–82.
34. Gask L, Klinkman M, Fortes S, Dowrick C. Capturing complexity: the case for a new classification system for mental disorders in primary care. Eur Psychiatry. 2008;23(7):469–76. https://doi.org/10.1016/j.eurpsy.2008.06.006.
35. Tractenberg RE, Futoshi Yumoto SJ, Morris JC. Sample size requirements for training to a kappa agreement criterion on clinical dementia ratings. Alzheimer Disase Assoc Disord. 2010;24(3):264–8.
36. Gwet K. Handbook of inter-rater reliability. The definitive guide to measuring the extent of agreement amongst raters 4th edition. Gaithersburg: Advanced Analytics LLC; 2014.
37. Cicchetti DV. Guidelines, criteria, and rules of thumb for evaluating normed and standardized assessment instruments in psychology. Psychol Assess. 1994;6(4):284–90.
38. Healthcare 2030: The Road to wellness. Western Cape Government. 2014 [cited 2014 Apr 20]. Available from: https://www.westerncape.gov.za/assets/departments/health/healthcare2030.pdf. Accessed 20 Apr 2014.
39. National Development Plan 2030. National Planning Commission, South African Government. [cited 2011 Nov 11]. Available from: http://www.gov.za/issues/national-development-plan-2030. Accessed 11 Nov 2011.
40. Clifford S, Barber N, Elliot R, Hartley E, Horne R. Patient-centred advice is effective in improving adherence to medicines. Pharm World Sci. 2006;28:165–70.
41. Epstein RM, Street RL. The values and value of patient-centered. Ann Fam Med. 2011;9(2):100–3.
42. Michie S, Miles J, Weinman J. Patient-centredness in chronic illness; what is it and does it matter? Patient Educ Couns. 2003;51(3):197–206.
43. Bauman AE, Fardy HJ, Harris PG. Getting it right: why bother with patient-centred care? Med J Aust. 2003;179:253–6.
44. Ambady N, Laplante D, Nguyen T, Rosenthal R, Chaumeton N, Levinson W. Surgeons' tone of voice: a clue to malpractice history. Surgery. 2002;132:5–9.
45. Rossouw L, Seedat S, Emsley R, Suliman S, Hagermeister D. The prevalence of burnout and depression in medical doctors working in the cape town metropolitan municipality community healthcare clinics and district hospitals of the provincial government of the western cape: a cross-sectional study. South African Fam Pract. 2014;55(6):567–73.
46. Bateman C. System burning out our doctors – study. SAMJ. 2012;102(7):593–4.
47. Malan Z, Mash B. Everett-murphy K. A situational analysis of training for behaviour change counselling for primary care providers, South Africa. Afr J Prm heal care. Fam Med. 2015;7(1):1–10.

48. Archer E. Engaging patient-centredness in an undergraduate curriculum (PhD thesis). Stellenbosch University; 2016. Available from: http://scholar.sun.ac.za/handle/10019.1/100338. Accessed 1 Sept 2017.

49. Mash R, Malan Z, Von Pressentin K, Blitz J. Strengthening primary health care through primary care doctors: the design of a new national postgraduate diploma in family medicine. South African Fam Pract 2016; 58(1):1–5. Available from: https://doi.org/10.1080/20786190.2015.1083719.

50. Tabler J, Scammon DL, Kim J, Farrell T, Tomoaia-Cotisel A. Patient care experiences and perceptions of the patient-provider relationship: A mixed method study. Patient Exp J. 2014;1(1):75–87.

51. Rodriguez HP, Marshall RE, Rogers WH, Safran DG. Primary care physician visit continuity: a comparison of patient-reported and administratively derived measures. J Gen Intern Med. 2008;23(9):1499–502.

52. Lee K, Wright SM, Wolfe L. The clinically excellent primary care physician: examples from the published literature. BMC Fam Pract. 2016;17(169):1–6. https://doi.org/10.1186/s12875-016-0569-x.

53. Haggerty JL, Reid RJ, Freeman GK, Starfield BH, Adair CE, McKendry R. Continuity of care: a multidisciplinary review. BMJ. 2003;327:1219–21. https://doi.org/10.1136/bmj.327.7425.1219.

54. Bresick G, Sayed A-R, Grange C, Bhagwan S, Manga N, Hellenberg D, et al. Western Cape Primary Care Assessment Tool (PCAT) study: Measuring primary care organisation and performance in the Western Cape Province, South Africa (2013). African J Prim Heal Care Fam Med. 2013;8(1):1–12. https://doi.org/10.4102/phcfm.v8i1.1057.

55. Wilson A, Zwart E, Everett I, Kernick J. The clinical effectiveness of nurse practitioners' management of minor injuries in an adult emergency department: a systematic review. Int J Evid Based Healthc. 2009;7:3):3–14.

56. Donald F, Kilpatrick K, Reid K, Carter N, Martin-misener R, Bryant-lukosius D, et al. A systematic review of the cost-effectiveness of nurse practitioners and clinical nurse Specialists : what is the quality of the Evidence ?. Vol. 2014, Nurs Res Pract. 2014 [cited 1BC Sep 1]. Available from: https://doi.org/10.1155/2014/896587. Accessed 1 Sept 2017.

57. Stanik-Hutt J, Newhouse R, White KM, Johantgen M, Bass EB, Zangaro G, et al. The quality and effectiveness of care provided by nurse practitioners. J Nurse Pract. 2013;9(8):492–500.

58. Kringos DS, Boerma WG, Hutchinson A, Van der Zee J, Groenewegen PP. The breadth of primary care: a systematic literature review of its core dimensions. BMC Health Serv Res. 2010;10(65) https://doi.org/10.1186/1472-6963-10-65.

9

Interpersonal continuity of primary care of veterans with diabetes: a cohort study using electronic health record data

Christine M. Everett[1*], Perri Morgan[1], Valerie A. Smith[2,3,4], Sandra Woolson[2], David Edelman[2,4], Cristina C. Hendrix[2,5], Theodore Berkowitz[2], Brandolyn White[2] and George L. Jackson[2,3,4]

Abstract

Background: Continuity of care is a cornerstone of primary care and is important for patients with chronic diseases such as diabetes. The study objective was to examine patient, provider and contextual factors associated with interpersonal continuity of care (ICoC) among Veteran's Health Administration (VHA) primary care patients with diabetes.

Methods: This patient-level cohort study ($N = 656,368$) used electronic health record data of adult, pharmaceutically treated patients (96.5% male) with diabetes at national VHA primary care clinics in 2012 and 2013. Each patient was assigned a "home" VHA facility as the primary care clinic most frequently visited, and a primary care provider (PCP) within that home clinic who was most often seen. Patient demographic, medical and social complexity variables, provider type, and clinic contextual variables were utilized. We examined the association of ICoC, measured as maintaining the same PCP across both years, with all variables simultaneously using logistic regression fit with generalized estimating equations.

Results: Among VHA patients with diabetes, 22.3% switched providers between 2012 and 2013. Twelve patient, two provider and two contextual factors were associated with ICoC. Patient characteristics associated with disruptions in ICoC included demographic factors, medical complexity, and social challenges (example: homeless at any time during the year $OR = 0.79$, $CI = 0.75–0.83$). However, disruption in ICoC was most likely experienced by patients whose providers left the clinic ($OR = 0.09$, $CI = 0.07–0.11$). One contextual factor impacting ICoC included NP regulation (most restrictive NP regulation ($OR = 0.79$ $CI = 0.69–0.97$; reference least restrictive regulation).

Conclusions: ICoC is an important mechanism for the delivery of quality primary care to patients with diabetes. By identifying patient, provider, and contextual factors that impact ICoC, this project can inform the development of interventions to improve continuity of chronic illness care.

Keywords: Continuity of care, Primary care, Diabetes

Introduction

A core function of primary care is continuity of care (CoC) [1, 2]. CoC is achieved when care is provided as an uninterrupted succession of events and can be achieved through a variety of mechanisms [1]. A cornerstone element of CoC in primary care is interpersonal continuity (ICoC), defined as a longitudinal relationship between a primary care provider (PCP) and patient that involves delivery of preventive care, treatment of multiple illness episodes, and a responsibility for care coordination [3]. ICoC may improve patient-provider communication, the delivery of preventive services and reduce hospitalizations, and may be particularly important for patients with chronic illnesses [4–6]. However, ICoC in the US is lacking, particularly for complex patients. One study suggested that approximately one-third of adults over 65 in the United States (i.e., Medicare beneficiaries) switch their PCP each year [7]. Similarly, staffing approaches which assign patients to a provider-led team do not guarantee ICoC [8].

Patient, organizational, and community factors have been shown to impact CoC. Older, female, more complex, and sicker patients are more likely to achieve CoC, as are

* Correspondence: Christine.everett@duke.edu
[1]Duke University School of Medicine, Physician Assistant Program|, 800 South Duke Street, Durham, NC 27701, USA
Full list of author information is available at the end of the article

patients who do not belong to a racial or ethnic minority [9–12]. Socioeconomic factors including insurance type can be a barrier to ICoC. Healthcare organization size also appears to impact continuity, but data on the direction of the relationship between large organizational size and continuity are contradictory [13–15]. Availability of providers, due to turn-over, training site or other work schedule issues, can lower patient satisfaction and diminish ICoC [15, 16]. In areas with few providers, such as rural settings, continuity may be higher due to fewer choices [17]. To our knowledge however, no study has simultaneously evaluated patient, organizational, and community factors, making it difficult to understand which factors might be the best points of intervention. This paper examines associations between patient, provider, organizational, and community factors with ICoC. Identifying factors that predict ICoC can assist in developing interventions to improve continuity.

Methods
Setting
The Veteran's Health Administration (VHA) is the largest integrated delivery system in the U.S. In 2012, the VHA provided primary care to over 6.33 million patients and had 990 outpatient clinics in 23 regionally defined integrated service networks (VISNs) [18, 19]. Patients who utilize the VHA for care tend to be sicker, older, and have lower incomes than the general population [20]. VHA's patient-centered medical home model, Patient-Aligned Care Team (PACT), aims to provide strong ICoC within a team-based setting [18, 21]. A panel of approximately 1200 primary care patients are assigned to a PACT, which consists of one PCP (physician, nurse practitioner (NP) or physician assistant (PA)), a registered nurse care manager, a clinical associate (licensed practical nurse, medical assistant or health technologist), and a clerk.

Data source and sample
This patient-level cohort study used centrally-available national VHA electronic health record data from fiscal years 2012 and 2013 (Fig. 1). The goal of the approach to the study cohort selection was to identify veterans with diabetes that have received a sufficient amount of primary care within the VHA system to impact diabetes outcomes. The sample included adult, pharmaceutically treated veterans with diabetes seen within VHA primary care clinics nationally. Specifically, veterans must have had a diabetes diagnosis (International Classification of Diseases 9th revision (ICD-9) codes 250.xx) associated with at least one VHA inpatient visit and/or at least two a primary care clinic visits (VHA stop codes 322,323,342, and 348) in fiscal year (FY) 2012 ($N = 1,049,638$) and a filled prescription for insulin and/or an oral hyperglycemic agent (VHA drug classes HS501 or HS502) the same year ($N = 830,602$). The combination of ICD-9 and medication criteria was chosen to

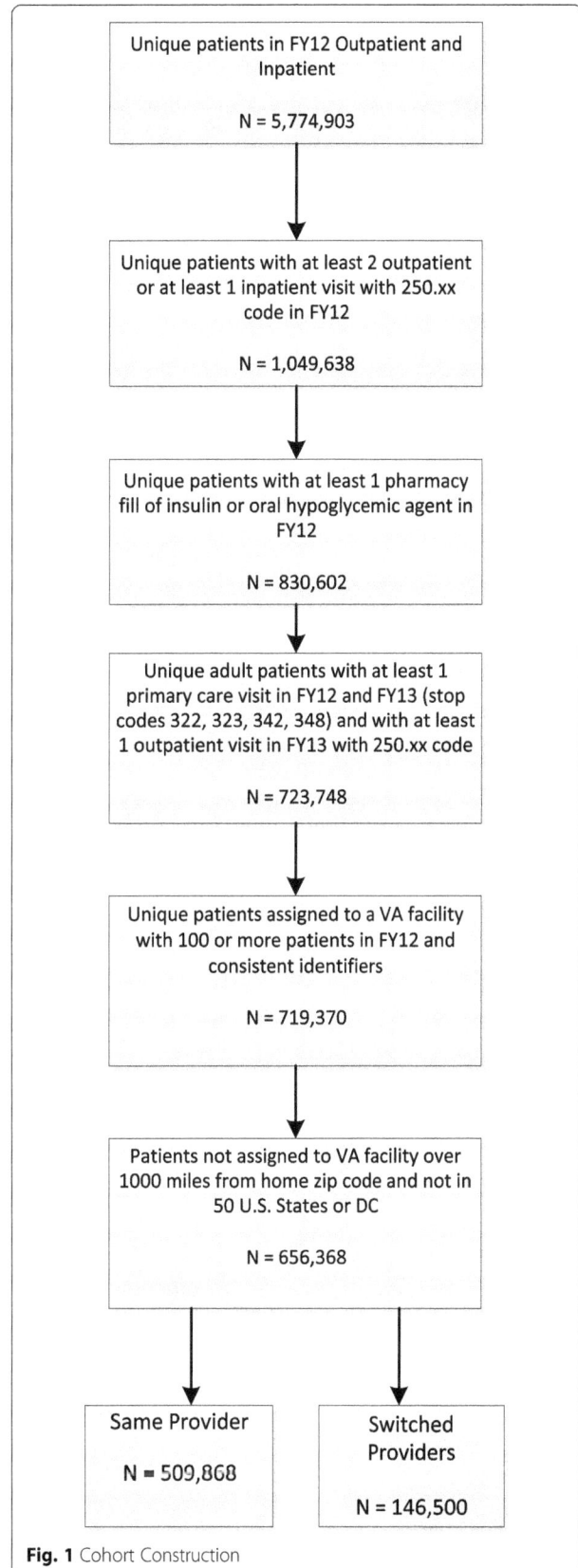

Fig. 1 Cohort Construction

maximize the likelihood that patients in the dataset have diabetes [22]. Similar algorithms in the VHA have a specificity approaching 100%. Patients were excluded if they did not also have an outpatient visit with a diabetes diagnosis in FY 2013 or were younger than 18. Each patient was assigned a "home" VHA facility as the clinic most frequently visited for primary care in FY 2012. To be retained in the cohort, patients had to have a "home" VHA facility with at least 100 diabetic patients in FY 2012 ($N = 719,370$). This was done to ensure that facilities have experience treating diabetes and provide an extra measure of patient confidentiality. The provider most often visited in the home VHA's primary care clinic in FY 2012 was considered to be the veteran's PCP. The same procedure was used to determine home clinic and PCP in FY 2013. We excluded patients whose home VHA facility was > 1000 miles from their home zip code or was not in one of the 50 U.S. states or the District of Columbia, did not have an assigned provider in FY 2012, or had missing information regarding body mass index ($N = 656,368$).

Community data used for explanatory variables was acquired from non-VHA sources. PA scope of practice (SOP) information by state was obtained from a tabulation of recommended key elements assembled by the American Academy of Physician Assistants [23]. NP SOP information was obtained from the 2012 Pearson Report [24]. Both data sources evaluate the extent to which SOP laws in a given state allow PAs or NPs to practice to the level of autonomy considered ideal by each profession's standards.

Measures

The outcome of interest was ICoC with a provider between 2012 and 2013. A binary variable was constructed to indicate whether patients switched providers between 2012 and 2013. Patients assigned to the same PCP in 2012 and 2013 were considered to have maintained ICoC. Patients assigned to different PCPs in 2012 and 2013 were considered to have interpersonal discontinuity.

Explanatory variables included patient, provider, organizational and community factors previously demonstrated to be related to ICoC and determined a priori. Patient level demographic factors included age, sex, race, ethnicity, marital status, distance of home address from assigned VHA primary care clinic, and change in home ZIP code between the two years. Patient-level variables suggesting social complexity included homelessness, whether or not the patient was exempt from VHA copayments on the basis of disability or low income, and presence of mental health diagnoses (separate variables for post-traumatic stress disorder (PTSD), mood disorders, substance abuse, and other mental health conditions), and diagnosis of dementia. Patient medical complexity was measured by the Diagnostic Cost Group (DCG) comorbidity measure, originally designed to predict cost of care but validated to measure

medical complexity within the VHA population [25, 26]. The algorithm uses demographic and diagnostic information to assign each patient a DCG score, normed so that the average Medicare patient (patients in the U.S. that are 65 years or older, are disabled, or have end stage renal disease) has a score equal to 1 [27]. All patient-level variables were constructed using VHA electronic health record data from FY 2012. Specific categories for each variable can be seen in Table 1.

Two provider-level variables were measured and assigned to each patient based on their assigned provider in 2012. Primary care provider type was represented by a categorical variable (staff physician, resident, NP, PA). A variable indicating provider turnover was also created. Since VHA providers can commonly take up to 3 months off work for health or professional issues, provider turn-over was considered to have occurred if a provider did not provide any visits within the clinic in a consecutive 4 month period. Primary care provider assignment to a clinic in FY 2012 was compared to visits performed at the same assigned station in FY 2013. If there was a 4 month or longer period in which a provider did not perform a single primary care visit at the station in FY 2013 then the provider was flagged as having left the clinic. If a PCP performed no visits in the final 4 months of year, they were also considered to have left the clinic (turn-over = 1).

Organizational level variables were assessed for each facility. The value for each facility variable was calculated based on the patient clinic assignment in 2012. Region of the country was categorized as West, Midwest, Northeast, South and rurality was indicated by rural urban commuting area (RUCA) of the facility location (metropolitan area core, micropolitan, other metropolitan area, small town or rural). If a facility had 500 or more clinic stops (visits) for 305 or 306 (VHA codes for an endocrinology visit) in FY 2012 then the facility was defined as having endocrinology referral capacity, designated with an indicator variable.

State level variables were identified based on the state in which the facility is located. State variables include the percent of primary care physicians who work with NPs or PAs within the state (lowest, middle and highest tertile), NP and PA SOP regulations (least restrictive, moderately restrictive, and most restrictive). The value for each state variable was based on the state of the patient's home clinic assignment in 2012.

Analysis

All analyses were conducted using SAS® 9.4 [28] and SAS Enterprise Guide 7.1 [29]. Descriptive statistics were calculated for all variables at the patient-level. The association between experiencing ICoC with a PCP and patient, provider, facility, and state contextual variables was evaluated using logistic regression fit with generalized

Table 1 Characteristics of VA Patients with Diabetes by Continuity of Care in Primary Care Provider[a] Type Assigned

Category	Switched Providers n = 146,500	Same Provider n = 509,868	Total n = 656,368
Patient-level factors			
Male	140,638 (96.0)	492,869 (96.7)	633,507 (96.5)
Female	5862 (4.0)	16,999 (3.3)	22,861 (3.5)
Age Group			
Less Than 40	2052 (1.40)	4862 (0.95)	6914 (1.05)
40 to Less Than 65	80,264 (54.8)	261,109 (51.2)	341,373 (52.0)
65 to Less Than 80	52,682 (36.0)	196,840 (38.6)	249,522 (38.0)
80 and Over	11,502 (7.85)	47,057 (9.23)	58,559 (8.92)
Race			
White	103,597 (70.7)	363,036 (71.2)	466,633 (71.1)
American Indian	1289 (0.88)	3678 (0.72)	4967 (0.76)
Asian	918 (0.63)	2832 (0.56)	3750 (0.57)
Black	26,975 (18.4)	91,991 (18.0)	118,966 (18.1)
Native Hawaiian	1599 (1.09)	5596 (1.10)	7195 (1.10)
Unknown or Missing	12,122 (8.27)	42,735 (8.38)	54,857 (8.36)
Hispanic	8561 (5.84)	24,157 (4.74)	32,718 (4.98)
Marital Status			
Currently Married	84,329 (57.6)	308,274 (60.5)	392,603 (59.8)
Never Married	17,016 (11.6)	54,421 (10.7)	71,437 (10.9)
Previously Married	44,772 (30.6)	145,689 (28.6)	190,461 (29.0)
Unknown Marital Status	383 (0.26)	1484 (0.29)	1867 (0.28)
Homeless at Any Time During Year	4549 (3.11)	8711 (1.71)	13,260 (2.02)
Copay Status			
No Copay Due to Disability	81,123 (55.4)	278,359 (54.6)	359,482 (54.8)
No Copay Due to Low Income	40,864 (27.9)	133,272 (26.1)	174,136 (26.5)
Must Pay Copay	22,502 (15.4)	91,157 (17.9)	113,659 (17.3)
Copay Status Unknown	2011 (1.37)	7080 (1.39)	9091 (1.39)
Mental Health Diagnoses			
Mood Disorder	39,135 (26.7)	121,321 (23.8)	160,456 (24.4)
Post-Traumatic Stress Disorder	22,683 (15.5)	72,896 (14.3)	95,579 (14.6)
Dementia	4957 (3.38)	15,236 (2.99)	20,193 (3.08)
Substance Abuse	13,689 (9.34)	38,160 (7.48)	51,849 (7.90)
Other Mental Health Diagnosis	8782 (5.99)	30,004 (5.88)	38,786 (5.91)
Diagnostic Cost Group (DCG) Score Category			
Less Than or Equal to 0.5	69,654 (47.5)	260,010 (51.0)	329,664 (50.2)
Greater Than 0.5 to 1	25,123 (17.1)	86,700 (17.0)	111,823 (17.0)
Greater Than 1 to 1.5	19,313 (13.2)	64,932 (12.7)	84,245 (12.8)
Greater Than 1.5 to 2	11,228 (7.66)	35,519 (6.97)	46,747 (7.12)
Greater Than 2	21,182 (14.5)	62,707 (12.3)	83,889 (12.8)
Distance from VHA Primary Care Clinic			
Less Than 5 Miles	31,941 (21.8)	119,774 (23.5)	151,715 (23.1)
5 to Less Than 25 Miles	71,412 (48.7)	265,553 (52.1)	336,965 (51.3)
25 to Less Than 50 Miles	24,976 (17.0)	83,394 (16.4)	108,370 (16.5)
50 Miles and Over	17,018 (11.6)	37,448 (7.34)	54,466 (8.30)

Table 1 Characteristics of VA Patients with Diabetes by Continuity of Care in Primary Care Provider[a] Type Assigned *(Continued)*

Category	Switched Providers n = 146,500	Same Provider n = 509,868	Total n = 656,368
Missing	1153 (0.79)	3699 (0.73)	4852 (0.74)
Baseline BMI			
Less Than 18.5	363 (0.25)	1152 (0.23)	1515 (0.23)
18.5 to Less Than 25	13,566 (9.26)	47,100 (9.24)	60,666 (9.24)
25 to Less Than 30	42,293 (28.9)	149,814 (29.4)	192,107 (29.3)
30 to Less Than 35	46,015 (31.4)	160,415 (31.5)	206,430 (31.5)
35 and Above	44,263 (30.2)	151,387 (29.7)	195,650 (29.8)
Number of PC Visits			
1 PC Visit	39,830 (27.2)	103,854 (20.4)	143,684 (21.9)
2 PC Visits	38,382 (26.2)	192,864 (37.8)	231,246 (35.2)
3 PC Visits	32,305 (22.1)	104,846 (20.6)	137,151 (20.9)
4 or More PC Visits	35,983 (24.6)	108,304 (21.2)	144,287 (22.0)
Pharmacy Fill of Insulin	65,784 (44.9)	216,765 (42.5)	282,549 (43.0)
Patient Had Same Zip Code in FY12 and FY13	127,158 (86.8)	478,420 (93.8)	605,578 (92.3)
Provider-level factors			
Assigned Provider Type in FY12			
Physician	104,395 (71.3)	394,959 (77.5)	499,354 (76.1)
Nurse Practitioner	25,616 (17.5)	79,588 (15.6)	105,204 (16.0)
Physician Assistant	10,185 (6.95)	30,798 (6.04)	40,983 (6.24)
Physician Resident	6304 (4.30)	4523 (0.89)	10,827 (1.65)
Assigned Provider Type in FY13			
Physician	87,706 (59.9)	395,286 (77.5)	482,992 (73.6)
Nurse Practitioner	20,564 (14.0)	79,464 (15.6)	100,028 (15.2)
Physician Assistant	7178 (4.90)	30,716 (6.02)	37,894 (5.77)
Physician Resident	5051 (3.45)	4402 (0.86)	9453 (1.44)
Unable to Assign	26,001 (17.7)		26,001 (3.96)
Provider Turnover from Station	24,512 (16.7)	8746 (1.72)	33,258 (5.07)
Facility-level factors			
Endocrinology Referral Capacity[b]	70,437 (48.1)	238,805 (46.8)	309,242 (47.1)
Rural Urban Commuting Area Status			
Metropolitan Area Core	106,700 (72.8)	377,339 (74.0)	484,039 (73.7)
Metropolitan Area Core - Remaining Levels	16,423 (11.2)	62,616 (12.3)	79,039 (12.0)
Micropolitan Area Core	18,003 (12.3)	53,501 (10.5)	71,504 (10.9)
Small Town or Rural	5374 (3.67)	16,412 (3.22)	21,786 (3.32)
State-level factors			
Percent of Primary Care Physicians Who Work With NPs/PAs			
Lowest Tertile	78,653 (53.7)	284,992 (55.9)	363,645 (55.4)
Middle Tertile	38,373 (26.2)	133,094 (26.1)	171,467 (26.1)
Highest Tertile	29,474 (20.1)	91,782 (18.0)	121,256 (18.5)
Nurse Practitioner Scope of Practice Regulations			
Least Restrictive	23,738 (16.2)	69,747 (13.7)	93,485 (14.2)
Moderately Restrictive	22,697 (15.5)	79,056 (15.5)	101,753 (15.5)
Most Restrictive	100,065 (68.3)	361,065 (70.8)	461,130 (70.3)

Table 1 Characteristics of VA Patients with Diabetes by Continuity of Care in Primary Care Provider[a] Type Assigned *(Continued)*

Category	Switched Providers n = 146,500	Same Provider n = 509,868	Total n = 656,368
Physician Assistant Scope of Practice Regulations			
Least Restrictive	20,774 (14.2)	69,521 (13.6)	90,295 (13.8)
Moderately Restrictive	36,532 (24.9)	113,202 (22.2)	149,734 (22.8)
Most Restrictive	89,194 (60.9)	327,145 (64.2)	416,339 (63.4)
VISN-LEVEL factors			
Region			
Northeast	16,522 (11.3)	75,920 (14.9)	92,442 (14.1)
West	32,865 (22.4)	91,014 (17.9)	123,879 (18.9)
Midwest	31,983 (21.8)	116,774 (22.9)	148,757 (22.7)
South	65,130 (44.5)	226,160 (44.4)	291,290 (44.4)

Data for patient-level variables are from the Veterans Administration electronic health record files. Other data sources are described in the Methods section
[a]Primary care provider (PCP) is assigned as the physician, NP, or PA seen most during FY 2012 and 2013
[b]Endocrinology referral capacity is defined as either present (endocrinology or other diabetes mellitus specialty clinics provided 500 or more visits to cohort patients in FY12) or absent (fewer than 500 visits to cohort patients)

estimating equations and an exchangeable correlation structure to account for clustering within facilities. Covariates were specified a priori and assessed for multicollinearity prior to being entered into the model. All analyses set statistical significance at $p < 0.05$.

IRB approval
This work was reviewed and approved by the Internal Review Board (IRB) of the Durham Veterans Affairs Health Care System. Reflecting that this is a secondary data study, the IRB approved a waiver of informed consent for this study.

Results
Patient characteristics
Approximately 18% (N = 1,049,638) of VHA patients had pharmaceutically treated diabetes mellitus (Fig. 1). Among the patients with diabetes that could be assigned to a PCP (N = 656,368) in 2012, 76% were assigned to an attending physician, 16% were assigned to an NP, 6.2% were assigned to a PA, and 1.7% were assigned to a resident physician. Approximately 22.3% of VHA patients with diabetes switched providers between 2012 and 2013. Switching providers occurred in 20.9% of patients assigned to physicians, 24.9% of patients assigned to PAs, 24.3% of patients assigned to NPs, and 58.2% of patients assigned to resident physicians.

Characteristics of the study population were similar to the general VHA population (Table 1). Patients with diabetes were predominantly older (mean age = 64.9 [standard deviation (SD) = 10.1]; less than 2% were under 40 years old), and were predominantly non-Hispanic (95%), white (71%), and male (97%). The study population was medically complex with approximately 20% of patients having at least 50% higher utilization (being at least 50% more complex) than the average Medicare

patient (i.e., the oldest and sickest patients in the U. S.) based on the DCG score and high rates of mental health disorders (mood disorders 24%, post-traumatic stress disorder 15%). Social complexity is also prevalent, with 55% of the sample having no copay due to disability, 27% having no copay due to income, and 2% experiencing homelessness during fiscal year 2012.

Facility and contextual characteristics
Primary care was delivered to the study sample in 831 facilities in all regions of the United States (22% in the West, 25% in the Midwest, 19% in the Northeast, and 34% in the South), with 53% located in metropolitan areas (Table 1). The mean number of providers with diabetes patients in the cohort per facility was 12.9 (SD = 20.2). The facilities had a range of staffing mixes, with the average percent of attending physicians, NPs, PAs, and residents at 74, 15, 6, and 1.4% respectively. Approximately 46% of the primary care facilities had provider turn-over between FY 2012 and FY 2013. Facilities were located in states with a range of SOP settings for NPs and PAs. Approximately 27% of facilities were in states with the most restrictive NP SOP regulation and 64% of facilities were in states with the most restrictive PA SOP regulation.

Factors associated with interpersonal continuity with a primary care provider
After adjustment for all other factors in the model, patient, provider, facility and contextual factors were associated with interpersonal continuity (Table 2). Demographic factors associated with increased odds of ICoC include male gender (OR = 1.14 CI 1.05–1.23), increasing age (age 40 to < 65 OR = 1.23 CI 1.16–1.30; age 65 to < 80 OR = 1.30 CI 1.23–1.38; age > 80 OR = 1.35 CI 1.27–1.44; reference age < 40), and living in the same zip code throughout

Table 2 Odds Ratios and 95% CI for Predicting Continuity of Care

Effect and Level	Odds Ratio	95% CI	P-Value
Patient-level factors			
Male	1.14	(1.05,1.23)	0.002
Age Group			
Less Than 40	Reference	Reference	
40 to Less Than 65	1.23	(1.16,1.30)	<.001
65 to Less Than 80	1.30	(1.23,1.38)	<.001
0 and Up	1.35	(1.27,1.44)	<.001
Race			
White	Reference	Reference	
American Indian	0.98	(0.91,1.05)	0.549
Asian	0.95	(0.88,1.04)	0.266
Black	1.02	(0.99,1.04)	0.124
Native Hawaiian	1.00	(0.95,1.06)	0.956
Unknown or Missing	1.02	(0.99,1.04)	0.188
Hispanic	0.96	(0.93,0.99)	0.011
Marital Status			
Currently Married	Reference	Reference	
Never Married	0.98	(0.96,1.00)	0.038
Previously Married	0.97	(0.96,0.98)	<.001
Unknown Marital Status	0.98	(0.90,1.08)	0.687
Homeless at Any Time During Year	0.79	(0.75,0.83)	<.001
Copay Status			
Must Pay Copay	Reference	Reference	
No Copay Due to Disability	0.98	(0.96,0.99)	0.010
No Copay Due to Low Income	0.95	(0.94,0.97)	<.001
Copay Status Unknown	0.93	(0.88,0.99)	0.013
Mental Health Diagnoses			
Mood Disorder	0.97	(0.95,0.98)	<.001
Substance Abuse	0.94	(0.92,0.96)	<.001
PTSD	0.99	(0.97,1.01)	0.399
Dementia	0.94	(0.90,0.97)	<.001
Other Mental Health Diagnosis	0.99	(0.96,1.02)	0.650
Diagnostic Cost Group (DCG) Score Category			
Less Than or Equal to 0.5	Reference	Reference	
Greater Than 0.5 to 1	0.95	(0.93,0.97)	<.001
Greater Than 1 to 1.5	0.93	(0.91,0.95)	<.001
Greater Than 1.5 to 2	0.91	(0.89,0.94)	<.001
Greater Than 2	0.89	(0.86,0.91)	<.001
Distance From VHA Primary Care Clinic			
Less Than 5 Miles	Reference	Reference	
5 to Less Than 25 Miles	0.97	(0.95,0.99)	0.001
25 to Less Than 50 Miles	0.85	(0.83,0.88)	<.001
50 Miles or Greater	0.62	(0.59,0.65)	<.001
Missing	1.15	(1.01,1.30)	0.034
Baseline BMI			
Less Than 18.5	Reference	Reference	

Table 2 Odds Ratios and 95% CI for Predicting Continuity of Care *(Continued)*

Effect and Level	Odds Ratio	95% CI	P-Value
18.5 to Less Than 25	0.97	(0.86,1.09)	0.611
25 to Less Than 30	0.98	(0.87,1.10)	0.723
30 to Less Than 35	0.97	(0.86,1.09)	0.600
Greater Than or Equal to 35	0.97	(0.86,1.09)	0.599
Number of PC Visits in FY12			
1 Visit	Reference	Reference	
2 Visits	1.78	(1.72,1.85)	<.001
3 Visits	1.25	(1.21,1.30)	<.001
4 or More Visits	1.23	(1.18,1.29)	<.001
Patient Had Same Zip Code	2.20	(2.12,2.28)	<.001
Provider-level factors			
Assigned Provider Type in FY12[a]			
Physician	Reference	Reference	
Nurse Practitioner	0.87	(0.78,0.97)	0.011
Physician Assistant	0.86	(0.73,1.02)	0.081
Physician Resident	0.18	(0.15,0.21)	<.001
Provider Turnover	0.09	(0.07,0.11)	<.001
Facility-level factors			
Presence of Endocrinology at Facility[b]	1.06	(0.89,1.25)	0.514
Rural Urban Commuting Area Status			
Metropolitan Area Core	Reference	Reference	
Other Metropolitan Area	1.07	(0.89,1.28)	0.467
Micropolitan	0.98	(0.82,1.16)	0.778
Small Town or Rural	0.81	(0.59,1.11)	0.193
State-level factors			
Percent of Primary Care Physicians Who Work With NPs/PA			
Lowest Tertile	Reference	Reference	
Middle Tertile	0.88	(0.72,1.07)	0.204
Highest Tertile	0.95	(0.74,1.22)	0.684
Nurse Practitioner Scope of Practice Regulations			
Least Restrictive	Reference	Reference	
Moderately Restrictive	0.92	(0.71,1.20)	0.545
Most Restrictive	0.79	(0.64,0.97)	0.027
Physician Assistant Scope of Practice Regulations			
Least Restrictive	Reference	Reference	
Moderately Restrictive	1.06	(0.83,1.36)	0.629
Most Restrictive	1.17	(0.93,1.46)	0.183
Visn-level factors			
Region			
Northeast	Reference	Reference	
West	0.85	(0.69,1.03)	0.100
Midwest	1.34	(1.06,1.70)	0.016
South	0.87	(0.73,1.04)	0.127

Data for patient-level variables are from the Veterans Administration electronic health record files. Other data sources are described in the Methods section
[a]Primary care provider (PCP) is assigned as the physician, NP, or PA seen most during FY 2012 and 2013
[b]Endocrinology referral capacity is defined as either present (endocrinology or other diabetes mellitus specialty clinics provided 500 or more visits to cohort patients in FY12) or absent (fewer than 500 visits to cohort patients)

both years ($OR = 2.20$ CI 2.12–2.28; reference changing zip codes) Demographic factors associated with slightly decreased odds of ICoC include copay status (no copay due to disability $OR = 0.98$ $CI = 0.96$–0.99; no copay due to low income $OR = 0.95$ CI 0.94–0.97; copay status unknown $OR = 0.93$ $CI = 0.88$–0.99; reference must pay copay), Hispanic ethnicity ($OR = 0.96$ $CI = 0.93$–0.99), marital status (never married $OR = 0.98$ $CI = 0.96$–1.00; previously married $OR = 0.97$ $CI = 0.96$–0.98; reference currently married) and distance from VHA primary care clinic (5 to < 25 miles $OR = 0.97$ CI 0.95–0.99; 25 to < 50 miles $OR = 0.85$ $CI = 0.83$–0.88; > 50 miles $OR = 0.62$ $CI = 0.59$–0.65; reference < 5 miles).

Patients with worse overall health status had modestly lower odds of ICoC from year to year. Higher DCG score categories in FY 2012 (i.e., complex patients with greater healthcare utilization) had lower odds of continuity (DCG 0.5–1.0 $OR = 0.95$ $CI = 0.93$–0.97; 1.0–1.5 $OR = 0.93$ $CI = 0.91$–0.95; 1.5–2.0 $OR = 0.91$ $CI = 0.89$–0.94; > 2.0 $OR = 0.89$ $CI = 0.86$–0.91; reference < 0.5). This is also seen for patients with a mental health diagnosis (mood disorder $OR = 0.97$ CI 0.95–0.98; substance abuse $OR = 0.94$ $CI = 0.92$–0.96; dementia $OR = 0.94$ $CI = 0.90$–0.97). Finally, a greater number of primary care visits in FY 2012 was associated with increased odds of ICoC (2 visits $OR = 1.78$ $CI = 1.72$–1.85; 3 visits $OR = 1.25$ $CI = 1.21$–1.30; 4+ visits $OR = 1.23$ $CI = 1.18$–1.29; reference = 1 visit).

Both provider variables were associated with decreased odds of ICoC. Patients who had a provider that left the clinic had a highly significant and large decrease in odds of ICoC ($OR = 0.09$, CI-0.07-0.11) when compared to patients assigned to providers that stayed in the clinic. Compared to patients assigned to an attending physician, patients with NPs ($OR = 0.87$ $CI = 0.78$–0.97) and resident physicians ($OR = 0.18$ $CI = 0.15$–0.21) as usual providers had decreased odds of ICoC.

Facility and contextual variables were also associated with ICoC. Compared to patients receiving primary care services in the Northeast, patients in the Midwest had increased odds of ICoC ($OR = 1.34$ $CI = 1.06$–1.70). Compared to patients that received primary care services at VHA clinics in states with the least restrictive NP SOP regulations, patients that received care in states with the most restrictive NP regulations had decreased odds of ICoC ($OR = 0.79$ $CI = 0.69$–0.97).

Discussion

Approximately 22% of VHA patients with diabetes experienced disruption in ICoC between 2012 and 2013, which is less than the one-third of Medicare patients in the US previously reported to change primary care providers from year to year [7]. Findings suggest that, when assessed simultaneously across the VHA, patient, provider, and contextual factors are associated with ICoC

for patients with diabetes. Patients with social and access challenges are less likely to experience ICoC. Similarly, region of the country and NP scope of practice regulation also impacted the likelihood of experiencing ICoC. However, the biggest impact appears to be associated with a provider-level variable: provider turn-over.

Even after adjustment for provider and contextual factors, patients with diabetes with medical complexity, social and access challenges were less likely to experience ICoC. Consistent with existing literature, patients with diabetes with sociodemographic factors including Hispanic ethnicity, female gender, marital status, low income, and living a greater distance from the clinic were less likely to experience ICoC [11, 12, 30]. Similarly, patients with greater medical complexity and mental health issues were less likely to experience ICoC. However, effect sizes for the aforementioned variables were small; the patient factors with the largest effect were patient living in the same zip code, age and primary care utilization. Older age groups and those with more primary care visits were more likely to experience ICoC. Since this effect was seen after controlling for patient complexity, this finding is less likely due to the medical needs of the patients and more likely due to patient preference [9, 10].

Contextual factors that impacted patient ICoC include region of the country and NP SOP regulations. Patients receiving care in the Midwestern US were more likely than those receiving care in the Northeast to experience ICoC. Several potential explanations exist. It could relate to regional differences in healthcare utilization patterns [31]. However, it is also likely that VHA expansion can explain at least some of the effect. For example, the VHA had 152,000 more patients in 2013 than 2012 [19]. Similarly, patients that lived in states with the most restrictive NP scope of practice regulations were less likely to experience ICoC. While the mechanism is unknown, this may be due to greater interdependence between NPs and physicians, resulting in more patient-sharing which appears like provider switching using our methodology.

Provider type and provider turn-over also appeared to impact ICoC for patients with diabetes. Compared to patients with attending physicians as usual providers, patients with physician residents and NPs were less likely to experience ICoC. The magnitude of effect was greatest with residents. Given the nature of physician training, in which trainees frequently rotate through other learning experiences, it is not unexpected that patients that receive the majority of their care from a resident physician would experience interpersonal discontinuity. However, the proportion of patients that receive care from resident physicians is small (1.7%). Patients with NPs as PCPs had only slightly lower odds of experiencing ICoC than those with physicians. This could be due to a variety of factors. It could be that patients with diabetes are dissatisfied with the care received from NPs and elect to switch providers. This explanation seems unlikely, given that existing literature suggests that satisfaction with and quality of care delivered by primary care NPs is as good as or better than satisfaction with physicians [32–35]. Alternatively, it could be due to policy changes regarding primary care NP roles within the VHA or to patient reassignent [18, 36–38]. The impact of provider turn-over appeared to have a far greater impact on continuity of care than provider type. Provider turn-over within the VHA has been high and increased after PACT implementation [37, 39]. Our data suggest that approximately 46% of primary care clinics had provider turn-over between 2012 and 2013, suggesting that turn-over has the potential to directly or indirectly impact a significant portion of VHA patients with diabetes.

This study has notable strengths and limitations. Unlike previous studies, our study has simultaneously evaluated patient, provider and contextual factors that can influence ICoC. This approach allows for a better understanding of the contribution of each factor to continuity. Unlike many commonly used data sources, our data also allows for accurate attribution of the performing provider of care for each patient with diabetes [40].

Several limitations must also be recognized. There is potential for misclassification of assignment to usual provider. Our methodology utilized only face-to-face visits with patients. Since PACT implementation, there has been a significant increase in the number of electronic encounters with patients such as phone and electronic communications, and could potentially disproportionately impact those patients living further away from their VHA facility [21]. However, many of these excluded encounters are provided by nurses other than NPs and other professionals that are not acting in usual provider roles [21]. Similarly, it is possible that patients could have had a minority of their primary care visits in 2013 with their PCP from 2012 even if they were assigned to a new PCP in 2013. However, including these patients in the "discontinuity" category would bias the findings toward the null; making any estimates provided conservative estimates of effect. Finally, despite the fact that our models included a large variety of variables that have been shown to predict ICoC, there is the potential for unmeasured confounding. For example, patient preferences were not addressed and may have provided some additional clarification [41].

Conclusion

ICoC of care is an important mechanism for the delivery of high quality primary care to patients with chronic illness such as diabetes. This paper contributes critical knowledge, by identifying patient, provider, and contextual factors that impact ICoC. Identification of factors associated with ICoC can assist with the development of interventions to improve chronic illness care. We found that patients with diabetes who are younger, with medical complexity, social and access challenges, are less likely to experience ICoC. This suggests that interventions to improve continuity may need to target these patients. Additionally, provider and contextual factors, especially provider turn-over, are reducing ICoC. These factors are likely sensitive to organizational policies, suggesting that VHA and other healthcare system administrators may wish to re-evaluate policies that impact NP roles and provider turn-over.

Abbreviations

CI: Confidence interval; CoC: Continuity of Care; DCG: Diagnostic cost group; FY: Fiscal year; ICD-9: International Classification of Diseases 9th revision; ICoC: Interpersonal continuity of care; NP: Nurse practitioner; OR: Odds ratio; PA: Physician assistant; PACT: Patient-Aligned Care Team; PCP: Primary care provider; PTSD: Post-traumatic stress disorder; RUCA: Rural urban commuting area; SOP: Scope of practice; VHA: Veteran's Health Administration

Funding

This research was supported by a grant from Department of Veterans Affairs (VA), Health Services Research and Development Service IIR 13–063.This work was also supported by the Center of Innovation for Health Services Research in Primary Care (CIN 13–410) at the Durham VA Health Care System. The grant funding source had no role in the design, conduct, collection, management, analysis, or interpretation of the data; or in the preparation, review, or approval of the manuscript.

Disclaimer

The views expressed in this article are those of the authors and do not reflect the position or policy of the Department of Veterans Affairs, United States government, or Duke University.

Authors' contributions

CE contributed to research design and was the primary author of the manuscript. PM collaborated on research design, interpretation of findings, and manuscript writing. VS collaborated on research design, oversaw dataset construction and analysis and contributed to writing the manuscript. SW and TB constructed the dataset, created variables, and performed analysis as well as contributed to manuscript writing. DE and CH collaborated on research design, interpretation of findings, and manuscript writing. BW contributed to project management and manuscript writing. GLJ was principle investigator of the project and contributed to research design, dataset construction, analysis, interpretation of findings, and manuscript writing. All authors read and approved the final manuscript.

Competing interests

The authors have no disclosures to report. With the exception of Drs. Everett and Morgan, all authors are employees of the Department of Veterans Affairs (VA). No VA author received compensation for preparation of this manuscript apart from his or her employment. Dr. Everett is a paid methodologic consultant on the research grant, and Dr. Morgan is supported through an interagency personnel agreement between the Durham Veterans Affairs Health Care System and Duke University.

Author details
[1]Duke University School of Medicine, Physician Assistant Program|, 800 South Duke Street, Durham, NC 27701, USA. [2]Center for Health Services Research in Primary Care, Durham Veterans Affairs Medical Center, Durham, NC, USA. [3]Department of Population Health Sciences, Duke University School of Medicine, Durham, NC, USA. [4]Division of General Internal Medicine, Duke University School of Medicine, Durham, NC, USA. [5]Clinical Health Systems & Analytics Division, Duke University School of Nursing, Durham, NC, USA.

References
1.   Starfield B. Primary care: balancing healthy needs, services, and technology. New York City: Oxford University Press; 1998.
2.   Institute of Medicine. Primary Care: America's Health in a New Era. Washington, DC: The National Academies Press; 1996. https://doi.org/10.17226/5152.
3.   Saultz JW. Defining and measuring interpersonal continuity of care. The Annals of Family Medicine. 2003;1:134–43.
4.   Saultz JW, Lochner J. Interpersonal continuity of care and care outcomes: a critical review. Ann Fam Med. 2005;3:159–66.
5.   van Servellen G, Fongwa M, Mockus D'EE. Continuity of care and quality care outcomes for people experiencing chronic conditions: a literature review. Nurs Health Sci. 2006;8:185–95.
6.   Katz DA, McCoy K, Sarrazin MV. Does improved continuity of primary care affect clinician–patient communication in VA? J Gen Intern Med. 2014;29:682–8.
7.   Pham HH, Schrag D, O'Malley AS, Wu BN, Bach PB. Care patterns in Medicare and their implications for pay for performance. N Engl J Med. 2007;356:1130–9.
8.   Rodriguez HP, Rogers WH, Marshall RE, Safran D. Multidisciplinary primary care teams: effects on the quality of clinician-patient interactions and organizational features of care. Med Care. 2007;45:19–27.
9.   Overland J, Yue DK, Mira M. Continuity of care in diabetes: to whom does it matter? Diabetes Res Clin Pract. 2001;52:55–61.
10. Nutting PA, Goodwin MA, Flocke SA, Zyzanski SJ, Stange KC. Continuity of primary care: to whom does it matter and when? Ann Fam Med. 2003;1: 149–55.
11. Stevens GD, Shi L. Racial and ethnic disparities in the primary care experiences of children: a review of the literature. Med Care Res Rev. 2003; 60:3–30.
12. Stevens GD, Seid M, Mistry R, Halfon N. Disparities in primary care for vulnerable children: the influence of multiple risk factors. Health Serv Res. 2006;41:507–31.
13. Baker R, Streatfield J. What type of general practice do patients prefer? Exploration of practice characteristics influencing patient satisfaction. Br J Gen Pract. 1995;45:654–9.
14. Parker G, Corden A, Heaton J. Experiences of and influences on continuity of care for service users and carers: synthesis of evidence from a research programme. Health & Social Care in the Community. 2011;19:576–601.
15. Alazri M, Heywood P, Neal RD, Leese B. Continuity of care: literature review and implications. Sultan Qaboos Univ Med J. 2007;7:197–206.
16. Smedby B, Smedby O, Eriksson EA, Mattsson L-G, Lindgren A. Continuity of care: an application of visit-based measures. Med Care. 1984;22:676–80.
17. Shortell SM. Continuity of medical care: conceptualization and measurement. Med Care. 1976;14:377–91.
18. Klein S. The Veterans Health Administration: Implementing Patient-Centered Medical Homes in the Nation's Largest Integrated Delivery System: The Common Wealth Fund; 2011. Report No.: 1537.
19. Selected VHA Statistics: FY 2012–2013 End of Year. In: Planning VHAOotADUSfHfPa, ed.December 19, 2013.
20. Oliver A. The veterans health administration: an American success story? Milbank Q. 2007;85:5–35.
21. Rosland AM, Nelson K, Sun H, et al. The patient-centered medical home in the veterans health administration. Am J Manag Care. 2013;19:e263–72.
22. Singh JA. Accuracy of veterans affairs databases for diagnoses of chronic diseases. Prev Chronic Dis. 2009;6:A126.
23. American Academy of Physician Assistnats. The Six Key Elements of Modern Physician Assistant Practice. AAPA Alexadria, VA March 2013.
24. Pearson LJ. The 2012 Pearson report: a National Overview of nurse practitioner legislation and health care issues. Monroe Township, N.J: NP Communications; 2012 February.
25. Ellis RP, Ash A. Refinements to the diagnostic cost group (DCG) model. Inquiry. 1995;32:418–29.
26. Maciejewski ML, Liu C-F, Derleth A, McDonell M, Anderson S, Fihn SD. The performance of administrative and self-reported measures for risk adjustment of veterans affairs expenditures. Health Serv Res. 2005;40:887–904.
27. Ash A, Porell F, Gruenberg L, Sawitz E, Beiser A. Adjusting Medicare capitation payments using prior hospitalization data. Health Care Financ Rev. 1989;10:17–29.
28. SAS 9.4. Cary, NC: SAS Institute, Inc.; 2002–2012.
29. SAS Enterprise Guide 7.1. Cary, NC: SAS Institute, Inc.; 2012.
30. Shen Y, Hendricks A, Zhang S, Kazis LE. VHA enrollees' health care coverage and use of care. Med Care Res Rev. 2003;60:253–67.
31. Ashton CM, Petersen NJ, Souchek J, et al. Geographic variations in utilization rates in veterans affairs hospitals and clinics. N Engl J Med. 1999;340:32–9.
32. Mundinger MO, Kane RL, Lenz ER, et al. Primary care outcomes in patients treated by nurse practitioners or physicians: a randomized trial. JAMA. 2000; 283:59–68.
33. Budzi D, Lurie S, Singh K, Hooker R. Veterans' perceptions of care by nurse practitioners, physician assistants, and physicians: a comparison from satisfaction surveys. J Am Acad Nurse Pract. 2010;22:170–6.
34. Jackson G, Lee S-Y, Edelman D, Weinberger M, Yano E. Employment of mid-level providers in primary care and control of diabetes. Primary Care Diabetes. 2011;5:25–31.
35. Everett CM, Morgan P, Jackson GL. Primary care physician assistant and advance practice nurses roles: patient healthcare utilization, unmet need, and satisfaction. Healthcare. 2016;4:327-333.
36. Edith Ramirez JB, Ohlhausen MK, Wright JD. In: Commission FT, editor. Policy Perspectives: Competition and the Regulation of Advanced Practice Nurses; 2014. p. 1–53.
37. Weeks WB. US department of veterans affairs primary care provider turnover and patient satisfaction. JAMA Internal Medicine. 2015;175:1870.
38. AP44 Proposed Rule - Advanced Practice Registered Nurses. Department of Veterans Affairs; 2016.
39. Sylling PW, Wong ES, Liu CF, et al. Patient-centered medical home implementation and primary care provider turnover. Med Care. 2014;52:1017–22.
40. Morgan PA, Strand J, Østbye T, Albanese MA. Missing in action: care by physician assistants and nurse practitioners in National Health Surveys. Health Serv Res. 2007;42:2022–37.
41. Dill MJ, Pankow S, Erikson C, Shipman S. Survey shows consumers open to a greater role for physician assistants and nurse practitioners. Health Aff. 2013;32:1135–42.

10

Factors contributing to the recognition of anxiety and depression in general practice

Henny Sinnema[1]* ⓘ, Berend Terluin[2], Daniëlle Volker[1], Michel Wensing[3] and Anton van Balkom[4]

Abstract

Background: Adequate recognition of anxiety and depression by general practitioners (GPs) can be improved. Research on factors that are associated with recognition is limited and shows mixed results. The aim of this study was to explore which patient and GP characteristics are associated with recognition of anxiety and depression.

Methods: We performed a secondary analysis on data from 444 patients who were recruited for a randomized trial. Recognition of anxiety and depression was defined in terms of information in the medical records, in patients who screened positive on the extended Kessler 10 (EK-10). A total of 10 patient and GP characteristics, measured at baseline, were tested and included in a multilevel regression model to examine their impact on recognition.

Results: Patients who reported a perceived need for psychological care (OR = 2.54, 95% CI 1.60–4.03) and those with higher 4DSQ distress scores (OR = 1.03; 95% CI 1.00–1.07) were more likely to be recognized. In addition, patients' anxiety or depression was less likely to be recognized when GPs were less confident in their abilities to identify depression (OR = 0.97; 95% CI 0.95–0.99). Patients' age, chronic medical condition, somatisation, severity of anxiety and depression, and functional status were not associated with the recognition of anxiety and depression.

Conclusions: There is room for improvement of the recognition of anxiety and depression. Quality improvement activities that focus on increasing GPs' confidence in the ability to identify symptoms of distress, anxiety and depression, as part of care according to guidelines, may improve recognition.

Keywords: Anxiety, Depression, Recognition, Primary care, General practitioner

Background

Anxiety and depression are highly prevalent, negatively impact everyday functioning, cause great suffering, and incur high healthcare costs and costs associated with reduced productivity [1–3]. Although clinical guidelines are available [4, 5], the management of these disorders in general practice is often suboptimal. Under-recognition of anxiety and depression has been reported, although more severe symptoms may be more easily recognized [6, 7]. Adequate recognition, diagnosis and treatment of anxiety and depression may decrease the burden of disease [8]. With approximately 75% of adult patients visiting their general practitioner (GP) at least once a year in the Netherlands, the GP is in a good position to detect anxiety and depression [9]. In the Netherlands more than 75% of patients diagnosed with psychological problems are treated in general practice [10]. Studies showed a wide range of recognition rates of depression and anxiety in primary care, also depending on the method of case ascertainment and the time allowed for GPs to recognize [11–13]. Recognition rates were higher when patient medical record extraction was used over an extended period compared to cross-sectional methods. In addition, when a less specific definition of recognition was used, recognition rates were higher. However, this may also result in more false positives [14].

Characteristics of both GPs and patients influence recognition of anxiety and depression. Many patients do not acknowledge that they suffer from anxiety or depression, and may present themselves in general practice with somatic symptoms [15–18]. Both patients and GPs may prioritise physical problems if they coexist with a (hidden) depression [19]. Even when a psychiatric diagnosis is made the patient or GP may not perceive a need

* Correspondence: hsinnema@trimbos.nl
[1]Netherlands Institute of Mental Health and Addiction, Trimbos Institute, Postbox 725, 3500, AS, Utrecht, The Netherlands
Full list of author information is available at the end of the article

for treatment [20]. Furthermore, some GPs find it difficult to distinguish between 'normal' distress and depression requiring treatment [21]. In the presence of chronic physical health problems GPs and patients tend to normalise distress [22]. In addition, there are barriers related to the access of care (e.g. stigma, lack of information about mental health and available services) [23].

Adequate recognition, and subsequent treatment, could improve outcomes for patients. Previous studies have examined different patient and GP characteristics as possible factors associated with the recognition of depression and anxiety, showing mixed results. Factors associated with recognition include female gender, advanced age, being single, severe depression, comorbid anxiety or depression, chronic somatic co-morbidity, history of depression, having disclosed mental health problems to the GP, and positive attitudes toward help seeking [7, 14, 24–29]. A few studies also examined whether primary care physician characteristics, such as years of experience, education, special interest, knowledge and skills, were associated with recognition of depression [7, 24] and anxiety [14]. Wittchen et al. (2001) found that physicians with more than 5 years of practice experience were more likely to recognize patients with a depression. Janssen et al. (2012) and Piek et al. (2012) concluded that there were no GP characteristics associated with recognition [7, 14]. Furthermore, GPs' attitudes likely constitute an important factor affecting the recognition of anxiety and depression [30–32].

Previous studies showed mixed results regarding factors associated with recognition and other factors are rarely studied. The factors include: (i) patient characteristics: age, married or living together, chronic medical condition, the perceived need for care, psychological symptoms and functional status, and (ii) GP characteristics: attitudes toward the management of anxiety and depression. The aim of the current study was to examine whether these factors are associated with the recognition of anxiety and depression in general practice.

Methods
Study design
This study is a secondary analysis of data from a cluster randomized controlled trial of tailored interventions, to improve the management of anxiety and depression in primary care (NTR1912) [33]. The aim of the trial was to determine the clinical and cost effectiveness of tailored interventions to improve compliance with guidelines for the recognition of anxiety and depression in general practice [34–37]. The trial compared training and feedback for GPs with training and feedback supplemented with a tailored intervention. Results showed that the tailored intervention resulted in increased recognition of anxiety and depression (42% versus 31%; OR =

1.60; 95% CI:1.01–2.53) [38].The identification of barriers to implementation of guidelines, the development of interventions targeting these barriers, and the application and perceived usefulness of the resulting tailored interventions have been described elsewhere [39]. The sample size was based on the primary trial objectives. The trial was approved by the medical ethics committee of the Institutions for Mental Health (METiGG; Utrecht, the Netherlands) in 2009.

Study population
The study population included 46 GPs in 23 general practices (12 practices were randomised to the intervention condition and 11 practices to the control condition), and all patients aged 18 years or older visiting one of the participating GPs between September 2010 and June 2011. A total of 7410 patients received an information letter and an invitation to participate and were asked to complete the extended Kessler 10 (EK-10), a validated screening tool for anxiety and depressive disorder in primary care [40]. The screening was returned by 1687 patients (response rate 23%) and 766 of them (45%) screened positive and were contacted by telephone. Based on predefined exclusion criteria 158 (21%) patients were excluded. Exclusion criteria were suicidal ideation and behavior, dementia or other severe cognitive disorders, psychotic disorder, bipolar disorder, dependence on alcohol or drugs, severe unstable somatic condition, insufficient knowledge of the Dutch language, GP diagnosis of anxiety or depression or psychological treatment in the six months before the start of the study. Of the remaining 608 patients, 164 (27%) patients did not provide informed consent. Therefore, 444 patients screening positive for anxiety and depression were included in the present study. GPs were blind to which patients had entered the study. For further details on recruitment and selection we refer to the study protocol [33].

Measures
Outcome measure
The outcome in the present study was GPs' recognition of anxiety or depression, as evidenced by information that was available in the patients' medical records, in the time period from 6 months before to 6 months after the EK-10 screening. Information that was deemed to be indicative of recognition was the presence of terms describing: (i) psychological complaints: anxiety, depression, worrying, sorrow or grief, stress, feeling down, disordered sleeping and unexplained somatic symptoms; (ii) International Classification of Primary Care-1 (ICPC-1) diagnostic codes [41] for anxiety, depression and related psychological problems i.e. acute stress, feeling anger or irritation, behaving irritably or

angrily, neurasthenia, or (iii) Four-Dimensional Symptom Questionnaire (4DSQ) scores. The 4DSQ can be used to help recognize anxiety and depressive disorders. This self-report instrument can be used to distinguish between stress-related syndromes (termed 'stress', 'burnout' and 'nervous breakdown') and psychiatric disorders (i.e. anxiety and depressive disorders) [42]. Recognition was operationalised this way because diagnostic coding alone strongly underestimates the accuracy of the GP [14, 43]. The medical records were retrospectively searched by two researchers. They assessed 50 medical records independently and weighted kappa statistics were calculated. The kappa yielded an inter-rater agreement of 96% (weighted kappa = 0.91; 95% CI: 0.79–1.00).

Patient and GP related factors

The independent variables investigated included patient and GP characteristics that might be associated with the recognition of anxiety and depression. The data were collected at baseline.

Patient characteristics were age, married or living together, presence of a chronic medical condition, psychological symptoms, perceived need for psychological care and functional status. Chronic medical condition was measured with the Dutch Central Bureau of Statistics (CBS) list, a questionnaire containing 28 conditions [44]. Psychological symptoms were measured with the Four-Dimensional Symptom Questionnaire (4DSQ). The 4DSQ has four subscales relating to common psychopathology: distress, depression, anxiety and somatisation; high scores correspond to high symptom levels. Perceived need for psychological care (henceforth "need for care") was measured with two questions after the 4DSQ: "Do you receive any help for these complaints" and "Do you need help to solve these complaints", answered with yes/no. Functional status was measured using the World Health Organisation's Disability Assessment Scale II (WHODAS II) which covers functional impairments in six domains over the past thirty days. The standardised total score, based on 32 items corrected for missing values was calculated [45, 46]. The domains are communication and understanding, getting around, self-care, getting along with people, life activities and participation in society. Scores range from 0 to 100; high scores indicate functional impairment.

GP characteristics were attitudes to anxiety and depression, measured with the Depression Attitude Questionnaire (DAQ) [47, 48] and with the REASON questionnaire [49]. The DAQ measures GPs' interest in and attitudes toward depressive disorders; respondents are asked to indicate the degree to which they agree or disagree (a 7-point Likert scale in which the discrete anchor points were converted to a 0–100 scale, where 0 means strongly disagree and 100 strongly agree) with 20

statements based on their day-to-day clinical experience. The DAQ consists of 4 components: treatment attitude (high scores indicate a preference for antidepressant drugs, low scores for psychotherapy); professional unease (high scores indicate discomfort in dealing with depressed patients, perception that treating depression is unrewarding and that patients would be better off being managed by a specialist); depression malleability (high scores indicate pessimism about one's ability to modify the course of depression) and depression identification (high scores indicate difficulty in differentiating depression from unhappiness, believes that it originates from recent misfortunes, and that there is likely to be little additional benefit beyond a GP's own treatment. The REASON measures GPs' attitudes to their role in the management of patients with depressive and anxiety disorders (scores can range from 1 to 7), and comprises two subscales: (i) professional comfort with and competence in care of mental health disorders (low scores indicate comfort and competence) and (ii) GPs' concerns about problems with the health care system for management of anxiety and depression (low scores indicate concerns about difficulties).

Statistical methods

Multiple imputation was used, creating 5 complete datasets to deal with missing values. The imputation model included recognition, condition (intervention or control), patient characteristics (gender, age, born in the Netherlands, married or living together, in paid employment, level of education, 4DSQ score, WHODAS II score, chronic medical condition, need for care, living conditions), and GP characteristics (attitude towards anxiety and depression). Missing values for recognition ($n = 24$), born in the Netherlands ($n = 8$), married or living together ($n = 5$), level of education ($n = 4$), living conditions ($n = 3$), 4DSQ score (4DSQ Distress $n = 11$, 4DSQ Depression n = 11, 4DSQ Anxiety $n = 12$, 4DSQ Somatization $n = 30$), WHODAS II score ($n = 17$), need for care ($n = 34$) were imputed.

The prediction of recognition was examined using multilevel logistic regression analyses. Logistic regression was used because of the binary character of the outcome variable (recognition yes/no). Multilevel analysis was used to account for the clustered design (i.e., patients were clustered within GPs and GPs were clustered within practices), which threatens the mutual independence of the observations [50]. Not taking into account the clustered nature of the data, results in under-estimation of standard errors and over-estimation of statistical significance. The analyses were performed using the Generalized Linear Mixed Models method as implemented in the Statistical Package for the Social Sciences (SPSS) 22 program. All analyses were conducted in the 5 imputed datasets and results were pooled using Rubin's rules [51]. We considered 15 potential predictors of recognition, ensuring not to exceed the limit of 10% of the number of events (i.e. recognition, $n = 160$) in the sample [52]. First, potential predictors (patients and GP characteristics) were tested through trivariate analyses using recognition as dependent (outcome) variable and condition as effect modifier. The reason to take the trial intervention (condition) into account as a possible effect modifier was that the intervention might have affected the effect of certain predictors on recognition. Predictors and interaction terms with p-values < 0.20 were selected for inclusion in a multivariate logistic regression model. Then stepwise backward selection was used to remove non-significant ($p > 0.05$) predictors and interaction terms one-by one from the model, starting with predictors and interaction terms with the highest p-value. To assess the extent to which the predictors and interactions retained in the final model actually explained the variance in recognition, a receiver operating characteristic (ROC) analysis was conducted using the model-predicted probabilities as test variable and recognition as the outcome variable. The area under the ROC curve (AUC) ranges from 0.5 and 1.0 with larger values indicating more variance explained [53].

Results

Characteristics of the study population

Baseline characteristics for patients and GPs are given in Table 1. The mean age of the 444 patients was 54 years, and 69% were female. The mean age of the 46 GPs was 49 years, and 54% were men.

The association of patient and GP characteristics with recognition

GPs recognized anxiety or depression in 160 patients (36%). Recognition rates were especially higher in patients who: were younger than 55 years, had a 4DSQ Distress score of ≥11, had a perceived need for psychological care, and a WHODAS II score of ≥21 (see Additional File 1). Table 2 shows the results of the trivariate and multivariate analyses. Ten predictors and/or their interaction terms with condition had p-values < 0.20 in the trivariate analyses and were entered in a multivariate model (in Table 2 indicated by a "‡" sign after the p-value). After the backward selection procedure only 4 predictors and one interaction term remained in the final model. Patients with higher 4DSQ distress scores (OR = 1.03; 95% CI 1.00–1.07) were significantly more likely to be recognized. Note that the OR of 1.03 is related to 1 point difference in the Distress score (range 0–32). To illustrate, if a person with 10 points on the Distress scale has a probability of 30% of being recognized, a person scoring 25 points has a probability of

Table 1 Baseline characteristics of primary care participants ($n = 444^*$) and general practitioners ($n = 46$). Values are numbers (percentages) unless stated otherwise

Patient characteristics	
Mean (SD) age (years)	54.3 (15.8)
Married or living together ($n = 439$)	294 (67.0%)
Number of chronic medical conditions[a](range: 0–28), mean (SD)	3 (2.1)
4DSQ[b] Distress score (range: 0–32), mean (SD) ($n = 433$)	12.2 (7.6)
4DSQ Depression score (range: 0–12), mean (SD) (n = 433)	1.7 (2.7)
4DSQ Anxiety score (range: 0–24), mean (SD) ($n = 432$)	3.0 (3.7)
4DSQ Somatisation score (range: 0–32), mean (SD) ($n = 414$)	8.4 (5.9)
Functional status[c]($n = 427$)	23.9 (15.7)
Need for care ($n = 410$)	201 (49%)
General Practitioner characteristics	
DAQ[d] mean score (SD)	
Treatment attitudes (range 0–100)	44.3 (7.2)
Professional unease (range 0–100)	44.9 (7.8)
Depression malleability (range 0–100)	40.1 (11.0)
Depression identification (range 0–100)	46.6 (11.1)
REASON[e] mean score (SD)	
Professional comfort with and competence in care of mental health problems (range 1–7)	3.2 (0.4)
GPs' concerns about problems with the health care system for treatment of anxiety and depression (range 1–7)	4.4 (0.8)

*n = 444 unless stated otherwise
[a]Chronic medical condition was measured with the Dutch Central Bureau of Statistics (CBS) list
[b]4DSQ = Four-Dimensional Symptom Questionnaire
[c]Functional status was measured with the WHODAS-II = World Health Organisation's Disability Assessment Scale II (excluding work)
[d]DAQ: Depression Attitude Questionnaire
[e]REASON questionnaire: GPs' attitudes to their role in the management of anxiety and depressive disorders

40%. Also patients who had reported a need for care (OR = 2.54, 95% CI 1.60–4.03) were significantly more likely to be recognized. In addition, patients' anxiety or depression was less likely to be recognized when GPs had less confidence in their abilities to identify depression (DAQ subscale depression identification; OR = 0.97; 95% CI 0.95–0.99). Married or living together was the only predictor showing an interaction with condition, suggesting that being married or living together was a predictor of recognition only in the intervention condition but not in the control condition. Actually, recognition was lowered in patients who were married or living together in the intervention condition (OR = 0.39; 95% CI 0.16–0.95). The ROC analysis showed an AUC of 0.698 (95% CI 0.645–0.751) suggesting that the amount of variance in recognition explained by the joint predictors in the final model was "poor" to "fair" [53]. Patients'

Table 2 Results of the trivariate and multivariate multilevel logistic regression analyses predicting recognition of anxiety and depression

Independent variables (predictors)	Trivariate analysis				Multivariate analysis		
	OR	95% CI	P		OR	95% CI	P
Condition (intervention/control)	1.50	0.94–2.39	0.087	‡	3.08	1.47–6.46	0.003
Age	0.98	0.96–1.00	0.060	‡			
Condition[a]Age	1.00	0.97–1.03	0.989				
Married or living together (ref. not married or living together)	1.40	0.77–2.52	0.268	‡	1.25	0.67–2.35	0.478
Condition[a]Married or living together	0.33	0.14–0.79	0.013	‡	0.39	0.16–0.95	0.039
Number of chronic medical conditions[a]	0.94	0.83–1.08	0.389				
Condition[a]Number of chronic medical conditions	1.03	0.85–1.25	0.784				
4DSQ[b]							
Distress	1.03	0.99–1.07	0.098	‡	1.03	1.00–1.07	0.024
Condition[a]Distress	1.04	0.99–1.10	0.153	‡			
Depression	1.04	0.95–1.15	0.393				
Condition[a]Depression	1.03	0.89–1.16	0.666				
Anxiety	1.02	0.94–1.10	0.615				
Condition[a]Anxiety	1.04	0.93–1.15	0.512				
Somatization	1.01	0.96–1.06	0.736				
Condition[a]Somatization	1.04	0.97–1.11	0.301				
Need for care (ref. no need for care)	2.77	1.56–4.91	0.001	‡	2.54	1.60–4.03	0.000
Condition[a]Need for care	1.18	0.49–2.85	0.719				
DAQ[c]							
Treatment Attitudes	1.02	0.97–1.06	0.508				
Condition[a]Treatment Attitudes	0.96	0.88–1.04	0.294				
Professional Unease	0.98	0.94–1.02	0.322	‡			
Condition[a]Professional Unease	1.05	0.99–1.11	0.137	‡			
Depression Malleability	0.98	0.95–1.00	0.084	‡			
Condition[a]Depression Malleability	1.03	0.99–1.07	0.150	‡			
Depression identification	0.96	0.94–0.99	0.003	‡	0.97	0.95–0.99	0.018
Condition[a]Depression identification	1.04	0.99–1.10	0.089	‡			
REASON[d]							
Comfort and competence with mental health care	0.52	0.27–1.03	0.060	‡			
Condition[a]Comfort and competence with mental health care	2.52	0.90–7.07	0.079	‡			
Concerns about difficulties with the health care system	1.26	0.85–1.88	0.253	‡			
Condition[a]Concerns about difficulties with the health care system	0.67	0.38–1.18	0.170	‡			
Functional status[e]	1.00	0.98–1.02	0.662	‡			
Condition[a]Functional status	1.03	1.00–1.05	0.055	‡			

Reference category: No recognition; OR = odds ratio; 95% CI = 95% confidence interval; P = p-value, ‡ variables entered in the multivariate model
[a]Interaction term
[b]4DSQ Four-Dimensional Symptom Questionnaire
[c]DAQ Depression Attitude Questionnaire
[d]REASON questionnaire: GPs' attitudes to their role in the management of anxiety and depressive disorders
[e]Functional status was measured with the WHODAS-II World Health Organisation's Disability Assessment Scale II

age, the presence of a chronic medical condition, the 4DSQ scores for somatisation, anxiety and depression, and patients' functional status were not associated with the recognition of anxiety and depression. In addition the DAQ subscales treatment attitude, professional unease and depression malleability were not associated with recognition. As well as the REASON subscales professional comfort with and competence in care of mental health disorders and GPs' concerns about problems with the health care system for management of anxiety and depression.

Discussion

Main findings

The results of this study indicate that patients with a perceived need for psychological care and those with high distress were more likely to be recognized by their GP as having anxiety or depression. This may not come as a big surprise. After all, it is very likely that patients who felt a need for care were more willing to disclose their mental health problems and express their need for care in the doctor's office, thereby obviously increasing the likelihood of subsequent recognition. Similarly, high distress is experienced as "having a difficult time" and this is probably close to having a need for support, advice or guidance. What is more surprising, is that high depression and anxiety were not associated with recognition after accounting for distress. It seems that the severity of psychological suffering (i.e. distress) is associated with recognition, rather than the severity of anxiety and depression. No association was found between somatization and recognition. The presentation of somatic complaints unexplained by physical illness (i.e. somatization) may hinder recognition of anxiety and depression, but this was not confirmed in our study. On the GP part, we found that GPs with confidence in their ability to identify depression were more inclined to recognize patients having anxiety or depression. Besides, GPs who had received the tailored intervention were relatively less likely to recognize anxiety and depression in patients who were married or living together. Possibly, GPs in the intervention group were more focused on the recognition of anxiety and depression particularly in high-risk groups, including people having little or no social support.

In our study the amount of variance in recognition explained by the joint factors in the final model was "poor" to "fair". Recognition seems to be largely determined by other factors, which we can only speculate about. On the part of the GP, we can think of experience with mental health problems, perceived professional responsibilities, sensitivity to emotions, and workload. On the patient part, we might think of past mental health problems, experience with mental health issues in relatives or friends, openness to own emotions, and stigma. On the part of the context of the doctor-patient encounter, we can think of the duration and quality of the doctor-patient relationship, the time available for a consultation (time pressure), and giving priority to one complaint after presentation of various complaints in one consultation.

Comparison with existing literature

Previous studies have identified patient and GP characteristics that are associated with the recognition or diagnosis of anxiety and depression. However, results are difficult to compare because different definitions of recognition were used, as well as different instruments for the assessment of anxiety and depression.

In our study high 4DSQ distress scores were associated with the recognition of anxiety and depression. Previous research showed that the 4DSQ distress scale turned out to be effective in detecting any depressive or anxiety disorder [54]. Remarkably, high 4DSQ scores on the subscales anxiety and depression were not associated with recognition. The finding is in line with the study of Marcus et al. (2011) [27]. Patients in this study completed four symptom severity self-report questionnaires (i.e. Penn State Worry Questionnaire, Beck Depression Inventory II, Anxiety Sensitivity Index and Mini Social Phobia Inventory) and no association was found with the detection of anxiety and depression. In contrast, other studies showed that patients with more anxiety or depressive symptoms were more likely to be recognized or diagnosed [7, 14, 24–26, 29, 55]. Although instruments used in these studies were different from our study (respectively the Beck Anxiety Inventory, the Depression Screening questionnaire, General Health Questionnaire, Center for Epidemiological Studies – Depression Scale, the Composite International Diagnostic Interview and the Patient Health Questionnaire 9), research showed that correlations between the 4DSQ scales and other symptom questionnaires were positive [42]. Furthermore, in keeping with the study of Piek et al. (2012), we found no association between the presence of chronic medical illness and recognition of anxiety and depression [7]. Coventry et al. (2011) found that in the presence of chronic physical health problems GPs and patients tend to normalise distress and depression. As a consequence, depression is less frequently recognized. In addition, Hermanns et al. (2013) concluded in a review that diagnosis and treatment of depression in people with chronic illness (i.e. diabetes) can be improved [56]. An estimated 50% of patients remain undiagnosed. Other studies, on the other hand, demonstrated a positive association between physical illnesses and recognition [25, 27]. Possibly, in these studies patients with chronic somatic diseases visited their GP more frequently and, as a consequence, were more likely to be recognized. Furthermore, in line with other studies, no association was found between age and recognition [7, 26, 27]. In contrast, a few studies found that patients of higher age were more likely to be recognized [14, 24]. An explanation for this finding might be that anxiety disorders are most common in people aged between 25 and 44 years [57]. In the study of Wittchen et al. (2001) most patients were older [24]. Finally, the finding that patients' need for care was a significant predictor of recognition was confirmed in previous research [27].

With respect to the GP characteristics, GPs' attitudes towards anxiety and depression and their ability to detect these disorders were rarely studied. One study examined the associations between attitudes, measured with the DAQ, and clinical behaviour, including depression identification [30]. When comparing both study populations, GPs score on the DAQ components 1, 2 and 4 are similar in our study. GPs score on component 3 'depression malleability' differs significantly between both studies (GPs score in our study was 40.1 and in the study of Dowrick 24.5). In the study of Dowrick et al. (2000) GP visitors completed the General Health Questionnaire 12 (GHQ-12) before the consultation and the GP rated each patient on the severity of their psychological disturbance ranging from 'no disorder' to 'severe disorder' after the consultation. Dorwick et al. (2000) found no association between GPs' confidence in their identification of depression and the accuracy in identifying it among their patients [30]. In contrast, our study showed that GPs having confidence in the ability to identify depression were more likely to recognize patients with anxiety or depression. Possibly, Dorwick et al. (2000) found no association because they used a less specific measurement instrument for the identification of depression, the GHQ-12 which measures general distress [30]. In our study we determined recognition in patient medical records and with several indicators.

Strengths and limitations

A strength of this study was that we identified recognition using multiple indicators in the medical records. Using diagnostic codes alone may underestimate the accuracy of GPs' recognition of anxiety and depression [14, 43]. In addition, data on recognition was gathered longitudinally, 6 months before and 6 months after patients completed the EK-10 and were included. Compared to cross-sectional methods, record extraction over an extended period may improve the accuracy of recognition [12, 13]. For example, because patients may express their psychological complaints in repeated consultations. However, there are inherent methodological limitations when using medical records: complexities in the definition of recognition, recording, assessment and in the exercise of clinical judgement in negotiating diagnoses. Another limitation was that a self-report questionnaire, the EK-10, was used as reference standard for including the participants in this study. Although the EK-10 is an instrument for screening for anxiety and depressive disorders in general practice, a more reliable instrument as reference standard for diagnosis would have been the Composite International Diagnostic Interview (CIDI) [58]. On the other hand, using the EK-10 can also be considered to constitute a strength of the study, providing a wide definition of anxiety and depression in keeping with the relatively non-specific, heterogeneous nature of mental health conditions in general practice.

Creating a regression model using a stepwise procedure to select independent variable in the final model, carries the risk of capitalizing on chance, i.e. the risk of inclusion of variables that coincidentally show significant associations with the outcome in a particular sample. The role of marital status in the recognition of anxiety and depression may have been a chance finding.

By design, by including only positively screened patients, our study did not provide any information on false-positive recognitions.

Practical implications and further research

Recognition of anxiety and depression is important because of its association with appropriate treatment according to guidelines [59]. Recognition could improve when GPs have more insight in factors associated with the recognition of anxiety and depression. Quality improvement activities may focus at increasing the confidence of GPs in their ability to identify symptoms of distress, anxiety and depression. Smolders et al. (2010) showed that GPs with strong confidence in their abilities to identify depression, treated their patients more often in accordance with guidelines than GPs who had difficulties with distinguishing depression from unhappiness [60]. The use of an instrument, such as the 4DSQ may be helpful to structure the dialogue with the patient, for a better understanding of the complaints and for coming to a shared understanding of the patient's problem [39]. In the presence of chronic physical health problems, GPs and patients have a tendency to normalise distress [18] and may prioritise physical problems [19]. Using the 4DSQ may prevent normalisation of distress. The instrument is helpful in informing the patient and GP about the distress level. A high score ($\geq$ 21) indicates a serious problem, such as a clinically significant psychiatric disorder. Hermanns et al. (2013) concluded that "self-assessment questionnaires can dramatically improve depression detection rates. Complementing such screening with assessments of psychological distress can have an additional and complementary impact on individual self-care" [56]. When using an instrument for recognition, it is important that the instrument fits the holistic focus of patient-centred consultation models favoured by GPs [61]. Certainly, recognition alone is not effective, it has to be part of care including accurate diagnosis, follow-up, and access to evidence based treatments [62, 63]. Patients have to be informed about their anxiety and depression, about evidence-based treatment options (including watchful waiting) and patients have to express their preferences. In case of major depressive disorders patients have to be convinced to initiate and continue treatment [63]. Furthermore, because patients with a perceived need for psychological care were more likely to be recognized, patients should be encouraged in disclosing their problems. Further research is needed into which strategies (individual- and societal level) are effective to disclose mental health problems.

In our study the focus was on factors contributing to the recognition of anxiety and depression in general practice, a small part of quality improvement in primary care. For sustainable improvements in primary mental health care integration with community engagement may contribute to a better recognition of anxiety and depression by the GP [64].

Conclusion

Patients with a perceived need for psychological care and those with high distress were more likely to be recognized by their GP as having anxiety or depression. In addition, GPs with confidence in their ability to identify depression were more likely to recognize patients with anxiety or depression. Educational efforts should concentrate on increasing GPs' confidence in the ability to identify symptoms of distress, anxiety and depression, as part of care according to guidelines. In addition, patients should be encouraged to disclose their mental health problems.

Abbreviations

4DSQ: Four-Dimensional Symptom Questionnaire; AUC: area under the curve; CBS: Central Bureau of Statistics; CIDI: Composite International Diagnostic Interview; DAQ: Depression Attitude Questionnaire; EK-10: extended Kessler 10; GHQ-12: General Health Questionnaire 12; GPs: general practitioners; ICPC-1: International Classification of Primary Care-1; ROC: receiver operating characteristic; SPSS: Statistical Package for the Social Sciences; WHODAS II: World Health Organisation's Disability Assessment Scale II

Acknowledgements

We thank the patients and general practitioners for their contribution to this study.
This study was funded by ZonMW, Organisation for Health Research and Development, the Netherlands.

Funding

This research project was funded by the Netherlands Organisation for Health Research and Development (ZonMW). The funder had no role in the study design, data collection and analysis, interpretation of data or in writing the manuscript.

Authors' contributions

HS contributed to the design of the study, performed the analysis and wrote this article. BT contributed to the design of the study, performed the analysis and co-authored this article. DV contributed to the design of the study and co-authored the article. MW contributed to the design of the study and co-authored the article. AVB contributed to the design of the study and co-authored the article. All authors have read and approved the final manuscript.

Competing interests

H Sinnema: None declared.
B Terluin: is the copyright owner of the 4DSQ and receives copyright fees from companies that use the 4DSQ on a commercial basis (the 4DSQ is freely available for non-commercial use in health care and research). BT received fees from various institutions for workshops on the application of the 4DSQ in primary care settings.
D Volker: None declared.
M Wensing: None declared.
A van Balkom: None declared.

Author details

[1]Netherlands Institute of Mental Health and Addiction, Trimbos Institute, Postbox 725, 3500, AS, Utrecht, The Netherlands. [2]Department of General Practice and Elderly Care Medicine, Amsterdam Public Health Research Institute, VU University Medical Centre, Van der Boechorststraat 7, 1081, BT, Amsterdam, The Netherlands. [3]Universitatsklinikum Heidelberg, Im Neuenheimer Feld 130.3, 69120 Heidelberg, Germany. [4]Department of Psychiatry, VU University Medical Centre and GGZinGeest, AJ Ernststraat 887, 1081, HL, Amsterdam, The Netherlands.

References

1. Demyttenaere K, Bruffaerts R, Posada-Villa J, Gasquet I, Kovess V, Lepine JP, et al. Prevalence, severity, and unmet need for treatment of mental disorders in the World Health Organization world mental health surveys. JAMA. 2004;291:2581–90.
2. Alonso J, Angermeyer MC, Bernert S, Bruffaerts R, Brugha TS, Bryson H, et al. Disability and quality of life impact of mental disorders in Europe: results from the European study of the epidemiology of mental disorders (ESEMeD) project. Acta Psychiatr Scand Suppl. 2004;420:38–46.
3. Gustavsson A, Svensson M, Jacobi F, Allgulander C, Alonso J, Beghi E, et al. Cost of disorders of the brain in Europe 2010. Eur Neuropsychopharmacol. 2011;21:718–79.
4. van Avendonk M, van Weel-Baumgarten E, van der Weele G, Wiersma T, Burgers JS. Summary of the Dutch College of General Practitioners' practice guideline 'Depression'. Ned Tijdschr Geneeskd. 2012;156:A5101.
5. van Avendonk MJ, Hassink-Franke LJ, Terluin B, van Marwijk HW, Wiersma T, Burgers JS. [Summarisation of the NHG practice guideline 'Anxiety']. Ned Tijdschr Geneeskd 2012, 156: A4509.
6. Lecrubier Y. Widespread underrecognition and undertreatment of anxiety and mood disorders: results from 3 European studies. J Clin Psychiatry. 2007;68:36–41.
7. Piek E, Nolen WA, van der Meer K, Joling KJ, Kollen BJ, Penninx BW, et al. Determinants of (non-)recognition of depression by general practitioners: results of the Netherlands study of depression and anxiety. J Affect Disord. 2012;138:397–404.
8. Andrews G, Issakidis C, Sanderson K, Corry J, Lapsley H. Utilising survey data to inform public policy: comparison of the cost-effectiveness of treatment of ten mental disorders. Br J Psychiatry. 2004;184:526–33.
9. Gijsen R, Poos M: *Zorggebruik:nadere uitwerking. In: Volksgezondheid Toekomstverkenning, Nationaal Kompas Volksgezondheid.* Bilthoven: RIVM; 2012.

10. Verhaak PF, van Dijk CE, Nuijen J, Verheij RA, Schellevis FG. Mental health care as delivered by Dutch general practitioners between 2004 and 2008. Scand J Prim Health Care. 2012;30:156–62.

11. Cepoiu M, McCusker J, Cole MG, Sewitch M, Belzile E, Ciampi A. Recognition of depression by non-psychiatric physicians–a systematic literature review and meta-analysis. J Gen Intern Med. 2008;23:25–36.

12. Mitchell AJ, Vaze A, Rao S. Clinical diagnosis of depression in primary care: a meta-analysis. Lancet. 2009;374:609–19.

13. Kessler D, Bennewith O, Lewis G, Sharp D. Detection of depression and anxiety in primary care: follow up study. BMJ. 2002;325:1016–7.

14. Janssen EH, van de Ven PM, Terluin B, Verhaak PF, van Marwijk HW, Smolders M, et al. Recognition of anxiety disorders by family physicians after rigorous medical record case extraction: results of the Netherlands Study of Depression and Anxiety. Gen Hosp Psychiatry. 2012;34:460–7.

15. Verhaak P, Prins MA, Spreeuwenberg P, Draisma S, van Balkom T, Bensing JM, et al. Receiving treatment for common mental disorders. Gen Hosp Psychiatry. 2009;31:46–55.

16. Wittkampf KA, van ZM, Smits FT, Schene AH, Huyser J, van Weert HC. Patients' view on screening for depression in general practice. Fam Pract. 2008;25:438–44.

17. Tylee A, Walters P. Underrecognition of anxiety and mood disorders in primary care: why does the problem exist and what can be done? J Clin Psychiatry. 2007;68(Suppl 2):27–30.

18. Chew-Graham C, Kovandzic M, Gask L, Burroughs H, Clarke P, Sanderson H, et al. Why may older people with depression not present to primary care? Messages from secondary analysis of qualitative data. Health Soc Care Community. 2012;20:52–60.

19. Overend K, Bosanquet K, Bailey D, Foster D, Gascoyne S, Lewis H, et al. Revealing hidden depression in older people: a qualitative study within a randomised controlled trial. BMC Fam Pract. 2015;16:142.

20. Prins MA, Verhaak PF, Smolders M, Laurant MG, van der Meer K, Spreeuwenberg P, et al. Patient factors associated with guideline-concordant treatment of anxiety and depression in primary care. J Gen Intern Med. 2010;25:648–55.

21. Barley EA, Murray J, Walters P, Tylee A. Managing depression in primary care: a meta-synthesis of qualitative and quantitative research from the UK to identify barriers and facilitators. BMC Fam Pract. 2011;12:47.

22. Coventry PA, Hays R, Dickens C, Bundy C, Garrett C, Cherrington A, et al. Talking about depression: a qualitative study of barriers to managing depression in people with long term conditions in primary care. BMC Fam Pract. 2011;12:10.

23. Kovandzic M, Chew-Graham C, Reeve J, Edwards S, Peters S, Edge D, et al. Access to primary mental health care for hard-to-reach groups: from 'silent suffering' to 'making it work. Soc Sci Med. 2011;72:763–72.

24. Wittchen HU, Hofler M, Meister W. Prevalence and recognition of depressive syndromes in German primary care settings: poorly recognized and treated? Int Clin Psychopharmacol. 2001;16:121–35.

25. Nuyen J, Volkers AC, Verhaak PF, Schellevis FG, Groenewegen PP, Van den Bos GA. Accuracy of diagnosing depression in primary care: the impact of chronic somatic and psychiatric co-morbidity. Psychol Med. 2005;35:1185–95.

26. Pfaff JJ, Almeida OP. A cross-sectional analysis of factors that influence the detection of depression in older primary care patients. Aust N Z J Psychiatry. 2005;39:262–5.

27. Marcus M, Westra H, Vermani M, Katzman M. Patient predictors of detection of depression and anxiety disorders in primary care. Journal of Participatory Medicine. 2011;

28. Rifel J, Svab I, Ster MP, Pavlic DR, King M, Nazareth I. Impact of demographic factors on recognition of persons with depression and anxiety in primary care in Slovenia. BMC Psychiatry. 2008;8:96.

29. Chin WY, Chan KT, Lam CL, Wong SY, Fong DY, Lo YY, et al. Detection and management of depression in adult primary care patients in Hong Kong: a cross-sectional survey conducted by a primary care practice-based research network. BMC Fam Pract. 2014;15:30.

30. Dowrick C, Gask L, Perry R, Dixon C, Usherwood T. Do general practitioners' attitudes towards depression predict their clinical behaviour? Psychol Med. 2000;30:413–9.

31. Ross S, Moffat K, McConnachie A, Gordon J, Wilson P. Sex and attitude: a randomized vignette study of the management of depression by general practitioners. Br J Gen Pract. 1999;49:17–21.

32. Robbins JM, Kirmayer LJ, Cathebras P, Yaffe MJ, Dworkind M. Physician characteristics and the recognition of depression and anxiety in primary care. Med Care. 1994;32:795–812.

33. Sinnema H, Franx G, Volker D, Majo C, Terluin B, Wensing M, et al. Randomised controlled trial of tailored interventions to improve the management of anxiety and depressive disorders in primary care. Implement Sci. 2011;6:75.

34. Terluin B, van Heest F, van der Meer K, Neomagus G, Hekman J, Aulbers L et al.: Dutch College of General Practitioners guideline: anxiety disorder, first revision [NHG-Standaard Angststoornissen, eerste herziening. In Dutch]. Huisarts en Wetenschap 2004, 47: 26–37.

35. Richtlijnwerkgroep Multidisciplinaire richtlijnen Angststoornissen en Depressie: Multidisciplinary guideline Anxiety Disord: guideline for diagnostics and treatment of adult clients with an anxiety disorder, first revision [Multidisciplinaire richtlijn Angststoornissen. Richtlijn voor de diagnostiek en behandeling van volwassen patiënten met een angststoornis, eerste revisie. In Dutch]. Utrecht:Trimbos-instituut; 2009.

36. Van Marwijk HWJ, Grundmeijer HGLM, Bijl D, Van Gelderen MG, De Haan M, Van Weel-Baumgarten EM. Dutch College of General Practitioners guideline: depression, first revision [NHG-Standaard Depressieve stoornis (depressie). Eerste herziening. In Dutch]. Huisarts & Wetenschap. 2003;46:614–23.

37. Richtlijnwerkgroep Multidisciplinaire richtlijnen Angststoornissen en Depressie: Multidisciplinary guideline depression: guideline for diagnostics and treatment of adult clients with a major depressive disorder, first revision [Multidisciplinaire richtlijn Depressie: richtlijn voor diagnostiek en behandeling van volwassen cliënten met een depressie, eerste revisie. In Dutch]. Utrecht: Trimbos-instituut; 2009.

38. Sinnema H, Majo MC, Volker D, Hoogendoorn A, Terluin B, Wensing M, et al. Effectiveness of a tailored implementation programme to improve recognition, diagnosis and treatment of anxiety and depression in general practice: a cluster randomised controlled trial. Implement Sci. 2015;10:33.

39. Sinnema H, Terluin B, Wensing M, Volker D, Franx G, van BA, et al. Systematic tailoring for the implementation of guideline recommendations for anxiety and depressive disorders in general practice: perceived usefulness of tailored interventions. BMC Fam Pract. 2013;14:94.

40. Donker T, Comijs H, Cuijpers P, Terluin B, Nolen W, Zitman F, et al. The validity of the Dutch K10 and extended K10 screening scales for depressive and anxiety disorders. Psychiatry Res. 2010;176:45–50.

41. Lamberts HWM. International classification of primary care (ICPC). Oxford: Oxford University Press; 1990.

42. Terluin B, van Marwijk HW, Ader HJ, de Vet HC, Penninx BW, Hermens ML, et al. The four-dimensional symptom questionnaire (4DSQ): a validation study of a multidimensional self-report questionnaire to assess distress, depression, anxiety and somatization. BMC Psychiatry. 2006;6:34.

43. Joling KJ, van Marwijk HW, Piek E, van der Horst HE, Penninx BW, Verhaak P, et al. Do GPs' medical records demonstrate a good recognition of depression? A new perspective on case extraction. J Affect Disord. 2011;133:522–7.

44. Hakkaart-van Roijen L: Manual Trimbos/iMTA questionnaire for costs associated with psychiatric illness [in Dutch]. Rotterdam: Institute for Medical Technology Assessment; 2002.

45. Chwastiak LA, Von Korff M. Disability in depression and back pain evaluation of the World Health Organization disability assessment schedule (WHO DAS II) in a primary care setting. J Clin Epidemiol. 2003;56:507–14.

46. Ustun TB, Chatterji S, Kostanjsek N, Rehm J, Kennedy C, Epping-Jordan J, et al. Developing the World Health Organization disability assessment schedule 2.0. Bull World Health Organ. 2010;88:815–23.

47. Botega N, Blizard R, Wilkinson G. General practitioners and depression-first use of the depression attitude questionnaire. Int J Methods Psychiatr Res. 1992;4:169–80.

48. Haddad M, Menchetti M, Walters P, Norton J, Tylee A, Mann A. Clinicians' attitudes to depression in Europe: a pooled analysis of depression attitude questionnaire findings. Fam Pract. 2012;29:121–30.

49. McCall L, Clarke DM, Rowley G. A questionnaire to measure general practitioners' attitudes to their role in the management of patients with depression and anxiety. Aust Fam Physician. 2002;31:299–303.

50. Twisk JWR. Applied multilevel analysis. Cambridge: Cambridge University Press; 2006.

51. Rubin DB. Multiple imputation for nonresponse in surveys. New York: John Wiley & Sons; 1987.

52. Harrell FE Jr, Lee KL, Matchar DB, Reichert TA. Regression models for prognostic prediction: advantages, problems, and suggested solutions. Cancer Treat Rep. 1985;69:1071–7.

53. Tape T: Interpreting Diagnostics Tests. Omaha: University of Nebraska Medical Centre; 2004.

54. Terluin B, Brouwers EP, van Marwijk HW, Verhaak P, van der Horst HE. Detecting depressive and anxiety disorders in distressed patients in primary care; comparative diagnostic accuracy of the four-dimensional symptom questionnaire (4DSQ) and the hospital anxiety and depression scale (HADS). BMC Fam Pract. 2009;10:58.

55. Kamphuis MH, Stegenga BT, Zuithoff NP, King M, Nazareth I, de Wit NJ, et al. Does recognition of depression in primary care affect outcome? The PREDICT-NL study. Fam Pract. 2012;29:16–23.

56. Hermanns N, Caputo S, Dzida G, Khunti K, Meneghini LF, Snoek F. Screening, evaluation and management of depression in people with diabetes in primary care. Prim Care Diabetes. 2013;7:1–10.

57. Flint AJ. Epidemiology and comorbidity of anxiety disorders in the elderly. Am J Psychiatry. 1994;151:640–9.

58. Wittchen HU. Reliability and validity studies of the WHO–composite international diagnostic interview (CIDI): a critical review. J Psychiatr Res. 1994;28:57–84.

59. Smolders M, Laurant M, Verhaak P, Prins M, van Marwijk H, Penninx B, et al. Adherence to evidence-based guidelines for depression and anxiety disorders is associated with recording of the diagnosis. Gen Hosp Psychiatry. 2009;31:460–9.

60. Smolders M, Laurant M, Verhaak P, Prins M, van Marwijk H, Penninx B, et al. Which physician and practice characteristics are associated with adherence to evidence-based guidelines for depressive and anxiety disorders? Med Care. 2010;48:240–8.

61. Mitchell C, Dwyer R, Hagan T, Mathers N. Impact of the QOF and the NICE guideline in the diagnosis and management of depression: a qualitative study. Br J Gen Pract. 2011;61:e279–89.

62. Gilbody S, Sheldon T, Wessely S. Should we screen for depression? BMJ. 2006;332:1027–30.

63. Baas KD, Wittkampf KA, van Weert HC, Lucassen P, Huyser J, van den Hoogen H, et al. Screening for depression in high-risk groups: prospective cohort study in general practice. Br J Psychiatry. 2009;194:399–403.

64. Dowrick C, Bower P, Chew-Graham C, Lovell K, Edwards S, Lamb J, et al. Evaluating a complex model designed to increase access to high quality primary mental health care for under-served groups: a multi-method study. BMC Health Serv Res. 2016;16:58.

11

Risk of opioid misuse in chronic non-cancer pain in primary care patients

Johannes Maximilian Just[1*] (iD), Linda Bingener[1], Markus Bleckwenn[1], Rieke Schnakenberg[1,2] and Klaus Weckbecker[1]

Abstract

Background: Efforts to improve treatment of pain using opioids have to adequately take into account their therapeutic shortcomings which involve addictiveness. While there are no signs of an "opioid epidemic" in Germany similar to that in the US, there is little data on the prevalence of prescription opioid misuse and addiction. Therefore, our objective was to screen primary care patients on long-term opioid therapy for signs of misuse of prescription opioids.

Methods: We recruited 15 GPs practices and asked all patients on long-term opioid therapy (> 6 months) to fill out a questionnaire including the "Current Opioid Misuse Measure" (COMM®), a self-report questionnaire. Patients with a malignant disease were excluded.

Results: $N = 91$ patients participated in the study (response rate: 75.2%). A third (31.5%) showed a positive COMM® - Score which represents a high risk of aberrant drug behaviour. A positive COMM® - Score showed a statistically significant correlation with a lifetime diagnosis of depression and neck pain.

Conclusions: While Germany does not face an "opioid eoidemic", addictiveness of opioids should be considered when using them in chronic non-tumor pain. In our study population, almost every third patient was at risk and should therefore be followed up closely. Co-prevalence of depression is a significant issue and should always be screened for in patients with chronic pain, especially thus with aberrant drug behaviour.

Keywords: Opioid, Misuse, Addiction, Prescription drugs, Prevalence

Background

Opioids are a cornerstone in the treatment of acute and chronic pain, still their therapeutic shortcoming have to be considered [1]. They involve risk of addiction, a narrow therapeutic ratio and lack of documented effectiveness in the treatment of several aspects of chronic non-cancer pain (CNCP) [2]. Misuse and addiction from prescription opioids is a serious public health issue in the US. The death toll has almost quadrupled in the 21st century, matching a similar increase in prescription rates [2, 3]. A meta-analysis calculated an average proportion of misuse between 21 and 29% (range, 95% confidence interval [CI]: 13–38%) for patients with CNCP [4].

Currently, significant effort is put into reversing these effects, including a new CDC guideline for "Prescribing Opioids for Chronic Pain" [2].

The increase of opioid prescription in the US is paralleled by an increase in all European countries [5]. A meta-analysis on medication misuse in the EU named prescription opioids as a main group of misuse but data on mortality directly linked to opioids does not exist in Germany [6]. The increase in opioid prescriptions in Germany is clearly less extreme than in the US. The percentage of persons with statutory health insurance who have been prescribed opioids at least once per year has increased from 3.3% in 2000 to 4.5% in 2010 [7]. An analysis of randomly selected claims records of 870,000 persons in a large German medical health insurance organization showed a pooled 1-year prevalence of abuse/addiction (defined as hospital stays related to

* Correspondence: johannes.just@ukbonn.de
[1]Institute of General Practice and Family Medicine, Bonn University Clinic, Sigmund-Freud-Street 25, 53127 Bonn, Germany
Full list of author information is available at the end of the article

addiction) of 0.008% in those on long-term opioid therapy (LTOT). Therefore, the authors concluded, that "there are no signals of an 'opioid epidemic' in Germany" [8].

Factors that may have contributed to the opioid epidemic in the US include higher doses of opioids per patient compared to other developed countries, a high individual health care cost burden, lesser regulatory restrictions for opioids and a "pro-profit" orientation of key elements of the health care system [9–11]. The German medical system on the contrary offers compulsory, high-quality health care with adequate regulatory restrictions for opioids including a ban on direct to consumer marketing by the pharmaceutical industry.

The lack of many society related contributing factors to opioid misuse in Germany is reassuring. Nevertheless addictive behaviour is a world-wide problem and more data on possible at-risk patients in Germany could help to keep rates of opioid misuse low. Therefore we conducted a study, screening primary care patients on LTOT for risk of misuse of prescription opioids, using a validated self-report measure [12].

Methods

We conducted a cross sectional study at GP's practices using the self-report questionnaire Current Opioid Misuse Measure (COMM®), adding items concerning the medical history as well as socio-economic information. COMM® Score results were the primary outcome criterion.

The COMM® Score is a self-report questionnaire for patients using opioids longer than six months. We used an existing German version of the COMM®. The questionnaire was translated from English to German by experienced translators using the "back-translation method". Then, a team of bilingual addiction experts fine-tuned the questionnaire in order to make sure that the meaning and intent of the original items were preserved [13]. Later, it was pre-tested for comprehensibility and acceptability with five representative patients by our study group, using cognitive interviewing techniques.

In order to recruit GPs, we contacted all GPs in the greater Bonn area (> 100) via fax and telephone. We stopped recruiting after having reached the planned number of 15 GPs. A total of four GPs refused to participate due to their high workload.

All patients on LTOT (> 6 months) for CNCP, who entered the practice to collect their prescription, were asked to fill in the questionnaire by the front desk staff. The study period was three months, as it represents the maximum duration of one prescription in Germany, making sure we included all relevant patients. Those who did not want to participate were asked to fill in

their age and sex to test for differences in participants and nonparticipants.

Inclusion criteria were LTOT (> 6 months) for CNCP and sufficient literacy. Excluded were patients with malignant disease, patients who could not collect their prescription themselves due to age or multimorbidity and patients on opioid-maintenance therapy.

The data management was performed at the Department of General Practice and Family Medicine in Bonn and included data entry, data validation by plausibility checks, frequency analyses and advanced statistics using IBM SPSS Statistics 22®. We used exploratory statistics and a multiple logistic regression model with a dichotomous dependent variable to describe data and to explore the relationship between dependent and independent variables. For comparison of participants and nonparticipants concerning age and sex, we used Student's t-test and Pearson's chi-squared test.

The anonymous survey received ethical approval by the Ethics Committee of the Medical Faculty of the University of Bonn (No. 243/16).

Results

The inclusion criteria were met by 121 patients from 12 GPs practices, of which 91 completed the questionnaire (response rate: 75.2%). Participants mean COMM® - Score was 7.26 (min-max: 0–41).

On average, we received nine (min - max: 0–17) questionnaires per practice. One practice claimed they did not have any patients matching our criteria, two practices did not proceed with the study due to "work overload" and were therefore considered "drop-outs" (rate: 13%).

All of the non-participants agreed to have their age and sex documented. Non-participants differed slightly from participants concerning age and sex, without differences being statistically significant (Table 1).

The mean age of participants was 69.70 years (SD 14.39), 62.4% were female. Most participants reported back and joint pain as the reason for taking opioid analgesics. The proportion of participants with a "high risk of aberrant drug behaviour" according to COMM® (meaning a score of nine or higher) was 31.5%. Of these patients, 64.3% had a high school education only. A statistically significant correlation with a positive COMM® - Score was present for the variables "lifetime diagnosis of depression" and "neck pain". A detailed description of all variables and the connected odds ratio for a positive COMM®-Score is given in Table 2.

We used a multiple regression model to control for statistically significant correlations between positive COMM® - Scores and the documented patient characteristics. The model was sound, showing a Nagelkerke's Pseudo-R^2 of 0.401. All tested variables are shown in Table 2.

Table 1 Age and sex distribution for participants and nonparticipants

Variable	All participants (n = 93)	Non participants (n = 28)	Difference significant
Age (mean)	69.70 (SD: 14.39; min/max: 25/93)	74.79 (SD: 14.06; min/max: 46/92)	No[a]
Sex: female	62.4%	60.7%	No[b]

[a]Student's t-test (df: 119)
[b]Pearson's chi-squared test (df: 2)

Discussion

Our study showed a high risk of aberrant drug behaviour in almost one third (31.5%) of the targeted patient group. With 75.2%, the response rate was good. Back and joint pain were the most commonly reported reasons for taking opioid painkillers. A statistically significant correlation with a positive COMM® - Score was present for the variables "lifetime diagnosis of depression" and "neck pain".

The proportion of "at risk patients" seems rather high, regarding the assumption that there is no opioid epidemic in Germany. In this context it needs to be emphasized, that we screened for patients how are at risk of developing misuse only. So there probably is potential for an opioid epidemic in Germany, but positive physician- and society related factors might have prevented such a development.

The proportion of "at risk" patients may have been overestimated in our study. The COMM® - Score uses several questions that target signs of emotional volatility that might be present in depression as well as in opioid misuse. As depression is more prevalent in patients with CNCP, this might explain the high proportion of COMM® - Score positive patients in the sample. Additionally, this may also explain the high proportion of patients with depression within the group of COMM® - Score positive patients. More than half of COMM® - Score positive participants reported a history of a diagnosis of depression (60.7%) with a statistically significant correlation between a positive score and the presence of depression. The average lifetime prevalence of depression in Germany in contrast is 11.6%, the prevalence of depression in a large European chronic pain patient cohort was 21% [14, 15]. So while the methodology does not allow us to make a statement concerning causality, and there might be a bias towards over-diagnosing risk of misuse in patients with depression, the high prevalence of depression should be kept in mind when treating patients with opioid misuse.

Some known risk factors connected to the opioid epidemic from prior studies in the US were not found in our study population (e.g. young age, male sex). [16, 17]. So the particularly alarming increase in opioid misuse in young, male subjects in the US seems not to be an issue in our sample group [18]. Numbers for "prior addiction diagnosis" and "addiction diagnosis in relatives" were very small (n < 5) in our study, which explains non-significant results for these well described risk factors.

The statistically significant correlation of neck pain and a positive COMM® - Score in the logistic regression model is

Table 2 Risk factors for positive COMM - Score (logistic regression analysis, n = 91, df = 14)

	CommScore positive	CommScore negative	OR (95% CI)	Sig.
N (%)	28 (31.5%)	65 (60.5%)	N/A	N/A
Gender, male	9 (32.1%)	25 (39.1%)	0.85 (0.25–2.87)	0.79
Age (mean (SD))	69.61 (17.2)	69.74 (13.2)	0.99 (0.95–1.04)	0.69
Headache	5 (17.9%)	6 (9.2%)	1.80 (0.27–12.19)	0.55
Back pain	23 (82.1%)	43 (66.2%)	1.45 (0.37–5.65)	0.60
Joint pain	17 (60.7%)	30 (46.2%)	2.70 (0.72–10.16)	0.14
Neck pain	10 (35.7%)	7 (10.8%)	9.23 (1.63–52.26)	0.01
Rheumatic pain	7 (25.0%)	11 (16.9%)	0.94 (0.20–4.53)	0.94
Postoperative pain	5 (17.9%)	10 (15.4%)	0.57 (0.12–2.75)	0.48
Other pain	4 (14.3%)	11 (16.9%)	0.28 (0.04–1.92)	0.19
Prior addiction diagnosis	2 (7.1%)	2 (3.1%)	1.34 (0.11–16.99)	0.82
Addiction diagnosis in family	3 (10.7%)	4 (6.2%)	5.55 (0.61–50.61)	0.13
Depression	17 (60.7%)	16 (25%)	6.84 (1.88–24.91)	0.004
Fear of Addiction	11 (39.3%)	18 (27.7%)	0.85 (0.24–3.06)	0.80
Education, high school or lower	18 (64.3%)	27 (41.5%)	3.13 (0.92–10.62)	0.07

N = absolute number of participants; (%) = percentage within variable COMM - Score; OR = Odds ratio; (95% CI) = 95% Confidence Interval for Odds ratio, Sig. = Significance of OR an interesting new finding. Psychosocial stress factors may have acted as a confounding factor, as they are contributing factors to both, substance abuse and neck pain [19–21]. Still, numbers are small and it would be interesting if our findings can be reproduced in larger samples for instance using secondary analysis of a large insurance database.

There are several further limitations to this study. It is difficult to control for bias that stems from different prescription patterns in doctors and we did only include patients from 12 different GPs practices. So we cannot claim that our sample is representative. Still they give a first hint at which proportion of opioid misuse in CNCP can be expected on a national level. The sample group of GP practices can be considered a convenience sample. While we did contact all GPs in the area, we did not randomly choose from those willing to participate. We did so to achieve higher numbers of participants but this could have led to a selection bias.

Generally, the Bonn area has a high socio-economic status, so we controlled for this factor using educational status as an indicator and tried to achieve socio-economic heterogeneity concerning the location of the participating practices. As shown in Table 2, there was no significant difference between COMM® - Score positive and negative patients in relation to their educational status. Furthermore, age adjusted average educational levels in Germany did not differ greatly when compared with the group of COMM® - Score positive patients (basic high school education or lower in COMM® - Score positive patients: 64.3%, age adjusted German average: 59.9%) [22].

The COMM® is a reliable and valid screening tool to help detect current aberrant drug-related behaviour among chronic pain patients [12]. We used a thorough method of translation and German language adaptation. Data from China suggests that the COMM® shows satisfactory reliability and validity, despite the arguably high cultural gap between China and the US [23]. Still it is a shortcoming of this study, that we did not perform tests for internal consistency, test-retest reliability, exploratory factor analysis and confirmatory factor analysis.

Conclusion

In summary, our study showed that 31.5% of patients with CNCP on LTOT in Germany might be at a high risk for aberrant drug behaviour. This does not signify that these patients are addicted yet, albeit their risk is probably increased. Considering opioids shortcomings (low therapeutic ratio, lack of documented effectiveness in the treatment of several aspects of chronic non-cancer pain), these at risk patients should be followed up regularly. Depression should always be screened for and treated in CNCP and the high co-incidence of addiction risk and depression should be acknowledged when doing so.

Abbreviations
CNCP: Chronic non-cancer pain; COMM®: Current opioid misuse measure; LTOT: Long-term opioid therapy

Acknowledgements
We thank Inflexxion™ for giving their consent to use the COMM® in this study. We thank Indivior Germany™ for allowing us to use their german translation of the COMM®.

Authors' contributions
JMJ designed the study with LB and drafted main parts of the paper. LB gathered data, performed statistical analysis and contributed to the development of the paper. MB contributed to the development of the paper. RS gave support in statistical analysis and helped drafting the paper. KW had the initial idea and helped drafting the final paper. All authors read and approved the final manuscript.

Ethics approval and consent to participate
The study was carried out under the declaration of Helsinki. It received ethical approval by the Ethics Committee of the Medical Faculty of the University of Bonn (No. 243/16). Participants received oral and written information on the study as well as the questionnaire. They were then given the option to put an empty or filled out anonymous questionnaire in a sealed box which was later handed over to the researchers. This procedure was used to give patients the opportunity of non-participation without being revealed. The return of a completed questionnaire was then interpreted as informed consent obtained from participants.

Competing interests
Indivior Germany™ gave us consent to use their translation of the COMM® thereby saving us the effort of high-quality translation. Klaus Weckbecker was a member of the advisory board of Indivior Germany™, manufacturer of Buprenorphine, a treatment option for opioid addiction. Additionally he received fees for lectures on addiction medicine from the same company. He has terminated these activities in 2015.
All other authors declare no conflict of interest.

Author details
[1]Institute of General Practice and Family Medicine, Bonn University Clinic, Sigmund-Freud-Street 25, 53127 Bonn, Germany. [2]Department for Health Services Research, Carl von Ossietzky Universität Oldenburg, Post office box 2503, 26111 Oldenburg, Germany.

References
1. WHO Model Lists of Essential Medicines [Internet]. [cited 2017 Jun 30]. Available from: http://www.who.int/medicines/publications/essentialmedicines/EML_2017_ExecutiveSummary.pdf?ua=1
2. Frieden TR, Houry D. Reducing the Risks of Relief — The CDC Opioid-Prescribing Guideline. N Engl J Med. 2016;374:1501–4.
3. National Institute on Drug Abuse: Overdose Death Rates [Internet]. [cited 2017 Jan 11]. Available from: https://www.drugabuse.gov/related-topics/trends-statistics/overdose-death-rates
4. Vowles KE, McEntee ML, Julnes PS, Frohe T, Ney JP, van der Goes DN. Rates of opioid misuse, abuse, and addiction in chronic pain: a systematic review and data synthesis. Pain. 2015;156:569–76.
5. Website [Internet]. [cited 2017 Aug 15]. Available from: Narcotic Drugs - Technical Reports [Internet]. International Narcotics Control Board. [cited 2017 Jun 7] ; Available from: https://www.incb.org/incb/en/narcotic-drugs/
6. Casati A, Sedefov R, Pfeiffer-Gerschel T. Misuse of medicines in the European Union: a systematic review of the literature. Eur Addict Res. 2012;18:228–45.

7. Schubert I, Ihle P, Sabatowski R. Increase in opiate prescription in Germany between 2000 and 2010: a study based on insurance data. Dtsch Arztebl Int. 2013;110:45–51.
8. Marschall U, L'hoest H, Radbruch L, Häuser W. Long-term opioid therapy for chronic non-cancer pain in Germany. Eur J Pain. 2016;20:767–76.
9. Fischer B, Keates A, Bühringer G, Reimer J, Rehm J. Non-medical use of prescription opioids and prescription opioid-related harms: why so markedly higher in North America compared to the rest of the world? Addiction. 2014;109:177–81.
10. Häuser W, Petzke F, Radbruch L, Tölle TR. The opioid epidemic and the long-term opioid therapy for chronic noncancer pain revisited: a transatlantic perspective. Pain Manag. 2016;6:249–63.
11. Sullivan MD, Howe CQ. Opioid therapy for chronic pain in the United States: promises and perils. Pain. 2013;154(Suppl 1):S94–100.
12. Butler SF, Budman SH, Fanciullo GJ, Jamison RN. Cross validation of the current opioid misuse measure to monitor chronic pain patients on opioid therapy. Clin J Pain. 2010;26:770–6.
13. Sperber AD. Translation and validation of study instruments for cross-cultural research. Gastroenterology. 2004;126:S124–8.
14. Busch MA, Maske UE, Ryl L, Schlack R, Hapke U. Prävalenz von depressiver Symptomatik und diagnostizierter Depression bei Erwachsenen in Deutschland. Bundesgesundheitsblatt - Gesundheitsforschung - Gesundheitsschutz. 2013;56:733–9.
15. Breivik H, Collett B, Ventafridda V, Cohen R, Gallacher D. Survey of chronic pain in Europe: Prevalence, impact on daily life, and treatment. Eur J Pain. 2006;10:287.
16. Edlund MJ, Martin BC, Fan M-Y, Devries A, Braden JB, Sullivan MD. Risks for opioid abuse and dependence among recipients of chronic opioid therapy: Results from the TROUP Study. Drug Alcohol Depend. 2010;112:90–8.
17. Turk DC, Swanson KS, Gatchel RJ. Predicting opioid misuse by chronic pain patients: a systematic review and literature synthesis. Clin J Pain. 2008;24:497–508.
18. National Institute on Drug Abuse. America's Addiction to Opioids: Heroin and Prescription Drug Abuse [Internet]. [cited 2017 Mar 29]. Available from: https://www.drugabuse.gov/about-nida/legislative-activities/testimony-to-congress.
19. Hush JM, Michaleff Z, Maher CG, Refshauge K. Individual, physical and psychological risk factors for neck pain in Australian office workers: a 1-year longitudinal study. Eur Spine J. 2009;18:1532–40.
20. Fricton JR, Kroening R, Haley D, Siegert R. Myofascial pain syndrome of the head and neck: a review of clinical characteristics of 164 patients. Oral Surg Oral Med Oral Pathol. 1985;60:615–23.
21. Cohen SP, Hooten WM. Advances in the diagnosis and management of neck pain. BMJ. 2017;358:j3221.
22. DESTATIS - German Statistics Agency [Internet]. [cited 2017 Aug 24]. Available from: https://www.destatis.de/DE/Publikationen/Thematisch/BildungForschungKultur/Bildungsstand/BildungsstandBevoelkerung5210002167004.pdf?__blob=publicationFile
23. Zhao Y, Li Y, Zhang X, Lou F. Translation and validation of the Chinese version of the Current Opioid Misuse Measure (COMM) for patients with chronic pain in Mainland China. Health Qual Life Outcomes. 2015;13:147.

12

Long-term impact of evidence-based quality improvement for facilitating medical home implementation on primary care health professional morale

Lisa S. Meredith[1,2]* (iD), Benjamin Batorsky[3], Matthew Cefalu[1], Jill E. Darling[4], Susan E. Stockdale[2,5], Elizabeth M. Yano[2,6] and Lisa V. Rubenstein[2,7]

Abstract

Background: Poor morale among primary care providers (PCPs) and staff can undermine the success of patient-centered care models such as the patient-centered medical home that rely on highly coordinated inter-professional care teams. Medical home literature hypothesizes that participation in quality improvement can ease medical home transformation. No studies, however, have assessed the impact of quality improvement participation on morale (e.g., burnout or dissatisfaction) during transformation. The objective of this study is to examine whether primary care practices participating in evidence-based quality improvement (EBQI) during medical home transformation reduced burnout and increased satisfaction over time compared to non-participating practices.

Methods: We used a longitudinal quasi-experimental design to examine the impact of EBQI (vs. no EBQI), a multi-level, interdisciplinary approach for engaging frontline primary care practices in developing evidence-based improvement innovations and tools for spread on PCP and staff morale following the 2010 national implementation of the medical home model in the Veterans Health Administration. The sample included 356 primary care employees (107 primary care providers and 249 staff) from 23 primary care practices (6 intervention and 17 comparison) within one Veterans Health Administration region. Three intervention practices began EBQI in 2011 (early) and three more began EBQI in 2012 (late). Three waves of surveys were administered across 42 months beginning in November 2011 and ending in January 2016 approximately 2 years 18 months apart. We used repeated measures analysis of the survey data on medical home teams. Main outcome measures were the emotional exhaustion subscale from the Maslach Burnout Inventory, and job satisfaction.

Results: Six of 26 approved EBQI innovations directly addressed provider and staff morale; all 26 addressed medical home implementation challenges. Survey rates were 63% for baseline and 48% for both follow-up waves. Age was associated with lower burnout among PCPs ($p = .039$) and male PCPs had higher satisfaction ($p = .037$). Controlling for practice and PCP/staff characteristics, burnout increased by 5 points for PCPs in comparison practices ($p = .024$) and decreased by 1.4 points for early and 6.8 points ($p = .039$) for the late EBQI practices.

Conclusions: Engaging PCPs and staff in EBQI reduced burnout over time during medical home transformation.

Keywords: Implementation, Evidence-based quality improvement, Patient-centered medical home, Primary care, Veterans

* Correspondence: lisa_meredith@rand.org
[1]RAND Corporation, 1776 Main Street, Santa Monica, CA 90407-2138, USA
[2]VA HSR&D Center for the Study of Healthcare Innovation, Implementation, and Policy, Los Angeles, CA, USA
Full list of author information is available at the end of the article

Background

Delivering patient-centered accountable care across enrolled populations requires high functioning primary care practice teams as the basis for prevention, chronic disease care, and links to specialty, hospital, and long-term care [1]. Burnout among primary care providers (PCPs) (defined here as internal medicine and family physicians, physician assistants, or nurse practitioners) and their team members (often referenced as staff) can impede achievement of high functioning primary care [2, 3]. High levels of burnout in clinical teams are associated with poorer quality healthcare and decreased patient safety [4, 5]. In the work presented here, we test an approach, termed evidence-based quality improvement (EBQI), for accelerating change and maintaining morale in six engaged primary care sites during large scale implementation of a new team-based, patient centered primary care model (the patient centered medical home).

Burnout is a complex multi-dimensional condition characterized by emotional exhaustion (EE, the sense of being overwhelmed and exhausted), cynicism (feeling depersonalized and detached from the job), and professional efficacy (the lack of a sense of personal accomplishment related to work goals) [6, 7]. EE is considered to be the most central of the three components, is the most widely reported, and in some studies is the first domain that manifests when the full burnout syndrome is developing [8]. Burnout, and its EE component in particular, can be associated with lowered job satisfaction and increased job turnover [9, 10]. We assess EBQI outcomes based on PCP and staff EE and job satisfaction; we refer to these two concepts as indicators of PCP and staff morale.

Patient-centered medical home models can improve both patient outcomes [11] and provider morale [12, 13]. The model enhances the capabilities of primary care practices by linking all patients to both a continuity PCP and the PCP's team. In the model, the patients work closely with their assigned PCP and team staff including e.g., a registered nurse, a health technician or licensed practical nurse, and a clerk. They also have access to extended team members that serve several PCP teams, such as a social worker, dietitian, and pharmacist. The model challenges traditional primary care disciplinary roles substantially by depending on strong team integration and functioning, with each member working "at the top of his or her license" [10, 11, 14].

Despite the enthusiasm for the medical home model, the stress inherent in transforming into high functioning, accountable primary care teams [10] runs the risk of increasing provider and staff burnout [9, 10] and reducing morale, thus impeding successful model implementation. The stresses are due not only to new working relationships, but to the many administrative challenges of adapting or replacing administrative systems such as scheduling, information systems, or performance monitoring. Yet it is particularly critical to maintain morale during transformation; falling levels can result in a vicious cycle of higher turnover within a primary care practice, less care continuity for patients, and greater burdens on continuing providers and staff. Just when expertise is most needed, trained team members may be replaced by less experienced professionals, causing continued turnover due to a poor work environment [6].

While much literature has examined the prevalence of burnout [15, 16] and its potential causes, very little has been written about how healthcare organizations might work to reduce it [9, 17]. Engagement in quality improvement has the potential to ease transformation by supporting development of local innovations for addressing transformation problems and for achieving needed care redesigns. Engagement might also empower teams to problem-solve in general, thus reducing feelings of stress, helplessness, and apathy [3] that can lead to burnout. Job satisfaction, in turn, is typically reduced when burnout occurs [18].

The Veterans Health Administration implemented its medical home model (termed Patient Aligned Care Teams, or PACT) nationally beginning in 2010 across its over 900 primary care sites [19, 20]. In addition to continuity team care, the implementation emphasized visit modalities other than face-to-face care, advanced or "open access" appointment scheduling, and new electronic performance measures accessible to sites on dashboards [21]. By engaging practices transforming into the new model in EBQI, a method tested both inside and outside the Veterans Health Administration [22], we aimed both to promote development of a high morale primary care quality improvement culture and to support systems re-engineering during transformation [22–30]. We previously documented high adherence to the EBQI model among the engaged sites [24]. We also found enhanced adoption of non-face-to-face care in EBQI compared to comparison sites [28]. We know of no prior work examining the impact of EBQI or similar approaches on morale.

EBQI aims to engage front-line clinical teams in developing innovations that reflect interdisciplinary input and are aligned with multi-level healthcare system leadership priorities. In this study, EBQI-engaged primary care sites developed quality councils [25] and participated in workgroups that generated proposals for innovations directed at medical home implementation; innovations are reviewed by regional leaders. Innovation teams discuss their approved projects in across-site telephone meetings and during yearly in person conferences that also engage regional leaders.

We addressed two questions: (1) Was transformation to the patient-centered medical home model associated with improved primary care practice morale (measured as emotional exhaustion and job satisfaction) over time? (2) Did engagement in EBQI improve morale among primary care practice's providers and staff?

Methods

Design and setting

We compared changes over time in primary care provider and staff morale in EBQI-engaged practices and non-EBQI-engaged practices within the desert Pacific administrative region of the Veterans Health Administration. The desert pacific region breaks into five distinct healthcare networks, each including a medical center and community-based outpatient clinics. Three of the five networks agreed to participate and each selected a specific clinic in which to employ a Veterans Administration Improvement Laboratory facilitated EBQI approach. Three distinct primary care practices implemented EBQI-PACT beginning shortly after national PACT implementation in August 2010. Three additional primary care practices from the same three medical center-based networks initiated EBQI 19 months later (May 2012), for a total of six intervention practices. The 17 remaining comparison practices in the region underwent PACT implementation without EBQI.

Exposure

EBQI promotes cross-discipline, data-driven problem solving in local primary care practices. EBQI aligns these local practices with organizational priorities to sustain successful QI innovations over time and spread them across teams and clinics. Specifically, the EBQI intervention focused on engaging and empowering front-line primary care teams with multi-level, interdisciplinary stakeholders in structured EBQI, and facilitated provider and staff initiated innovation projects. For EBQI practices, we engaged regional and local health system leaders and two frontline primary care practices from each of three of five local medical center-based Veterans Health Administration healthcare systems in the region.

The EBQI intervention included a proposal review and approval process that solicited brief innovation proposals from front-line providers and staff and provided approved innovation projects with additional support. Innovations could be proposed through either the EBQI practice's quality council (supported by a quality council coordinator) [25] or through an across-EBQI site workgroup. The three medical center based networks supported the approved innovations with limited release time for the leaders of approved innovation projects, based on a prior Memorandum of Understanding initiated through the improvement laboratory with support of regional leaders. Regional leaders (administrative, quality, medical care, information technology, patient advocacy, pharmacy experts) served to set QI priorities by reviewing and rating the submitted proposals (a total of 71 during the time period reported here). We also convened yearly collaborative learning sessions across EBQI practices. We provided quality councils with local primary care site audit and feedback [25] comprised of practice level data on their patients, providers and staff, including provider and staff burnout, and assisted them in learning to access practice administrative data themselves.

Approved proposals (a total of 26) received a responsive innovation evidence review [31, 32] a budget based on the proposal budget request (average $12,000), and QI facilitation for project management and measures. Successful projects generated tools; if the innovation showed spread to at least one other site, the improvement laboratory assisted in formatting the tool and posting it on a Veterans Health Administration accessible SharePoint site (a total of 12 tools). An example of a tool is a step-by-step guide for enrolling and authenticating Veteran patients to use the online health portal for Veterans Health Administration. Additional volunteer projects could be undertaken by practices as well. All innovations addressed specific PACT-based problems or challenges. For example, one project addressed reducing homelessness among Veterans and another aimed to reduce unscheduled visits. There were six PACT team member-initiated, quality council approved projects designed to address provider and staff burnout and six volunteer projects addressing burnout completed during the reported time period.

Participants

Our survey sample included all PACT PCPs (physicians, nurse practitioners, and physician assistants) and core PACT team staff (nurses, care/case managers, health educators, health technicians, medical assistants), as well as axillary staff such as dietitians/nutritionists, integrated mental health professionals, social workers, and pharmacists in EBQI and comparison sites, identified based on Veterans Health Administration's electronic Primary Care Management Module. We excluded trainees from all disciplines.

Data collection

We developed two versions of a survey: one for PCPs (Additional file 1) and one for staff (Additional file 2) that were identical in content where relevant. At each of three survey waves, we invited all PCPs and staff to complete the surveys online or to request a mail version. Surveys were administered from November 30, 2011 to March 30 2012 (wave 1), August 1, 2013 to January 15, 2014 (wave 2), and September 10, 2015 to January 8, 2016 (wave 3). We informed potential participants in an initial email request for participation that included consent language which made it clear that clicking the button to start the survey indicated that they have consented. All individuals who visited the web site or requested a mail version were entered into a drawing to win one of two iPad Air 2 s (in each wave).

Measures

We examined two outcome measures. Emotional exhaustion burnout was the primary outcome, assessed with the 9-item subscale of the original Maslach Burnout Inventory ($\alpha = .92$) [33, 34]. We scored the subscale by summing across the items rated on a 7-point (0–6) frequency scale (never, a few times a year, every month, a few times a month, every week, a few times a week, every day). Because of the overall burden of the study survey, we were unable to include items for the other two subscales (cynicism and professional efficacy). We measured past month job satisfaction with a single item, "Overall, I am satisfied with my job," rated on a 5-point Likert scale.

We specified our 3-category *independent variable* using two binary variables to indicate each of the two EBQI intervention groups (early and late implementation) with the comparison group as the omitted category.

Covariates

We controlled for age in years, gender with a binary indicator for male (vs. female), race/ethnicity (with binary indicators Latino and non-white/non-Latino relative to white as the omitted category), and number of years at the study clinic.

Analysis

For the analysis, we included PCPs/staff who completed at least two of the three waves of surveys administered at baseline, approximately 20 and approximately 42 months later. We used three-wave repeated measures analyses in the form of a linear mixed model to estimate the total effect of EBQI vs. the comparison practice providers and staff on the emotional exhaustion subscale of burnout and the single item measure of job satisfaction [35]. We included main effects for survey wave and intervention group, their interaction, and random effects to account for the repeated measures within individual and the clustering of individuals within clinics controlling for covariates.

Results

Survey and sample characteristics

The overall response rates were 63% for baseline, and 48% for both follow-up waves. Response rates for professionals in EBQI practices were the same as professionals in comparison practices at waves 1 and 2 but were higher in wave 3 (38% vs. 55%). The analysis sample included 356 professionals (107 PCPs and 249 staff).

Response rates were higher for staff compared with PCPs for all three waves. There were no significant differences between the groups of providers (Table 1) with the exception of years in the clinic; EBQI providers spent 8 years on average in their assigned practices compared with 5.2 years for providers in comparison practices ($p = .011$).

Effect of EBQI-PACT on EE burnout over time

Figure 1 illustrates the unadjusted findings for EE over time for each of the three groups (early EBQI, late EBQI, and comparison practices) separately for PCPs and staff. We found large intervention effects over time for PCP burnout, particularly by wave 3, but little or no change over time in staff EE.

Table 2 shows the estimated effect of EBQI and the changes over time based on difference in differences analyses in each of the three groups stratified by provider type after adjusting for covariates. From wave 1 to wave 3, relative to the comparison practices and accounting for each practices' baseline EE score, the early EBQI-PACT practices had lower EE scores over time by 1.42 points (not significant) and the late implementation EBQI-PACT practices had significantly lower EE scores by 6.82 points ($p = .039$), a difference equivalent to one-half a standard deviation.

Table 2 also shows absolute change over time between wave 1 and wave 3 within each of the three groups after adjusting for covariates. PCPs in comparison practices had increased EE scores over time of 4.96 points ($p = .024$). This five-point increase is equivalent to 0.40 of a standard deviation on the 0–54 point EE scale. Though not significant, scores also increased for PCPs in early EBQI-PACT practices (by 3.54 points) but decreased by 1.86 points for late EBQI-PACT practices.

Table 2 further shows the absolute differences in EE between the comparison group and the early and late EBQI groups by survey wave, after adjusting for covariates (i.e., without taking account of baseline practice differences). There were no significant differences between the comparison practices and the early EBQI-PACT practices at any survey wave. However, the late EBQI-PACT practices showed a marginally significant difference in EE by wave 3 of 6.23 points lower than comparison practices ($p = .073$). Among the set of covariates, only age was significantly associated with EE over time for PCPs; older PCPs had lower EE scores by 0.29 points ($p = .039$).

Effect of EBQI on job satisfaction over time

The unadjusted patterns of effects for job satisfaction (Fig. 2), and adjusted estimates appear in Table 2. We found no significant differences in the difference in differences analyses, and no significant changes in PCP job

Table 1 Demographic and Professional Characteristics of Primary Care Employees by Study Group

Characteristic	EBQI (n = 181)[a]	Comparison (n = 175)[a]	Full Sample (n = 356)[a]
Female, no. (%)	124 (67)	121 (70)	245 (69)
Latino, no. (%)	20 (11)	15 (9)	35 (10)
Non-white non-Latino, n (%)	87 (47)	71 (41)	158 (44)
Age, mean (SD), y	47.4 (10.0)	47.6 (11.0)	46.8 (10.9)
Years in clinic, mean (SD)	8.0 (8.1)	5.2 (7.1)	7.0 (7.7)*
Job type, no. (%)			
Physician			75 (21)
General practice/family medicine	3 (2)	7 (4)	10 (3)
Internal medicine	39 (22)	20 (11)	59 (17)
Other specialty[a]	3 (2)	3 (2)	6 (2)
Nurse practitioner	12 (7)	16 (9)	28 (8)
Physician assistant	2 (1)	2 (1)	4 (1)
Registered nurse	48 (27)	49 (28)	97 (27)
Licensed practical/vocational nurse	37 (20)	41 (23)	78 (22)
Mental health professional	4 (2)	4 (2)	8 (2)
Social worker	1 (1)	5 (3)	6 (2)
Dietician or nutritionist	5 (3)	3 (2)	8 (2)
Pharmacist	11 (6)	12 (7)	23 (6)
Health/medical technician/assistant/clerk	8 (4)	2 (1)	10 (3)
Clerk	8 (4)	11 (6)	19 (5)

*$p < .01$, where EBQI and comparison employees differ significantly for these variables
[a]Other specialties include rheumatology, geriatrics, and infectious diseases

satisfaction in EBQI versus comparison practices. In adjusted results testing absolute within group differences over time, we observed a significant decrease in satisfaction over time for staff in comparison practices and no change over time for staff in early EBQI practices or for change over time for staff in late EBQI practices. Specifically, staff in comparison practices had significantly reduced job satisfaction by 0.39 points ($p = .008$), but for those in early implementation of EBQI group, this effect was near zero, and in

the late EBQI group, burnout decreased by 0.31 points though not significantly. Of the covariates, only gender for staff was significantly associated with satisfaction for PCPs; men had satisfaction scores 0.39 points higher ($p = .037$), approximately 35% of a standard deviation.

Discussion

Experts agree that high functioning primary care teams, such as those featured in patient-centered medical home

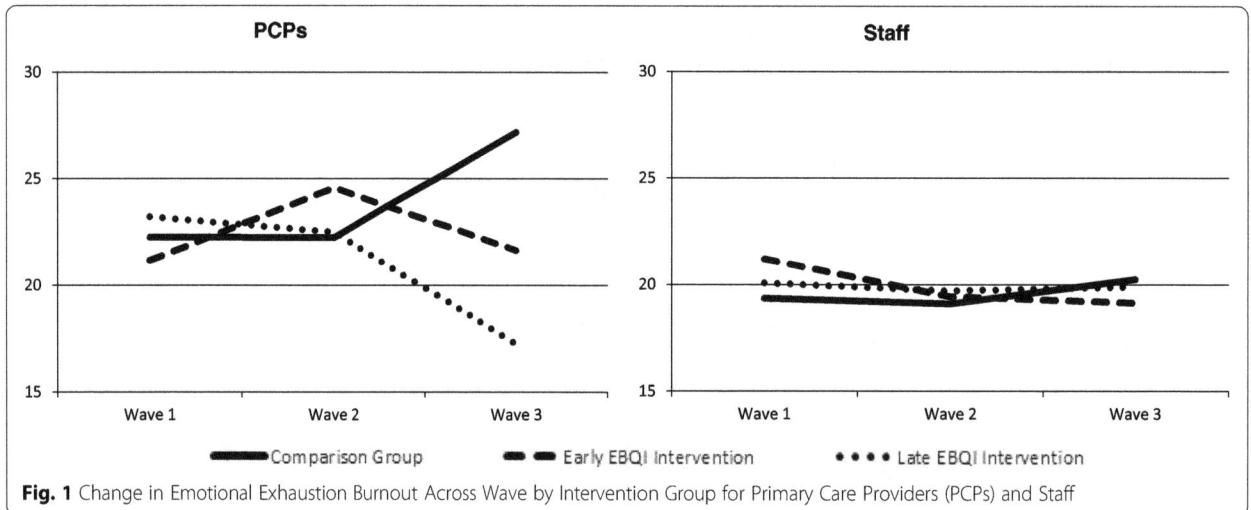

Fig. 1 Change in Emotional Exhaustion Burnout Across Wave by Intervention Group for Primary Care Providers (PCPs) and Staff

Table 2 Results from Regression Models for Change in Emotional Exhaustion Burnout and Job Satisfaction, Score (CI)

Variable	Emotional Exhaustion Burnout		Job Satisfaction	
	PCPs	Staff	PCPs	Staff
Intercept	40.38 (25.81, 54.94)	14.88 (7.34, 22.43)	2.38 (1.23, 3.54)	4.26 (3.72, 4.80)
Difference in Differences (Wave 3 – Wave 1)				
Early EBQI-PACT vs. Comparison	−1.42 (−8.74, 5.90)	−1.44 (−7.02, 4.15)	−0.12 (−0.77, 0.54)	0.36 (−0.16, 0.88)
Late EBQI-PACT vs. Comparison	−6.82 (−13.29, −0.35)*	−1.30 (−6.72, 4.11)	0.22 (−0.38, 0.82)	0.08 (−0.43, 0.60)
Change within Group (Wave 3 – Wave 1)				
Comparison Group	4.96 (0.66, 9.25)*	0.84 (−2.28, 3.96)	−0.21 (−0.61, 0.18)	−0.39 (−0.68, −0.10)**
Early EBQI-PACT Intervention	3.54 (−2.53, 9.60)	−0.60 (−5.28, 4.08)	−0.33 (−0.86, 0.20)	−0.03 (−0.47, 0.40)
Late EBQI-PACT Intervention	−1.86 (−6.84, 3.11)	−0.46 (−4.98, 4.06)	0.01 (−0.45, 0.47)	−0.31 (−0.74, 0.12)
Change from Wave 1 (Comparison Group)				
Wave 1 (Reference group)	–	–	–	–
Wave 2	1.75 (−2.18, 5.69)	0.03 (−2.77, 2.83)	−0.09 (−0.43, 0.26)	−0.22 (−0.48, 0.05)
Wave 3	4.96 (0.66, 9.25)*	0.84 (−2.28, 3.96)	−0.21 (−0.61, 0.18)	−0.39 (−0.68, −0.10)**
Covariates				
Age, y	−0.29 (−0.57, −0.01)*	0.06 (−0.08, 0.21)	0.02 (0.00, 0.04)	0.00 (−0.01, 0.01)
Male	−3.71 (−8.30, 0.89)	−1.17 (−4.78, 2.43)	0.39 (0.02, 0.75)*	0.08 (−0.17, 0.33)
Latino	−5.50 (−13.16, 2.15)	−2.25 (−6.72, 2.22)	0.36 (−0.26, 0.97)	0.00 (−0.33, 0.33)
Non-white, Nor-Latino	0.64 (−4.38, 5.66)	2.79 (−0.41, 5.99)	−0.19 (−0.59, 0.20)	−0.18 (−0.40, 0.04)
Years at clinic	−0.11 (−0.37, 0.16)	0.11 (−0.13, 0.36)	0.01 (−0.01, 0.03)	0.00 (−0.01, 0.02)

*$p < .05$; **$p < .01$

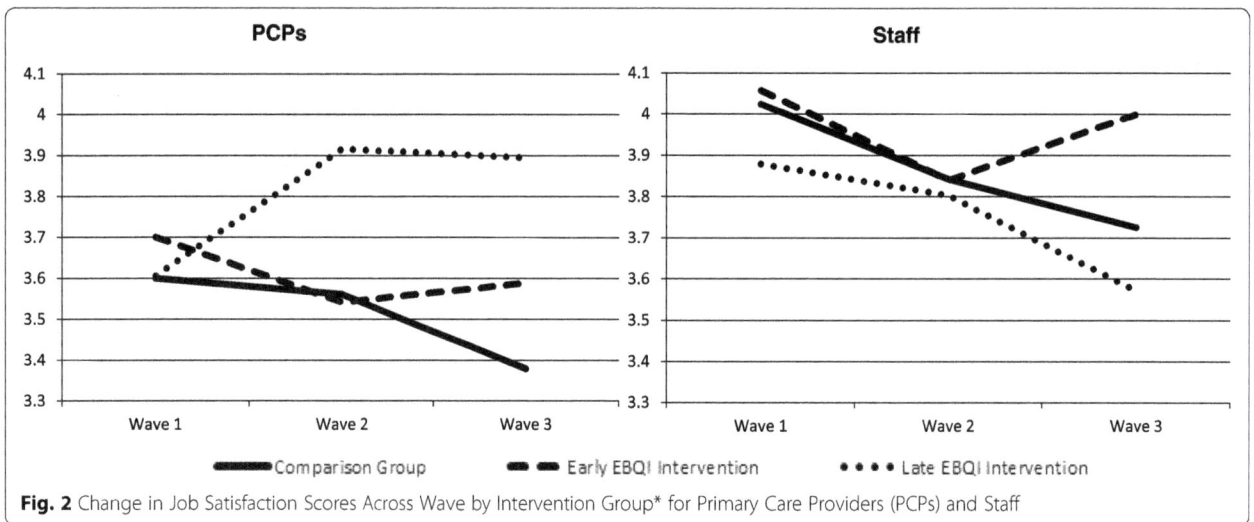

Fig. 2 Change in Job Satisfaction Scores Across Wave by Intervention Group* for Primary Care Providers (PCPs) and Staff

models, are essential for delivery of high value accountable care across enrolled patient populations. Yet achieving transformation to these models is challenging. We examined whether EBQI [24] was effective in reducing PCP/staff burnout [33, 34] or increasing satisfaction during national transformation to the Veterans Health Administration's medical home model. We used a rigorous quasi-experimental design that compared change over time in intervention clinics (EBQI in the context of the medical home) vs. comparison clinics (medical home alone) within the first five years of transformation. We found a significant EBQI effect on reducing burnout among PCPs, but no significant effect for early EBQI-PACT practices or for late EBQI-PACT practices relative to comparison practices.

Our findings are important because burnout and dissatisfaction are associated with adverse consequences for patient care [21, 36] and with increased job turnover across industries [2, 15, 37, 38]. Worsened burnout and job satisfaction can become acute during transformation to the patient-centered medical home [2], threatening the success of the new model. Only PCPs had significantly reduced EE burnout but not staff. Conversely, job satisfaction was better over time only for staff but not for PCPs. A possible explanation for this finding is that because PCPs have overall responsibility for creating and leading functional teams, their role in PACT is inherently more stressful than for staff which makes them more prone to burnout. This longitudinal observational study is the first to test whether a systematic approach to engaging front-line primary care practices in inter-professional medical home-related quality improvement innovation might ameliorate or reduce burnout and increase job satisfaction during the difficult work of implementing the medical home model.

This study followed PCPs and staff for nearly five years after national patient-centered medical home

implementation in Veterans Health Administration, far longer than in previous studies of change in burnout and satisfaction, and began over a year after medical home implementation was nationally mandated in Veterans Health Administration. The study thus spanned the initial five years of medical home transformation. Additionally, unlike most prior work, this study assessed PCPs and staff separately, given that medical home implementation role and task changes are substantially different for PCPs compared to staff [39, 40]. Further, we do not know if the innovation efforts were initiated by PCPs, other types of providers and staff, or with equal input across type of provider/staff. It is possible that the reason we found a positive impact on PCP burnout but not staff burnout is that because most of the innovations were spearheaded by PCPs, the psychological investment was greater for them. Greater psychological investment is likely associated with more engagement in change. Heavier investments, particularly by enthusiastic employees, have been found to have positive associations with a number of work characteristics including less role ambiguity and greater autonomy [41]. Although a few studies have found reductions in burnout over time post-medical home implementation, these have been limited to one or two years [11, 13]. Two years may be too short; one study found that practices that were relatively more successful at implementing the medical home model did so only after more than two years of implementation [42]. Adopting new models of care requires changing the culture of practice and getting past initial change fatigue as well as having an infrastructure that enables transformation [43]. Health systems should consider tracking provider engagement and well-being (including burnout levels) along with standard institutional measures such as cost, quality, and patient satisfaction) [17] following medical home implementation.

Major change takes time and resources, particularly at the organizational level. This is possibly why we did not observe a statistically significant difference between early EBQI and the comparison group for either EE or job satisfaction. National Veterans Health Administration PACT implementation, experienced by both intervention and comparison groups in this study, included a well-documented care model, mandated changes in staffing, time-limited increases in special funding for implementation, data resources including a national dashboard with primary care practice level PACT process measures, web-based tools, redesign collaboratives, and substantial PACT training opportunities for providers and staff. Nevertheless, without EBQI, burnout increased for comparison practices. EBQI appeared to have a protective effect, avoiding significant worsening of morale (burnout and satisfaction) among the early EBQI group and improving it in the late EBQI group.

In a recent meta-analysis of interventions to prevent and reduce physician burnout, West and colleagues [44] identified a total of 15 randomized trials and 37 cohort studies that were relevant. They found that interventions that were focused on the individual as well as interventions that were focused on structural changes or at the organizational-level were associated with clinically meaningful reductions in burnout. The statistical review of these studies is the first step toward understanding how to engage the healthcare workforce in strategies to boost morale and prevent or minimize burnout and improve morale under hyperkinetic circumstances. The EBQI approach used here includes both individual and organizational strategies (i.e., interdisciplinary leadership participation, management assistance from quality council coordinators, and technical assistance from improvement laboratory researchers) by engaging individual providers as well as administrators and leadership in the transformation process. The approach emphasizes psychological factors that can make adaptation to change a more positive experience [45, 46]. It also emphasizes using systematic, interdisciplinary, organizationally aligned redesign to solve the inevitable issues arising from transformation. The redesign efforts used local innovation, formal quality improvement methods, outcome measures, and tool-based spread. Our findings suggest that the EBQI approach holds promise for putting the joy back into practice [3], as well as for more rapid implementation of medical home features [28].

Our study has a number of important limitations warranting caution in interpreting results. First, our design was quasi-experimental; participating medical center-based network leaders chose EBQI practices for a variety of reasons. Our repeated measures analyses and covariates control for major differences between EBQI and comparison practices at baseline. However, our sample size limited our ability to control for all possible differences and effects of unmeasured variables cannot be ruled out. Our restricted sample size also prevented disaggregating the sample staff to examine specific experiences of mental health providers or pharmacists. Also, while our self-report burnout measure could be biased, we would expect this effect to influence baseline as well as follow-up results. Additionally, we measured burnout based on only the emotional exhaustion subscale of the Maslach burnout inventory; we did not administer the other two subscales at waves 2 and 3. Our previous analyses of wave 1 data indicated that the emotional exhaustion subscale was highly correlated with the other two Maslach subscales (cynicism and professional efficacy) and more sensitive to variations in PACT.

Conclusion

Engaging PCPs and staff in EBQI reduced burnout over time during medical home transformation. Observed effects may have been due to more rapid solving of medical home-related problems and challenges through system redesign or the other types of quality improvement innovations undertaken by EBQI practices, including innovations directly aimed at addressing burnout. They may also have been due to increased engagement of PCPs and staff in medical home implementation. Healthcare systems should consider EBQI as a systematic method for assisting with large organizational changes, such as medical home implementation.

Abbreviations
EBQI: Evidence-based quality improvement; EE: Emotional exhaustion; medical home: PACT: Patient Aligned Care Teams; Patient-Centered Medical Home; PCP: Primary Care Providers; VA: Veterans Administration; VHA: Veterans Health Administration

Acknowledgements
The authors wish to acknowledge the contributions made by Adeyemi Okunogbe, M.D. MPhil, Yan Wang, MPhil, and Gulrez Azhar, MPhil, for assistance with data preparation, Barbara Simon, M.A., for survey methods expertise, the RAND Multimode Interviewing Capability (MMIC) team (Tania Gutsche, Bas Veerman, Julie Newell, and Bart Orriens, Diana Malouf, and Alerk Amin), and Karleen Giannitrapani, Ph.D. for providing comments on the draft manuscript. We also thank Rosie Velasquez for her assistance with manuscript preparation. We appreciate Bing Han, Ph.D. and Martin Lee, Ph.D., for early statistical guidance.

Funding
Funding for the PACT Demonstration Laboratory initiative, which includes the Veterans Administration Improvement Laboratory, was provided to Drs. Rubenstein, Yano, and Altman from the VA Office of Patient Care Services. Dr. Yano's effort was contributed through a VA HSR&D Senior Research Career Scientist award (Project #05–195).

Authors' contributions

LM, Survey design, data analysis, data interpretation, and manuscript preparation. BB, Data analysis, data interpretation, and manuscript preparation. MC, Data weighting, imputation, analysis, and interpretation; manuscript preparation. JD, Survey design, data interpretation, and manuscript preparation. SS, Survey design, data interpretation and manuscript preparation. EY, Study conceptualization/design; data interpretation and manuscript preparation. LR, Study conceptualization/design; data interpretation, and manuscript preparation. All authors have read and approved the manuscript.

Ethics approval and consent to participate

The study protocol, including ethics and consent to participate, was reviewed and approved by both the VA and RAND Institutional Review Boards (the Veterans Health Administration (VHA) Greater Los Angeles IRB and the Human Subjects Protection Committee, respectively). We informed potential participants in an initial email request for participation that included consent language which made it clear that clicking the button to start the survey indicated that they have consented.

Competing interests

The authors declare that they have no competing interests.

Author details

[1]RAND Corporation, 1776 Main Street, Santa Monica, CA 90407-2138, USA. [2]VA HSR&D Center for the Study of Healthcare Innovation, Implementation, and Policy, Los Angeles, CA, USA. [3]TriveHive, Boston, MA, USA. [4]USC Center for Economic and Social Research, Los Angeles, CA, USA. [5]Department of Psychiatry and Biobehavioral Medicine, UCLA School of Medicine, Los Angeles, CA, USA. [6]Department of Health Policy and Management, UCLA Fielding School of Public Health, Los Angeles, CA, USA. [7]UCLA Schools of Medicine and Public Health, Los Angeles, CA, USA.

References

1. Sevin C, Moore G, Shepherd J, Jacobs T, Hupke C. Transforming care teams to provide the best possible patient-centered, collaborative care. J Ambul Care Manage. 2009;32:24–31.
2. Helfrich CD, Dolan ED, Simonetti J, Reid RJ, Joos S, Wakefield BJ, et al. Elements of team-based care in a patient-centered medical home are associated with lower burnout among VA primary care employees. J Gen Intern Med. 2014;29(Suppl 2):S659–66.
3. Sinsky CA, Willard-Grace R, Schutzbank AM, Sinsky TA, Margolius D, Bodenheimer T. In search of joy in practice: a report of 23 high-functioning primary care practices. Ann Fam Med. 2013;11:272–8.
4. Salyers MP, Bonfils KA, Luther L, Firmin RL, White DA, Adams EL, et al. The relationship between professional burnout and quality and safety in healthcare: a meta-analysis. J Gen Intern Med. 2017;32(4):475–82.
5. Hall LH, Johnson J, Watt I, Tsipa A, O'Connor DB. Healthcare staff wellbeing, burnout, and patient safety: a systematic review. PLoS One. 2016;11:e0159015.
6. Maslach C, Schaufeli WB, Leiter MP. Job burnout. Annu Rev Psychol. 2001;52:397–422.
7. Maslach C, Leiter MP, Jackson SE. Making a significant difference with burnout interventions: researcher and practitioner collaboration. J Organ Behav. 2012;33:296–300.
8. Maslach C, Jackson SE, Leiter MP. Maslach Burnout Inventory Manual. Palo Alto: Consulting Psychologists Press; 1996.
9. Meredith LS, Schmidt Hackbarth N, Darling J, Rodriguez HP, Stockdale SE, Cordasco KM, et al. Emotional exhaustion in primary care during early implementation of the VA's medical home transformation: patient-aligned care team (PACT). Med Care. 2015;53:253–60.
10. Nutting PA, Miller WL, Crabtree BF, Jaen CR, Stewart EE, Stange KC. Initial lessons from the first national demonstration project on practice transformation to a patient-centered medical home. Ann Fam Med. 2009;7:254–60.
11. Reid RJ, Fishman PA, Yu O, Ross TR, Tufano JT, Soman MP, et al. Patient-centered medical home demonstration: a prospective, quasi-experimental, before and after evaluation. Am J Manag Care. 2009;15:E71–87.
12. Parker LE, de Pillis E, Altschuler A, Rubenstein LV, Meredith LS. Balancing participation and expertise: a comparison of locally and centrally managed health care quality improvement within primary care practices. Qual Health Res. 2007;17:1268–79.
13. Reid RJ, Coleman K, Johnson EA, Fishman PA, Hsu C, Soman MP, et al. The group health medical home at year two: cost savings, higher patient satisfaction, and less burnout for providers. Health Aff (Millwood). 2010;29:835–43.
14. Crabtree BF, Nutting PA, Miller WL, McDaniel RR, Stange KC, Jaen CR, et al. Primary care practice transformation is hard work insights from a 15- year developmental program of research. Med Care. 2011;49:S28–35.
15. Shanafelt T, Sloan J, Satele D, Balch C. Why do surgeons consider leaving practice? J Am Coll Surg. 2011;212:421–2.
16. Shanafelt TD, Boone S, Tan L, Dyrbye LN, Sotile W, Satele D, et al. Burnout and satisfaction with work-life balance among US physicians relative to the general US population. Arch Intern Med. 2012;172:1377–85.
17. Shanafelt TD, Dyrbye LN, West CP. Addressing physician burnout: the way forward. JAMA. 2017;317:901–2.
18. Bodenheimer T, Sinsky C. From triple to quadruple aim: care of the patient requires care of the provider. Ann Fam Med. 2014;12:573–6.
19. Klein S. The Veterans Health Administration: implementing patient-centered medical homes in the nation's largest integrated delivery system. New York: The Commonwealth Fund; 2011. https://www.commonwealthfund.org/publications/case-study/2011/sep/veterans-health-administration-implementing-patient-centered.
20. Rosland AM, Nelson K, Sun H, Dolan ED, Maynard C, Bryson C, et al. The patient-centered medical home in the veterans health administration. Am J Manag Care. 2013;19:e263–72.
21. Friedberg MW, Chen PG, Van Busum KR, Aunon FM, Pham C, Caloyeras JP, et al. Factors affecting physician professional satisfaction and their implications for patient care, health systems, and health policy. Rand health and American Medical Association. Santa Monica: RAND Corporation; 2013.
22. Rubenstein LV, Meredith LS, Parker LE, Gordon NP, Hickey SC, Oken C, et al. Impacts of evidence-based quality improvement on depression in primary care: a randomized experiment. J Gen Intern Med. 2006;21:1027–35.
23. Fortney J, Enderle M, McDougall S, Clothier J, Otero J, Altman L, et al. Implementation outcomes of evidence-based quality improvement for depression in VA community based outpatient clinics. Implement Sci. 2012;7:30.
24. Rubenstein LV, Stockdale SE, Sapir N, Altman L, Dresselhaus T, Salem-Schatz S, et al. A patient-centered primary care practice approach using evidence-based quality improvement: rationale, methods, and early assessment of implementation. J Gen Intern Med. 2014;29(Suppl 2):S589–97.
25. Stockdale SE, Zuchowski J, Rubenstein LV, Sapir N, Yano EM, Altman L, et al. Fostering evidence-based quality improvement for patient-centered medical homes: initiating local quality councils to transform primary care. Health Care Manag Rev. 2018;43(2):168–80.
26. Yano EM, Darling JE, Hamilton AB, Canelo I, Chuang E, Meredith LS, et al. Cluster randomized trial of a multilevel evidence-based quality improvement approach to tailoring VA patient aligned care teams to the needs of women veterans. Implement Sci. 2016;11:101.
27. Yano EM, Rubenstein LV, Farmer MM, Chernof BA, Mittman BS, Lanto AB, et al. Targeting primary care referrals to smoking cessation clinics does not improve quit rates: implementing evidence-based interventions into practice. Health Serv Res. 2008;43:1637–61.
28. Yoon J, Chow A, Rubenstein LV. Impact of medical home implementation through evidence-based quality improvement on utilization and costs. Med Care. 2016;54:118–25.
29. Chaney EF, Rubenstein LV, Liu CF, Yano EM, Bolkan C, Lee M, et al. Implementing collaborative care for depression treatment in primary care: a cluster randomized evaluation of a quality improvement practice redesign. Implement Sci. 2011;6:121.

30. Cohen AN, Chinman MJ, Hamilton AB, Whelan F, Young AS. Using patient-facing kiosks to support quality improvement at mental health clinics. Med Care. 2013;51:S13–20.

31. Danz MS, Hempel S, Lim YW, Shanman R, Motala A, Stockdale S, et al. Incorporating evidence review into quality improvement: meeting the needs of innovators. BMJ Qual Saf. 2013;22:931–9.

32. Hempel S, Shekelle PG, Liu JL, Sherwood Danz M, Foy R, Lim YW, et al. Development of the quality improvement minimum quality criteria set (QI-MQCS): a tool for critical appraisal of quality improvement intervention publications. BMJ Qual Saf. 2015;24:796–804.

33. Maslach C, Jackson SE. The measurement of experienced burnout. J Organ Behav. 1981;2:99–113.

34. Schaufeli WB, Leiter MP, Maslach C, et al. Maslach Burnout Inventory - General Survey (MBI-GS). In: Maslach C, Jackson SE, Leiter MP, eds. MBI Manual (3rd ed.). Palo Alto, CA: Consulting Psychologists Press. All versions of the MBI, including MBI-GS, are now published online by Mind Garden, mindgarden.com; 1996.

35. Abadie A. Semiparametric difference-in-differences estimators. Rev Econ Stud. 2005;72:1–19.

36. Shipman SA, Sinsky CA. Expanding primary care capacity by reducing waste and improving the efficiency of care. Health Aff (Millwood). 2013;32:1990–7.

37. Hinami K, Whelan CT, Wolosin RJ, Miller JA, Wetterneck TB. Worklife and satisfaction of hospitalists: toward flourishing careers. J Gen Intern Med. 2012;27:28–36.

38. Linzer M, Manwell LB, Williams ES, Bobula JA, Brown RL, Varkey AB, et al. Working conditions in primary care: physician reactions and care quality. Ann Intern Med. 2009;151:28–36. W6-9

39. Giannitrapani KF, Soban L, Hamilton AB, Rodriguez H, Huynh A, Stockdale S, et al. Role expansion on interprofessional primary care teams: barriers of role self-efficacy among clinical associates. Healthc (Amst). 2016;4:321–6.

40. Ladebue AC, Helfrich CD, Gerdes ZT, Fihn SD, Nelson KM, Sayre GG. The experience of patient aligned care team (PACT) members. Health Care Manag Rev. 2016;41:2–10.

41. Salanova M, Del Libano M, Llorens S, Schaufeli WB. Engaged, workaholic, burned-out or just 9-to-5? Toward a typology of employee well-being. Stress Health. 2014;30:71–81.

42. Sugarman JR, Phillips KE, Wagner EH, Coleman K, Abrams MK. The safety net medical home initiative: transforming care for vulnerable populations. Med Care. 2014;52:S1–10.

43. Wagner EH, Gupta R, Coleman K. Practice transformation in the safety net medical home initiative: a qualitative look. Med Care. 2014;52:S18–22.

44. West CP, Dyrbye LN, Erwin PJ, Shanafelt TD. Interventions to prevent and reduce physician burnout: a systematic review and meta-analysis. Lancet. 2016;388:2272–81.

45. Epstein RM, Privitera MR. Doing something about physician burnout. Lancet. 2016;388:2216–7.

46. Privitera MR, Rosenstein AH, Plessow F, LoCastro TM. Physician burnout and occupational stress: an inconvenient truth with unintended consequences. J Hosp Adm. 2014;4:p27.

13

Not a magic pill: a qualitative exploration of provider perspectives on antibiotic prescribing in the outpatient setting

Traci D. Yates[1*], Marion E. Davis[1], Yhenneko J. Taylor[1], Lisa Davidson[2], Crystal D. Connor[1], Katherine Buehler[1] and Melanie D. Spencer[1]

Abstract

Background: Inappropriate prescribing of antibiotics poses an urgent public health threat. Limited research has examined factors associated with antibiotic prescribing practices in outpatient settings. The goals of this study were to explore elements influencing provider decisions to prescribe antibiotics, identify provider recommendations for interventions to reduce inappropriate antibiotic use, and inform the clinical management of patients in the outpatient environment for infections that do not require antibiotics.

Methods: This was a qualitative study using semi-structured interviews with key informants. Seventeen outpatient providers (10 medical doctors and 7 advanced care practitioners) within a large healthcare system in Charlotte, North Carolina, participated. Interviews were audio recorded, transcribed, and analyzed for themes.

Results: Primary barriers to reducing inappropriate antibiotic prescribing included patient education and expectations, system-level factors, and time constraints. Providers indicated they would be interested in having system-wide, evidence-based guidelines to inform their prescribing decisions and that they would also be receptive to efforts to improve their awareness of their own prescribing practices. Results further suggested that providers experience a high demand for antibiotic prescriptions; consequently, patient education around appropriate use would be beneficial.

Conclusions: Findings suggest that antibiotic prescribing in the outpatient setting is influenced by many pressures, including patient demand and patient satisfaction. Training on appropriate antibiotic prescribing, guideline-based decision support, feedback on prescribing practices, and patient education are recommended interventions to improve levels of appropriate prescribing.

Keywords: Qualitative research, Antibiotic prescribing, Patient-provider relationships, Outpatient setting, Primary care, Antibiotic prescribing decisions, Patient antibiotic education

Background

Antibiotic resistant organisms and the infections they cause are an urgent public health threat worldwide [1]. Inappropriate antibiotic prescribing is the most significant factor behind increasing resistance that causes more than two million illnesses annually in the United States [1, 2]. Outpatient settings account for more than 154 million antibiotic prescriptions each year [3]. As much as 50% of antibiotics prescribed for acute respiratory infections and 30% of oral antibiotics prescribed across all conditions in the outpatient setting may be unnecessary or inappropriate [4]. This misuse of antibiotics is a major contributor to antibiotic resistant infections that cause over 23,000 deaths annually [5]. While several strategies to improve outpatient antibiotic prescribing have been proposed, challenges to the success of these interventions include variations across settings and geography, levels of clinician acceptance, and issues of sustainability [6–13].

* Correspondence: Traci.Yates@atriumhealth.org
[1]Center for Outcomes Research and Evaluation, Atrium Health, Charlotte, NC, USA
Full list of author information is available at the end of the article

Research on the specific factors that impact antibiotic prescribing practices in outpatient settings [4] and how patient-provider dynamics play a role in influencing care decisions made in those environments is limited. Given that most antibiotic prescriptions originate in the out-patient setting [14], these interactions may be crucial to clinical outcomes. Indeed, previous research has shown that physicians are more likely to prescribe medications in-appropriately (e.g., opiates and antipsychotics) in the face of real or perceived expectations from patients [15–18]. If the same pattern is true for antibiotics in the outpatient setting, addressing these dynamics has the potential to im-prove practice and reduce inappropriate prescribing.

This study was part of a larger project focused on redu-cing inappropriate antibiotic prescribing in the outpatient setting. The goals of this study were to explore factors in-fluencing provider decisions to prescribe antibiotics, iden-tify provider recommendations for interventions to reduce inappropriate antibiotic use, and inform the clinical man-agement of patients in the outpatient environment for in-fections that do not require antibiotics. This study adds to available evidence regarding how and why providers de-cide to prescribe antibiotics by incorporating the perspec-tives not only of physicians, but also of advanced care practitioners [19–21]. Moreover, it responds to a previous call for updated studies of antibiotic utilization among pri-mary care providers within the United States [21].

Methods
Setting
This study was conducted at Atrium Health, a large, inte-grated healthcare network in the Southeastern United States. Atrium Health is a comprehensive, not-for-profit, healthcare organization comprised of over 900 care locations including hospitals, doctors' offices, urgent care clinics, emergency de-partments, and long-term care facilities, with over twelve million patient encounters annually. This study focused on providers in outpatient primary care settings (i.e., doctors' offices, urgent care clinics).

Ethical considerations
The Atrium Health Institutional Review Board reviewed this study and classified it as quality improvement, therefore determining that project activities were not re-quired to act in accordance with research policies and regulations. Still, an information sheet detailing the pur-pose of the study, how the study would work, and par-ticipants' role in the research, including risks, benefits, reimbursement for time, costs, and confidentiality was reviewed at the beginning of each interview. Verbal con-sent to participate in the study and to record the inter-view was also obtained prior to the interview start. Participants received a pair of movie tickets to thank them for their time.

Participants
Doctors and advanced care practitioners (i.e., nurse practitioners and physician assistants) who were actively involved in delivering care in the outpatient setting within Atrium Health were eligible to participate. The physician leading the study sent a recruitment letter to clinic medical directors, who then invited their providers to participate in the key informant interviews. Providers were contacted in person by Atrium Health quality im-provement coordinators familiar with these individuals through their prior collaborative work. The study team received a list of 24 providers who indicated interest in participating. All 24 individuals received either an email message or phone call. Of these, 17 providers were suc-cessfully contacted, agreed to participate, and completed the interview (Table 1). None of the 24 providers refused an invitation to interview; the remaining 7 providers did not respond to emails or phone calls.

Data collection
A phenomenological perspective was used in designing a qualitative study to explore providers' experiences with making decisions about the use of antibiotics in the treatment of patients; the types of factors that motivate their treatment decisions regarding the use of antibiotics; their experiences as a part of a healthcare system in which decisions are made regarding the use of antibi-otics; and their perceptions of patient experiences with provider decisions regarding the use of antibiotics to treat their illnesses [22]. Data were collected using semi-structured interviews that allowed for exploration of provider perceptions. The interview guide included questions developed around several areas of interest identified by project stakeholders: a) key factors in anti-biotic prescribing; b) communicating with patients about

Table 1 Demographics of providers participating in interviews regarding antimicrobial stewardship ($n = 17$)

Characteristic	Number of providers
Sex	
Male	5
Female	12
Credentials	
MD[a]	10
ACP[b]	7
Practice Setting	
Family Medicine	9
Pediatrics	3
Urgent Care	4
Pediatric Urgent Care	1

[a]Doctor of Medicine
[b]Advanced Care Practitioner

antibiotics; c) helping patients to feel better; d) patient knowledge and experiences; e) the problem of antibiotic resistance; f) barriers to appropriate prescribing; and g) education, training, and reporting. Interviews were conducted on weekdays between the hours of 7:00 a.m. and 5:00 p.m. during November and December 2016 and lasted less than one hour. All providers elected to participate via telephone and all interviews were conducted by the same experienced qualitative researcher. Each interview was audio recorded and transcribed for analysis. Data collection continued until saturation was achieved as indicated by the researcher (TDY) responsible for both conducting the interviews and the primary analysis. To confirm, we conducted two additional interviews with providers beyond our original goal of 15. Data production followed a quality control process whereby transcripts were created by a transcriptionist (KB), quality checked by a trained member of the research team (CDC), and finalized by the original transcriptionist prior to analysis. No identifying information was included in the production of the texts.

Data analysis

Key areas of focus addressed in the interview guide informed an inductive analysis of the data. Transcripts were initially open-coded at the descriptive level. Second-level coding involved identifying salient categories and condensing initial coding classifications to reflect emerging patterns and relationships among the data. Thematic analysis of the data proceeded from an in vivo (i.e., in their own words) and descriptive level interpretation to more abstracted categories [23]. Written notes taken by the researcher during interviews were also expanded into analytic memos and included as an intermediate component of the analysis process that documented early and emerging interpretations of the data [24]. Major themes were identified based upon patterns evident across provider responses. NVivo Version 10 was used to assist with data management and analysis. Data were analyzed by the same qualitative researcher who conducted all provider interviews.

Efforts to ensure quality

As previously described, all participants were employed by one healthcare system in the Southeast United States at the end of 2016, and our study design assumed that these practitioners had experiences with and opinions regarding antibiotic prescribing in the outpatient setting. During interviews with these providers, we frequently asked participants to confirm the researcher's understanding of their responses. Throughout data analysis and report preparation, portions of the transcript were reviewed and discussed with the primary transcriptionist (KB). In the case of contradicting interpretations,

consensus was achieved. Preliminary findings were reported to and discussed internally with the larger research team and key stakeholders, including interview participants. While all data were included for analysis, results presented in this manuscript are excerpts reflecting major themes that emerged. The lead author (TDY), who also served as the interviewer, claims no bias regarding the subject matter.

Results

Interviews with providers revealed several key elements impacting their discussions with patients regarding appropriate use of antibiotics as well as some primary barriers to reducing inappropriate prescribing. These included patient education and expectations, system-level factors, and time constraints.

Current antibiotic prescribing practices

To better understand current antibiotic prescribing patterns, we asked providers about key factors they consider when making antibiotic prescribing decisions, how they communicate with patients about antibiotics, and strategies they use to help patients feel better when an antibiotic is not prescribed (Table 2).

The providers who participated in this study indicated that they focus on several items including acute clinical presentation (e.g., presence of fever, evidence of bacterial infection); best practices in the form of guidelines and decision support tools; patient level factors such as age, treatment history and social considerations; as well as workflow (i.e., time per patient and patient volume) when making treatment decisions. One physician elaborated on time constraints:

> Definitely. If you're seeing patients in 10–15 min intervals, it's very hard. It's easier to write the prescription for an antibiotic than it is to have the discussion about why they may not need that. (MD, Interview 10)

Regarding communication with their patients about antibiotics, providers indicated that they often need time to explain the difference between viral and bacterial infections while simultaneously offering measures to relieve symptoms, advising of signs to watch for (e.g., presence of fever, prolonged duration of symptoms) and indicating when and how to follow up if the patient's condition does not improve. The same provider also shared:

> So I usually try to explain what an antibiotic does because a lot of people don't understand virus versus bacteria... Antibiotics themselves are really geared towards bacteria. And if you don't have [a] bacterial infection, you know, antibiotics [are] not going to help your viral infection at all. (MD, Interview 10)

Table 2 Interview topics, categories, and themes from discussions with outpatient care providers regarding antibiotic prescribing

Interview Topics	Categories	Themes
Key Factors in Decision Making about Prescribing Antibiotics	Acute clinical presentation	Current Antibiotic Prescribing Practices
	Best practices	
	Patient level factors (e.g., age)	
	Workflow	
Communicating with Patients about Antibiotics	Understanding viral and bacterial infections	
	Disease course	
	Symptomatic relief	
	Signs to watch for	
	Follow up	
Helping Patients to Feel Better	Over-the-counter medications	
	Personal care	
	Rest	
Perceptions of Patient Knowledge and Experiences	Expectations are high	Provider Perceptions of Patient Knowledge and Awareness
	Want to feel better	
	A quick fix	
Perceptions of the Problem of Antibiotic Resistance	Largely unaware	
	Some peripheral knowledge	
	Often disassociate	
	Can vary based on demographics	
Perceptions of Barriers to Appropriate Prescribing	Patient education	
	Patient expectations	
	System-level concerns	
	Time constraints	
Education and Training for Providers	System-wide, evidence-based guidelines	Recommendations for Education, Training, and Reporting
	Decision support tools	
Reporting Antibiotic Use to Providers	Multiple forms of delivery (i.e., in person, electronic)	
	Align with current reporting practices	

Providers aimed to acknowledge and attend to their patients' feelings while at the same time communicating reasons for not prescribing an antibiotic. The physician summarized:

When you try to explain to them that what they have is viral and self-limited...and by self-limited I don't mean shortened. I don't mean not a pain...or that you don't feel well, but that an antibiotic is not going to serve any purpose. (MD, Interview 10)

We also asked providers to describe how they help patients feel better if not prescribing an antibiotic. Providers suggested that in these circumstances they focus discussions on over-the-counter medications that provide symptomatic relief, as well as on rest and personal care (e.g., warm baths and tea) for their patients.

And [I] just tell them to care for themselves, take a little extra time and care for yourself. Take a hot shower. Take a hot bath. Put your sweat pants on and go home. Take it easy. ...I think sometimes people just need that encouragement to take care of themselves a little bit better instead of thinking, well, if I take a Z-pak I can be back at work in 24 h. (ACP, Interview 4)

Provider perceptions of patient knowledge and awareness
When asked to share their perceptions of patients' expectations of when to obtain an antibiotic prescription, providers explained that patient expectations are high for receiving something at their visit to help them feel better.

They're showing up in the office. They're paying for something, and they expect something in return. And my advice isn't enough. (MD, Interview 13)

I think that's one of the barriers that we have to overcome because patients come into this outpatient setting wanting something. That's why they spent their money. That's why they spent their time. And they have an expectation, which we may or may not be able to meet. (MD, Interview 1)

You know, an antibiotic is not a magic pill, which I think a lot of people feel it is. (ACP, Interview 6)

Moreover, providers characterized patients as being mostly unaware of antibiotic resistance, indicating that some may have only a peripheral knowledge (e.g., they have heard of superbugs).

I think most patients have a peripheral awareness. I think they know it exists. They know that it could be a problem but they don't realize how severe, how much resistance is out there. So, they have it in their mind[s]. They hear about it every once in a while but they don't realize that it's likely affecting lots of people around them. (ACP, Interview 5)

Providers further suggested that patients often disassociate themselves from the problem of antibiotic resistance, perceiving it as something that happens to others, but not directly affecting them or their immediate family.

...there's a lot of disassociation between the patient and antibiotic resistance. Yeah, but that's not me. Except for, you know, the Vac-resistant enterococcus and the methicillin-resistant staph. Those are all things that become real problems for people, but only if it's affecting them at that moment. (MD, Interview 13)

Finally, providers cited the overall education of the population, health literacy, and socioeconomic status as factors impacting patient awareness of antibiotic resistance.

I don't really think that very many people are aware of how significant that problem is. Um, I'm not, I'm not really sure that with the population that I deal with here that is rural, I don't really think there's much awareness. In a higher educated population that does their reading, that does their research, that's, that's different. ...But a lot of folks who are not well educated as far as that, they don't really understand what resistance is and they don't understand how devastating that can be until it's them. (ACP, Interview 4)

Barriers to appropriate prescribing of antibiotics

In provider interviews, we specifically asked, "What do you think are some of the primary barriers to reducing inappropriate prescribing of antibiotics?" As follow-up,

we also probed for thoughts regarding several distinct elements including patient and provider education and awareness as well as institutional level factors. A key patient level factor identified in provider responses was patients' expectations for a tangible return on their investment of time and money. One provider described the expectations patients have for immediate relief from their symptoms as follows:

I think they have a high expectation for an antibiotic. Very high. Very high. I've had patients call over the phone: "Can you call me in [an] antibiotic?" "No, I can't. Not. Nope. Nope because I don't know what you have." (ACP, Interview 4)

Limited provider time with patients was highlighted as a key clinician level factor. Providers explained that they often did not have enough time to spend with a patient in any one visit, even though repeat visits facilitated education around antibiotics over time.

I need to be seeing patients on an average of every 7 ½ minutes. So it does not give me much time to talk to them about the merits of the treatment plan or what options they have. (MD, Interview 13)

A lack of patient education regarding the appropriate use of antibiotics was identified as an important education and awareness barrier, and concerns about discontinuity of care as well as patient satisfaction were emphasized as primary institutional level barriers. In terms of education and awareness, providers indicated that most patients do not understand the nature of viral infections, how long the associated symptoms are likely to last, and/or the treatment measures recommended to combat them. This patient level factor creates obstacles to appropriate prescribing.

I do think a big barrier is patient education. Um, public education. And even just the damage of antibiotics, what we have been doing with antibiotics... I shouldn't give you an antibiotic because of XYZ but every time I give you an antibiotic and you don't need one, we're contributing to this bigger problem. Um and that's the thing, that you know when someone is not feeling well, they don't care about the bigger problem. (MD, Interview 10)

Institutional level barriers that impact antibiotic prescribing practices included concerns about lack of continuity in care and low confidence that different providers would make consistent treatment decisions. Providers mentioned they may see patients only once, especially in urgent care settings. In this scenario, one provider within the healthcare system may not choose antibiotic treatment for a patient, while a different provider may prescribe an antibiotic for the same set of indications.

Lack of continuity, when you don't see somebody...all the time, that trust isn't built. So I think that helps, if you have continuity that helps improve judicious use of antibiotics. (MD, Interview 3)

Because they think that you know, they were sick on day three they came in and saw somebody who did the right thing and did not give them an antibiotic and then three days later they're still sick so they go to urgent care. ...And they're like, "We're going to go ahead and give you this antibiotic that way it doesn't turn into something worse." So it's a lot of, you know, some of it is being done to ourselves by different colleagues in different situations. (MD, Interview 10)

Other institutional factors included provider concerns about patient satisfaction and organizational support for their decisions not to prescribe an antibiotic.

Well the concerns are patient satisfaction is not necessarily quality of care. You're being judged on what someone's expectations were when they came in and if they don't get what they think they should have got, they're not happy. And that's gonna affect your patient satisfaction scores. ...It's counter-productive to the whole theory about antibiotic stewardship but that's part of the thing providers are getting judged on. It's not quality of care; that's patient satisfaction. (MD, Interview 14)

Recommendations for education, training, and reporting

When asked, "What suggestions, if any, do you have for how to inform clinicians about their use of antibiotics to treat patients," participating providers indicated that they would be interested in having system-wide, evidence-based guidelines to inform practice and support decision-making. When explicitly asked for suggestions on how to equip providers with current training and educational information regarding appropriate prescribing, providers emphasized a desire for guidelines that would allow them to be "on the same page" with their colleagues.

I think we do need to have educational training. I think we need to be very clear on the guidelines, evidence-based guidelines on when an antibiotic is appropriate and when it's not appropriate. (MD, Interview 8)

They further expressed a desire for decision support tools that would facilitate decision-making at the point of care.

I am a big proponent of decision support because I don't think any of us can keep it all in our brains anymore....Maybe input a couple of criteria regarding your patient's situation and then it could give you some choices that are all evidence-based but then you would select with your patient the most appropriate option for them. (ACP, Interview 12)

Beyond promoting consistent and competent care, providers suggested that these resources may empower a provider to confidently deny a request for an unnecessary antibiotic.

...guidelines that are geared for the providers really liberate the provider[s] to say, "No, I have criteria that says I did the right thing." (MD, Interview 15)

Many providers in this study indicated they would like to be informed about their prescribing practices, acknowledging they may not be aware of how often they prescribe when an antibiotic may not be indicated.

I think if you get really busy you may not even realize how many prescriptions you're writing in a certain day or a certain week. I mean, I can[not] tell you how many prescriptions I write in any given day, just off the top of my head. So that would be something interesting to see, you know, out of this many patients, this is how many I'm seeing that were acute that I did write an antibiotic on. (ACP, Interview 6)

Providers recommended delivering information about antibiotic prescribing practices both electronically and in-person, utilizing reporting practices already in place.

I think it would be helpful to have reporting the way we have with other quality metrics. Have a percentage of times that you have a URI [upper respiratory infection] with antibiotics or bronchitis with antibiotics. And some sort of baseline bar or metric. (MD, Interview 9)

Of note, while providers were largely in favor of reporting antibiotic prescribing practices, they also expressed concerns about the types of information that would be reported, how widely it would be shared, and what impact it might have upon prescribing behaviors. For example, one provider expressed:

I don't know that just telling a provider they gave an antibiotic to a patient is helpful. But maybe if there's some sort of chart review…it was likely inappropriate in this situation, you could learn from that. But that would require a lot of work. (ACP, Interview 12)

Discussion

This study examined provider experiences with antibiotic prescribing and perceptions of ways to reduce inappropriate prescribing of antibiotics in the outpatient setting. Providers indicated that they consider several key factors when deciding whether to administer antibiotics (i.e., clinical presentation, best practices). Within the constraints of appointment times, providers aimed to help their patients find ways to manage symptoms while simultaneously explaining the differences between viral and bacterial infections with respect to appropriate treatments. Additionally, providers noted that patient expectations for relief were high whereas both patient awareness of antibiotic resistance and appropriate use of antibiotics remained low. This lack of awareness was attributed to sociocultural factors along with a tendency for individual patients to disassociate themselves from what they perceived to be a more global issue. Finally, providers identified institutional concerns (e.g., discontinuity of care and patient satisfaction) together with provider time constraints, patient expectations, and a lack of patient education as key barriers to appropriate prescribing.

As in previous research, the results presented here suggest that system-wide, evidence-based guidelines to support decision-making and efforts to improve providers' awareness of their own prescribing practices would be well received [25]. Consequently, consistent system-level training and prescribing guidelines as well as regular reporting of providers' antibiotic use may improve levels of appropriate prescribing and has been previously noted in the literature [19, 21, 26]. Educational materials that are concise, easy to access, evidence-based, consistent across practice settings, and utilize both push (e.g., email, text) and pull (e.g., system website) technologies in the dissemination of this information may be most effective. Recommendations for reporting antibiotic use to providers include providing information on a regular basis (e.g., monthly, quarterly), in an easy-to access electronic format. Individual, yet comparative, reporting that remains sensitive in delivery is further proposed and aligns with previous research [27].

Providers recommended patient and public education efforts that occur prior to care delivery (e.g. public service announcements, internet resources, waiting room videos), are reinforced through conversation at patient encounters, and repeated in patient handouts (print outs, pamphlets). This finding is consistent with prior research that suggests that regular and ongoing patient-specific and general public education around appropriate antibiotic use could reduce pressures that providers feel to provide antibiotics [28, 29]. Reducing this burden may in turn have a multiplicative effect as previous research has shown that patient expectation for antibiotics is strongly related to provider overprescribing [30, 31]. Additional recommendations for improving patient education include using multiple media forms, engaging imagery, and language that is easy to understand [32]. One example of this is the Center for Disease Control's *Get Smart: Know When Antibiotics Work* program [33]. This campaign's webpage provides materials (e.g., fact sheets, social media messages, graphics, and quizzes) aimed at educating both patients and providers. Moreover, offering tangible items (e.g., tip sheets, symptomatic care kits) to patients that represent a return on their investment may be worth consideration. Consequently, these insights have been used to inform the development of patient education materials, provider scripting, and a reporting dashboard for use at Atrium Health.

Our findings suggest that multiple factors impact antibiotic prescribing practices in the outpatient setting. These include the education and experience of patients, as well as the education and experience of providers [34]. Consistent with prior research, our results also suggest that decision-making is affected by both cultural and system level factors and the dynamics of the patient-provider relationship, influences formerly identified in the literature [35–37]. Research has examined the social context within which prescribing decisions are made, as well as the social norms that guide them, and previously highlighted the impact of these elements on practice [16, 18, 19]. A growing body of literature further suggests that provider characteristics and patient-provider dynamics both impact clinical decision making [34, 35, 38–41]. Thus, a provider's decision to prescribe can be influenced by numerous factors beyond what is known to be best practice. Any one of these facets, or several in combination, may lead to an increased likelihood of inappropriate prescribing.

Study limitations

Although multiple coders are preferred in qualitative data analysis, only one researcher coded the data for this study. In addition, all participants in this research were employed by the same healthcare system and their perspectives may not be representative of providers in other settings. Additionally, the results of this study are based on a small convenience sample of providers; this may further limit the generalizability of the findings. Another limitation is that individuals volunteered to participate in the study. Therefore, self-selection bias may have had some impact on the range of attitudes and perceptions provided by the respondents. Notwithstanding, the pressures and challenges related to antibiotic prescribing expressed by providers in this study aligned with those from prior studies in other settings [16–18, 38, 39]. Our convenience sample included primary and urgent care providers. While primary care and urgent care settings have high volumes of antibiotic prescriptions, additional research with providers in other outpatient settings may be useful.

Conclusion

A myriad of factors including patient expectations and limitations on providers' time influence providers' decisions to prescribe antibiotics in the outpatient setting. Our research suggests that both patient and provider education may be key elements of any successful antibiotic stewardship program.

Abbreviations

Vac-resistant: vancomycin resistant; Z-pak: Zithromax (azithromycin)

Acknowledgements

We would like to thank Ryan Burns and Whitney Rossman for their assistance with project management as well as Elizabeth Handy and Marque Macon for their role in connecting us with providers.

Funding

The study was funded by a grant received from The Duke Endowment (Grant Number 6577-SP). The funders had no role in study design, data collection and analysis, decision to publish, or preparation of the manuscript.

Authors' contributions

TDY conducted the semi-structured interviews, analyzed and interpreted the qualitative research data, and drafted the manuscript. MED led the design of the study and developed the interview guides. LD and MDS conceived the study. YJT helped to interpret the data. KB transcribed all audio recordings and assisted with data analysis along with CDC. All authors critically revised the manuscript for important intellectual content and approved the final version.

Ethics approval and consent to participate

This study was reviewed and approved by the Atrium Health Institutional Review Board. The Atrium Health Institutional Review Board determined that the project activities described in a quality improvement vs. research screening form fell into the category of quality improvement. The grant application outlining the study activities was also reviewed and deemed to be quality improvement. Per Atrium Health IRB policy, the project and all activities therein were therefore not required to act in accordance with research policies and regulations. Although it was deemed to be a quality improvement project, subjects were verbally consented to provide confirmation that there was an understanding of the objectives of the interview, that the subjects themselves were willing and able to participate, and that they could decline to participate further at any time.

Competing interests

M.D.S. reports a research grant from Eli Lilly and Company. The authors have no other relationships or activities that could appear to have influenced the submitted work.

Author details

¹Center for Outcomes Research and Evaluation, Atrium Health, Charlotte, NC, USA. ²Division of Infectious Disease, Atrium Health, Charlotte, NC, USA.

References

1. The White House. National action plan for combating antibiotic-resistant bacteria. https://obamawhitehouse.archives.gov/sites/default/files/docs/national_action_plan_for_combating_antibotic-resistant_bacteria.pdf (2015). Accessed 12 June 2017.
2. Centers for Disease Control and Prevention. About antimicrobial resistance. 2017. https://www.cdc.gov/drugresistance/about.html. Accessed 12 June 2017.
3. Centers for Disease Control and Prevention. CDC: 1 in 3 antibiotic prescriptions unnecessary. 2016 May. https://www.cdc.gov/media/releases/2016/p0503-unnecessary-prescriptions.html. Accessed 12 June 2017.
4. Fleming-Dutra KE, Hersh AL, Shapiro DJ, Bartoces M, Enns EA, File TM, et al. Prevalence of inappropriate antibiotic prescriptions among US ambulatory care visits, 2010-2011. JAMA. 2016;315:1864–73.
5. Centers for Disease Control and Prevention. Antibiotic resistance threats in the United States, 2013. 2013. https://www.cdc.gov/drugresistance/threat-report-2013/. Accessed 12 June 2017.
6. Arnold SR, Straus SE. Interventions to improve antibiotic prescribing practices in ambulatory care. Cochrane Database Syst Rev. 2005:CD003539.
7. Drekonja DM, Filice GA, Greer N, Olson A, MacDonald R, Rutks I, et al. Antimicrobial stewardship in outpatient settings: a systematic review. Infect Control Hosp Epidemiol. 2015;36:142–52.
8. Gerber JS. Improving outpatient antibiotic prescribing: another nudge in the right direction. JAMA. 2016;315:558–9.
9. Hicks LA, Bartoces MG, Roberts RM, Suda KJ, Hunkler RJ, Taylor TH, et al. US outpatient antibiotic prescribing variation according to geography, patient population, and provider specialty in 2011. Clin Infect Dis Off Publ Infect Dis Soc Am. 2015;60:1308–16.
10. McDonagh M, Peterson K, Winthrop K, Cantor A, Holzhammer B, Buckley DI. Improving antibiotic prescribing for uncomplicated acute respiratory tract infections. 2016. http://www.ncbi.nlm.nih.gov/books/NBK344270/. Accessed 10 Aug 2017.
11. Ranji SR, Steinman MA, Shojania KG, Gonzales R. Interventions to reduce unnecessary antibiotic prescribing: a systematic review and quantitative analysis. Med Care. 2008;46:847–62.
12. Smith RA, M'ikanatha NM, Read AF. Antibiotic resistance: a primer and call to action. Health Commun. 2015;30:309–14.
13. Vanden Eng J, Marcus R, Hadler JL, Imhoff B, Vugia DJ, Cieslak PR, et al. Consumer attitudes and use of antibiotics. Emerg Infect Dis. 2003;9:1128–35.
14. Pakyz AL, Harpe SE. Takin' it to the streets: antimicrobial stewardship in the outpatient setting. J Am Pharm Assoc JAPhA. 2016;56:608–9.
15. McKay R, Mah A, Law MR, McGrail K, Patrick DM. Systematic review of factors associated with antibiotic prescribing for respiratory tract infections. Antimicrob Agents Chemother. 2016;60:4106–18.
16. Westanmo A, Marshall P, Jones E, Burns K, Krebs EE. Opioid dose reduction in a VA health care system–implementation of a primary care population-level initiative. Pain Med Malden Mass. 2015;16:1019–26.
17. Calcaterra SL, Drabkin AD, Doyle R, Leslie SE, Binswanger IA, Frank JW, et al. A qualitative study of hospitalists' perceptions of patient satisfaction metrics on pain management. Hosp Top. 2017;95:18–26.
18. Lohr WD, Brothers KB, Davis DW, Rich CA, Ryan L, Smith M, et al. Providers' behaviors and beliefs on prescribing antipsychotic medication to children: a qualitative study. Community Ment Health J. 2017;54:1–10.
19. Charani E, Birgand G. Managing behaviours: social, cultural, and psychological aspects of antibiotic prescribing and use. In: Laundy M, Gilchrist M, Whitney L, editors. Antimicrob Steward. 1st ed. Oxford: Oxford University Press. p. 20–8.
20. Suda KJ, Roberts RM, Hunkler RJ, Taylor TH. Antibiotic prescriptions in the community by type of provider in the United States, 2005-2010. J Am Pharm Assoc JAPhA. 2016;56:621–626.e1.
21. Sanchez GV, Roberts RM, Albert AP, Johnson DD, Hicks LA. Effects of knowledge, attitudes, and practices of primary care providers on antibiotic selection, United States. Emerg Infect Dis. 2014;20:2041–7.

22. Creswell JW, Poth CN. In: Fourth, editor. Qualitative Inquiry and Research Design: Choosing among five approaches. Washington DC: SAGE; 2018.

23. Merriam SB. Qualitative research: a guide to design and implementation. 2nd ed. San Francisco, CA: Jossey-Bass; 2009.

24. Saldana J. The coding manual for qualitative researchers. 2nd ed. Washington DC: SAGE; 2016.

25. Anthierens S, Tonkin-Crine S, Cals JW, Coenen S, Yardley L, Brookes-Howell L, et al. Clinicians' views and experiences of interventions to enhance the quality of antibiotic prescribing for acute respiratory tract infections. J Gen Intern Med. 2015;30:408–16.

26. Gerber JS, Prasad PA, Fiks AG, Localio AR, Bell LM, Keren R, et al. Durability of benefits of an outpatient antimicrobial stewardship intervention after discontinuation of audit and feedback. JAMA. 2014;312:2569–70.

27. Meeker D, Linder JA, Fox CR, Friedberg MW, Persell SD, Goldstein NJ, et al. Effect of behavioral interventions on inappropriate antibiotic prescribing among primary care practices: a randomized clinical trial. JAMA. 2016;315:562–70.

28. Carter RR, Sun J, Jump RLP. A survey and analysis of the American public's perceptions and knowledge about antibiotic resistance. Open Forum Infect Dis. 2016;3

29. Michael CA, Dominey-Howes D, Labbate M. The antimicrobial resistance crisis: causes, consequences, and management. Front Public Health. 2014;2

30. Sirota M, Round T, Samaranayaka S, Kostopoulou O. Expectations for antibiotics increase their prescribing: causal evidence about localized impact. Health Psychol Off J Div Health Psychol Am Psychol Assoc. 2017;36:402–9.

31. Stivers T. Non-antibiotic treatment recommendations: delivery formats and implications for parent resistance. Soc Sci Med 1982. 2005;60:949–64.

32. Davis ME, Liu T-L, Taylor YJ, Davidson L, Schmid M, Yates T, et al. Exploring patient awareness and perceptions of the appropriate use of antibiotics: a mixed-methods study. Antibiot Basel Switz. 2017;6

33. Centers for Disease Control and Prevention. Get smart: know when antibiotics work in the doctor's offices. 2015. https://www.cdc.gov/getsmart/community/materials-references/print-materials/everyone/index.html. Accessed 12 June 2017.

34. Schmidt ML, Spencer MD, Davidson LE. Patient, Provider, and Practice Characteristics Associated with Inappropriate Antimicrobial Prescribing in Ambulatory Practices. Infect Control Amp Hosp Epidemiol. 2018;39:1–9.

35. Williams J. Effect of patient antibiotic education on provider perceived patient expectation for antibiotics [Doctoral Thesis]. [Kansas City]: University of Missouri-Kansas City; 2017. https://mospace.umsystem.edu/xmlui/handle/10355/60380. Accessed 12 June 2017.

36. May L, Gudger G, Armstrong P, Brooks G, Hinds P, Bhat R, et al. Multisite exploration of clinical decision making for antibiotic use by emergency medicine providers using quantitative and qualitative methods. Infect Control Hosp Epidemiol. 2014;35:1114–25.

37. Heid C, Knobloch MJ, Schulz LT, Safdar N. Use of the health belief model to study patient perceptions of antimicrobial stewardship in the acute care setting. Infect Control Hosp Epidemiol. 2016;37:576–82.

38. Cullinan S, O'Mahony D, Fleming A, Byrne S. A meta-synthesis of potentially inappropriate prescribing in older patients. Drugs Aging. 2014;31:631–8.

39. Johnson CF, Williams B, MacGillivray SA, Dougall NJ, Maxwell M. "Doing the right thing": factors influencing GP prescribing of antidepressants and prescribed doses. BMC Fam Pract. 2017;18:72.

40. Caplow J, Cluzet V, Mehta JM, Degnan K, Hamilton K. Targets for antimicrobial stewardship: a study of variability in antibiotic prescribing practices among outpatient care providers. Open Forum Infect Dis. 2016;3:1903.

41. Dempsey PP, Businger AC, Whaley LE, Gagne JJ, Linder JA. Primary care clinicians' perceptions about antibiotic prescribing for acute bronchitis: a qualitative study. BMC Fam Pract. 2014;15:194.

14

Job satisfaction and stressors for working in out-of-hours care – a pilot study with general practitioners in a rural area of Germany

R. Leutgeb[1*], J. Frankenhauser-Mannuß[1], M. Scheuer[2], J. Szecsenyi[1] and Katja Goetz[1,3]

Abstract

Background: Challenging work environment, high workload, and increasing physician shortages characterize current rural general practice in Germany and in most European Countries. These factors extend into Out-Of-Hours Care (OOHC). However, little research about potential stressors for general practitioners (GPs) in OOHC settings is available. This pilot study aimed to evaluate workload, different elements of job satisfaction and stressors for GPs in OOHC and to analyze whether these aspects are associated with overall job satisfaction.

Methods: Cross-sectional survey with a sample of 320 GPs who are working in OOHC was used to measure workload in OOHC, job satisfaction (using the Warr-Cook-Wall scale) and stressors with the effort-reward imbalance questionnaire. In order to assess associations between workload, job satisfaction and stressors at work we performed descriptive analyses as well as multivariable regression analyses.

Results: The response rate was 40.9%. Over 80% agreed that OOHC was perceived as a stressor and 79% agreed that less OOHC improved job satisfaction. Only 42% of our sample were satisfied with their overall job satisfaction. The regression analysis showed that the modification of current OOHC organization was significantly associated with overall job satisfaction.

Conclusions: Our results suggest that OOHC in the current form is a relevant stressor in daily work of rural GPs in Germany and one of the reasons for a decreasing overall job satisfaction. Strategic changes such as the implementation of structural reforms e.g. reducing frequency of OOHC duties for each GP and improving continuing professional development options related to OOHC are needed to address current workload challenges experienced by GPs providing OOHC in Germany.

Keywords: Effort-reward imbalance, General practitioner, Health services research, Out-of-hours care, Job satisfaction

Background

Significant demographic changes in age distribution in the German population along with the desire of Generation Y physicians (millennium generation, born between 1980 and 2000) for a balanced work-life situation and the high workloads of general practitioners (GP) are all factors influencing the shortage of GPs, especially in rural areas. Health policy makers in Europe increasingly recognize that 'primary care, the backbone of a nation's health care, is at grave risk of collapse' a statement of the American College of Physicians in 2006 [1]. In the Netherlands, the United Kingdom and in Scandinavian countries health reform at the end of the 1990s and the early 2000s created more attractive working conditions for doctors working in primary care and providing Out-of-Hours Care (OOHC). In Germany, OOHC reforms are only just being begun at a political level [2–5].

In Germany, under the National Health Insurance Scheme, there are physicians who are assigned a

* Correspondence: ruediger.leutgeb@med.uni-heidelberg.de
[1]Department of General Practice and Health Services Research, University Hospital Heidelberg, Marsillus-Arcades, Western Tower, Im Neuenheimer Feld 130.3, 69120 Heidelberg, Germany
Full list of author information is available at the end of the article

catchment area to provide care for insured patients (in German: *Vertragsarzt*). In 2015, approximately 110,000 of these physicians who worked in regular care -thereof 35,100 GPs and 11,500 internists worked additional in OOHC, except for doctors' with chronic diseases and in-patient physicians [6]. A recent study with German GPs views on the situation in OOHC reported on critical issues, in particular highlighting that OOHC is one primary factor making the role as a GP in Germany unattractive [7]. Unfortunately, there are no data available which show the workload of physicians who worked in OOHC and regular care.

Little published research has reported on working conditions and occupational demands in the workplace of OOHC physicians. Mc Loughlin et al. conducted a study in 2005 with GPs who were working in newly founded OOHC-Co-operatives in comparison to GPs not working in such Co-operatives. No differences were found regarding mental health and job stress between these two groups [8]. Two other studies revealed an improvement of quality of life for GPs working in Co-Operatives [8, 9].

Workload, job satisfaction and working conditions of physicians are crucial aspects for provided the quality of care [10]. This is an aspect not only in regular care but also in OOHC. Because of the shortage of GPs in many European countries (and in oversea countries like Australia) and the overcrowding of emergency departments in hospitals it is essential to improve the job satisfaction and working conditions of physicians [2, 11–14]. However, to date, only a few studies have explored workload, job satisfaction and stressors at work of GPs in primary care OOHC settings in Europe. Therefore, the aim of the study was to evaluate the workload, different elements of job satisfaction and stressors at work of GPs in OOHC with established survey instruments and to analyze whether these aspects are associated with overall job satisfaction concerning GPs working in OOHC rotation groups.

Methods
Setting
OOHC is defined as care during out-of-hours periods where regular medical ambulatory services are not available. In Hesse, a federal state of Germany where this study was performed, these periods extend from 7:00 p.m. to 7:00 a.m. on Monday, Tuesday and Thursday, and from 2:00 p.m. to 7:00 a.m. on Wednesday and Friday and also on weekends and public holidays [15]. The OOHC periods, especially on Wednesdays and Fridays, are scheduled as an agreement between the licensed physicians and the Association of Statutory Health Insurance Hesse. Since introduction of the national emergency number 116117 in 2015 the OOHC periods were adapted in

all federal states of Germany. The characteristics of OOHC in rural areas of Germany in the year 2012 are cited in Table 1 [16]. The Organization for Economic Co-operation and Development (OECD) methodology classifies local administrative units (LAU) with a population density below 150 inhabitants per km^2 as rural. It is defined intermediate, if the share of population living in rural LAU is between 15 and 50% and predominantly rural, if the share of population living in rural LAU is higher than 50%. Our survey was sent to all panel doctors in the specific local district 'Landkreis Bergstraße' of the federal state of Hesse. This LAU is 'intermediate rural' in terms of the OECD-definition [17].

Study design and participants
This exploratory study was based on a written questionnaire survey in one rural region in Germany. Data were collected from GPs who worked in OOHC. Between August 2012 and November 2012 all 320 GPs of the region were contacted to participate on the postal questionnaire survey. Addresses were selected via an address register of the Association of Statutory Health Insurance of Hesse, Germany. The GPs were invited to participate by mail. The return of the anonymous paper-based questionnaire was classified as informed consent. No reminder was sent out.

Table 1 Out-Of-Hours Care (OHHC)-services in rural areas of different federal states of Germany in 2012 [16]

Service obligation for all panel physicians to do on-call duty but not to maintain registration as a GP or (as another specialist discipline)
• Approximately 110,000
Most frequent model of OOHC in Germany in rural areas
• OOHC rotation groups 30–50 physicians
OOHC care centre
• OOHC practices predominantly in the middle of the local district respectively care provision in GP practices
• Either GPs of the region or hired clinicians work in the OOHC care centres
Opening hours in OOHC centre
• On weekdays From 07:00 pm to 07:00 am
• On Wednesday already at 2:00 pm
• From Friday 07:00 pm to Monday 7:00 am
• On holidays
Catchment area
• Local districts with 40,000–80,000 inhabitants
• Distance of patients to OOHC-centre 15-20 km
Accessibility
• Access via regional telephone numbers
• about 10–15% walk in without a call in advance
Telephone triage
• In 2012 no triage model was implemented
• The doctor himself answered the phone calls, rarer a nurse
Provision of care
• Telephone advice
• Consultation-hours
• Home visits.

Measurements
Workload in OOHC
The workload of GPs in OOHC was measured with a self-developed questionnaire based on qualitative interviews with GPs in OOHC and literature review. The interviews focused on the experiences of GPs who worked in OOHC. All GPs were interviewed with the same semi structured interview guideline. Theme saturation reached after 8 interviews. Within the 8 interviews the statements were categorized to individual stress, general conditions of care and present situation of care. The categories were transformed to items in an interactive process by an interdisciplinary team consisted of GPs who worked in OOHC, a sociologist and a health service researcher This questionnaire consists of 7 items rated on a four-point Likert scale (from 1 = fully disagree to 4 = fully agree). Cronbach's α was 0.772 for the items of workload. The questionnaire was not validated before.

Job satisfaction
For evaluation of job satisfaction a modified Warr-Cook-Wall job satisfaction scale was used, which has been already used in previous studies with GPs [18, 19]. The instrument consists of 9 items to different aspects on job satisfaction and 1 item to overall job satisfaction. These 10 items rated on a seven-point Likert scale (from 1 = extreme dissatisfaction to 7 = extreme satisfaction). A higher overall mean score indicates higher job satisfaction. An example item is: 'How satisfied are you with your income? ' Cronbach's α was 0.855 for the job satisfaction scale without the general question of job satisfaction.

Stressors at work
Stressors at work were measured with effort-reward imbalance (ERI) developed by Siegrist [20]. It is a well-known instrument which was validated in different human service settings and has been already used in previous studies with physicians [21, 22].This measurement consists of three scales: effort (6 items), reward (11 items) and overcommitment (6 items). Effort and reward as extrinsic components constitute the ERI. It means an imbalance between professional overspending and reward. The scale effort evaluates the professional overspending (e.g. working under high time pressure) and reward scale measures the reward at workplace like recognition for work or adequate remuneration. All questions could be rated on a five-point Likert scale ranging from 1 = low stress to 5 = high stress. The reward scale is subdivided in three subscales: 'esteem' (5 items), 'job security' (2 items), and 'job promotion' (4 items). The effort-reward ratio (ER-ratio) was calculated based on the following equation: ER-ratio = 11 × effort/6 × reward. Values of ER-ratio over 1.0, a high amount of effort not

met with adequate reward is indicated. The scale overcommitment as intrinsic component is independently from the ER-ratio and was assessed with 6-item on a four-point rating scale, from agree to disagree with the given statement. The Cronbach's α was 0.830 for the effort-reward imbalance scale.

Data analysis
Analyses were performed using SPSS version 22.0 (SPSS Inc., IBM). A descriptive analysis was performed concerning the 7 items of workload and the 10 items of the job satisfaction scale. Means, standard deviation and 95% confidence intervals as well as a summarization of the percentage of fully agree and agree respectively extreme satisfied, rather satisfied and satisfied of workload and job satisfaction were reported. The descriptive analysis of the scales of effort, reward and its subscales and overcommitment included means and standard deviation. Moreover, sum scores of the ERI as well the ER-ratio was calculated. The sum score of effort varies between 6 (no stress) and 30 (very stressful). The sum score of reward ranges between 11 (lowest reward) and 55 (high level of reward) [20]. For further analyses the full range of answer options and not the summarization from the variables were used. The dependent variable 'overall job satisfaction' as well as the independent variables were handled as linear variables. Pearson's correlation was used to find out which the independent variables individual characteristics, workload, aspect of job satisfaction and effort, reward and overcommitment showed a significant correlation with the dependent variable 'overall job satisfaction'. Afterwards, a linear regression analyses were used to explore potential associations between the dependent variable 'overall job satisfaction with OOHC' and independent variables which correlated significantly with the dependent variable. An alpha level of $P < 0.05$ was used for tests of statistical significance.

Results
Three hundred and twenty questionnaires were handed out to GPs who worked in OOHC, 131 participated on the survey. The response rate was 40.9%.

Table 2 shows the characteristics of the participating OOHC physicians.

Moreover, 26% of our sample stated that they felt 'extreme stress due to care for people in retirement or nursing homes within OOHC'.

Evaluation of workload and job satisfaction
The evaluation of workload in OOHC and job satisfaction scale is presented in Table 3. 79.4% of GPs agreed that job satisfaction could improve due to less OOHC, 80.9% agreed that working in OOHC was a general

Table 2 Summary of the basis characteristics of the physicians involved in Out-Of-Hours Care (OOHC)

Characteristics			Our sample (n = 131)
Gender, n (%)	Male		99 (75.6)
	Female		32 (24.4)
Age, years; mean (SD), range (min – max)			51.8 (8.1), 32–70
OOHC-duties in the quarter; mean (SD)			4.4 (4.6)
Home visits during OOHC; mean (SD)			4.0 (4.0)
Number of patient during OOHC; mean (SD)			7.3 (7.9)
Telephone calls during OOHC; mean (SD)			7.4 (8.0)
Attending retirement homes during OOHC; mean (SD)			2.1 (3.1)
Attending nursing homes during OOHC; mean (SD)			1.9 (2.1)
Kilometer distance during OOHC; mean (SD)			19.6 (21.3)
Participating OOHC physicians within the district; mean (SD)			26.1 (17.2)
Quarterly contact group[a], n (%)	< 500 patients		9 (6.6)
	500–1000 patients		19 (14.5)
	1001–1500 patients		55 (42.0)
	> 1500 patients		47 (35.9)

[a]n = varies due to missing data; *SD* standard deviation, *OOHC* Out-Of-Hours Care

stressor. Furthermore, 72.5% of GPs were satisfied with 'colleagues and fellow workers' and 69.5% were satisfied with 'freedom of working method' but 27.5% were satisfied with 'hours of work' and 30.6% were satisfied with 'income'.

The effort-reward imbalance

The different scores of the ERI and their scales are presented in Table 4. The scale 'effort' was high (mean = 21.0) in contrast to a low level of 'reward' (mean = 23.6). Also low levels of the subscales of 'reward' were

Table 3 Descriptive statistics of workload and job satisfaction of the physicians involved in in Out-Of-Hours Care (n = 131)

Items of workload in OOHC[a]	Mean (SD)	CI 95%	Percentage of answers to fully agree and agree
Negative effects on job satisfaction due to OOHC	2.83 (1.0)	2.7–3.0	68.7
Psychosocial stress due to OOHC	3.06 (0.9)	2.9–3.2	73.3
Negative effects on the following day after OOHC	3.11 (0.9)	3.0–3.3	77.1
Improvement of general job satisfaction due to less OOHC	3.28 (0.9)	3.1–3.4	79.4
OOHC as a general stressor	3.19 (0.9)	3.0–3.3	80.9
Financial incentive to work more in the OOHC centre of the rotation groups	2.21 (1.0)	2.0–2.4	32.8
Modification of current OOHC-organization	3.14 (1.0)	3.0–3.3	72.5
Items of job satisfaction[b]	Mean (SD)	CI (95%)	Percentage of answers to extreme, rather and satisfied
Amount of variety in job	4.88 (1.5)	4.6–5.1	62.6
Opportunity to use abilities	4.89 (1.5)	4.6–5.2	64.2
Freedom of working method	5.05 (1.5)	4.8–5.3	69.5
Amount of responsibility	4.85 (1.5)	4.6–5.1	63.4
Physical working condition	4.58 (1.3)	4.4–4.8	48.9
Hours of work	3.60 (1.6)	3.3–3.9	27.5
Income	3.69 (1.6)	3.4–4.0	30.6
Recognition for work	4.76 (1.3)	4.5–5.0	60.4
Colleagues and fellow workers	5.28 (1.2)	5.1–5.5	72.5
Overall job satisfaction	3.98 (1.6)	3.7–4.3	42.0

[a]ranged from 1 "fully disagree" to 4 "fully agree"
[b]ranged from 1 "extreme dissatisfaction" to 7 "extreme satisfaction"
OOHC Out-Of-Hours Care, *SD* standard deviation, *CI* Confidence interval

Table 4 Effort-reward imbalance of physicians involved in Out-Of-Hours Care ($n = 131$)

Scales (range; minimum to maximum)	Mean (SD)
Effort (6–30)	21.0 (5.2)
Reward (11–55)	23.6 (7.1)
Overcommittment (6–24)	14.7 (3.0)
Subscales of reward-scale (range; minimum to maximum)	Mean (SD)
Job promotion (4–20)	8.9 (3.5)
Esteem (5–25)	10.0 (3.0)
Security (2–10)	4.7 (2.0)
ER-Ratio[a]	1.7

[a]value > 1.0: imbalance between high effort and low reward
SD standard deviation, *ER-Ratio* Effort-reward ratio

observed. The mean score of the ER-ratio was 1.7. Over 127 (94.7%) of the GPs in OOHC showed an ER-ratio over 1.0.

Factors associated with overall job satisfaction

The correlation showed that the variables of workload with the exception of the variable "financial incentive to work more often in the OOHC centre of the rotation groups" correlated strong with the dependent variable "overall job satisfaction". For the different aspects of job satisfaction, a strong correlation to the dependent variable with exception of variable "colleagues and fellow workers" was also found. The scales 'effort', 'reward' and 'overcommitment' correlated strongly with the dependent variable "overall job satisfaction".

No correlation was found for the different individual characteristics which were presented in Table 2.

The linear regression analysis of the independent variables workload and job satisfaction on the dependent variable overall job satisfaction of working in OOHC is shown in Table 5. The linear regression model explained more than 46% ($R^2 \sim 0.462$) of the variance of the dependent variable 'overall job satisfaction'. A higher agreement to modification of current OOHC-organization was associated with more job satisfaction. More variety in the job was associated with more job satisfaction.

Discussion

The aim of the current study was to evaluate workload, different elements of job satisfaction and stressors at work of GPs in OOHC and to explore potential associations to overall satisfaction. A comparison between our sample of participating GPs and the whole sample of GPs in Germany show similar results concerning age but differs slightly by gender, 24.4% women in our sample comparing to 43.9% in the whole sample of GPs in Germany [23]. It can be assumed that more men than women working as GP in OOHC which is comparable to studies concerning after-hours care in Australia [14, 24]. Our results showed

that our participants were mostly satisfied with their colleagues but dissatisfied with their income and working hours. Over 80% of our sample agreed that working in OOHC was perceived as a general stressor. Moreover, GPs highly agreed with the statement: 'less OOHC-duties could improve general job satisfaction', which was also observed within the regression model and was strongly associated with overall job satisfaction. It could be assumed that the modification of current OOHC-organization could have an impact on a positive feeling at working in OOHC.

Our findings concerning workload and job satisfaction of GPs are in agreement with previous studies not only in different European countries but also in the USA and Australia [14, 19, 24–26]. In contrast to our study with low income satisfaction rate a study in Australia show a high level of income satisfaction in after-hours care; it can be explained as physicians were paid per patient [14].

A survey conducted by the Commonwealth Fund evaluated that German GPs have the highest workload with the most working hours per day, the shortest consultation time with their patients and were most unsatisfied with own professional situation in comparison to GPs in other Western European countries and the USA [26]. Additional, it was found that German physicians felt more in control of their working hours than British physicians but the impact on job satisfaction is unclear [27].

It could be assumed that high workload, dissatisfaction with income and obligations for duty in OOHC could be a reason for reducing the overall satisfaction of Germans GPs.

The health policy consequences of this assumption are potentially severe. The shortage of GPs, particularly in rural areas could be exacerbated. This is already a problem in many European countries [3, 4, 9, 28]. Considering our results about workload and job satisfaction, it could be assumed that our sample of physicians is increasingly less motivated to do the OOHC-duties. In the Netherlands, 85% of the GPs delegate 25% of their shifts, so most of the GPs do their shifts solely in GP- cooperatives. Like German physicians, they also complain about the high workload because of the large number of patients with minor ailments. However, they feel responsible to deliver continuity of primary care. Unlike the situation in Germany, GPs in the Netherlands have to provide OOHC to maintain their registration as a GP. This could be an additional explanation to the high quota of GPs in the Netherlands doing their shifts in OOHC [29].

The development in Germany is different, a high percentage of OOHC duties –exact figures are not available- are transferred to assistant doctors of hospitals and locum doctors. A key element, the continuity of care with experienced GPs in OOHC, is lost, which could

Table 5 Associations of workload, different aspects of job satisfaction and scales of effort-reward imbalance of of physicians involved in Out-Of-Hours Care to outcome variable 'overall job satisfaction' (results of the linear regression analysis, under specification of standardized beta coefficient, $\alpha = 5\%$)

	Variables	β (p-value)
Items of workload in OOHC	Negative effects on job satisfaction due to OOHC	−0.111 (0.274)
	Psychosocial stress due to OOHC	−0.066 (0.601)
	Negative effects on the following day after OOHC	−0.020 (0.876)
	Improvement of general job satisfaction due to less OOHC	−0.043 (0.755)
	OOHC as a general stressor	−0.117 (0.410)
	Modification of current OOHC-organization	−0.278 (0.008)
Items of job satisfaction	Amount of variety in job	0.226 (0.048)
	Opportunity to use abilities	0.001 (0.994)
	Freedom of working method	0.068 (0.515)
	Amount of responsibility	0.162 (0.145)
	Physical working condition	0.006 (0.950)
	Hours of work	0.017 (0.861)
	Income	0.067 (0.503)
	Recognition for work	−0.033 (0.754)
Scales of effort-reward imbalance	Effort	−0.019 (0.860)
	Reward	0.077 (0.499)
	Overcommitment	−0.045 (0.647)
	Extreme stress due to care for people in retirement or nursing homes while OOHC	0.014 (0.877)
R^2	0.462	

have an impact on quality of care and should be examined in further studies. Campbell et al. argued that GPs have to lead OOHC services because of their generalized skills and experiences. Patients' satisfaction with OOHC increases if they are treated by GPs [30]. In contrast to this statement, it can be assumed that patients would visit hospital emergency departments if they are dissatisfied with the treatment in primary OOHC because of the inexperience of the assistant doctors working there. The consequences would be further inefficiencies and overcrowding in the emergency departments and potentially rising costs for the health care system [31].

Kjaer et al. showed the importance of continuing professional development programmes for GPs to improve professional standards in general practice [32]. Therefore, in our opinion investment in continuing professional development related to OOHC could improve the quality of treatment in OOHC. For example, an interactive learning program including updates of new knowledge in clinical practice could be implemented for the medical staff (GPs, assistant physicians and nurses) and others practicing in OOHC. Additional training in the competencies related to triage, reasons of encounter in OOHC and the resulting therapy options would be desirable [33]. It can be assumed that continuing professional development, especially concerning collaborative

skills between health professionals, in the implementation of validated triage systems and in the implementation of error managements in OOHC could increase the quality of care and could potentially positively affect workload and job satisfaction of physicians and other health care professionals working in OOHC. Experts of the European research network for out-of-hours primary health care (EurOOHnet) have discussed such strategies during their conferences in the recent years and highlighted their potential impact on job satisfaction in OOHC [34]. In particular, an international study (SAFE-EUR-OOH) started in 2014 under the leadership of the Norwegian colleagues' to prove the safety attitudes questionnaire in OOHC in different member countries [35–37].

In our study population, a high imbalance between effort and reward could be observed, nearly 95% of the GPs in OOHC showed an ER-ratio over 1.0 (mean score 1.7). It was found that GPs from Sweden and Norway have a significant lower effort-reward-ratio as physicians in Germany explained by better working conditions in these countries [38, 39]. Finnish GPs feel more distressed than the Finnish specialists because of the perceived increasing demands in the subject of general practice [40]. Furthermore, in Japan it was observed that effort-reward imbalance of GPs was significant associated with depression [41]. Interestingly, for primary care physicians who work in after-hours care in Australia a low level of stress was observed [42]. Concerning the special situation of OOHC in the region of Germany examined, our results could indicate that the high ER-ratio of GPs working in OOHC is associated with low satisfaction regarding income, higher frequency of home and nursing home visits, and psychosocial stressors like the misusing of health care utilization in OOHC through non-urgent complaints. These aspects should be considered for potential health policy reforms in OOHC. It can be concluded that more research is needed to identify potential risk factors as reference points, which could be improved through reforms. It is evident that organizational and structural reforms should be developed to improve the balance between effort and reward and to reduce the health risks of GPs in OOHC. Unfortunately, studies about health risks of GPs in OOHC are rare. One study with GPs showed that higher job satisfaction is associated with good health behavior. It was also demonstrated that support from colleagues influences positively the work and health of GPs [43]. Therefore, it could be assumed that working in OOHC with support from colleagues as a source of social support prevents mental or physical illness [44]. Moreover, it has been observed that surveys of patient experiences with OOHC provide additional data about quality of care and working situation of GPs [45].

To our knowledge there are few research studies about workload, job satisfaction and potential stressors in a primary care OOHC setting that have been published to date. The present study used well-proven instruments, the Warr-Cook-Wall scale and the ERI, which enables comparison of results as they have been both validated and have often been used in other studies [18, 20]. However, the survey tools were not piloted and validated for this study. We only measured the internal consistency for each of the three survey tools: workload of GP's in OOHC, job satisfaction and effort-reward-imbalance. Our sample may not be representative for all OOHC physicians in Germany because we only involved physicians in one rural area who were willing to participate voluntarily on the survey. But a response rate of 40.9% is notably high and one of the strength of this study in comparison to the statement by Kelley et al. [46]. They assumed for postal questionnaire surveys a response rate of 20% as normal for such surveys [46].

A limitation is that we could not evaluate all possible key factors like family situation, leisure opportunities or infrastructure in the local district 'Landkreis Bergstraße', which could contribute to GPs perceptions of overall job satisfaction. Furthermore, the demographic data presenting in Table 2 are subjective statements made by the participating physicians. Official data from the

"Association of Statutory Health Insurance Physicians" are not available. Unfortunately, we did not define clearly within the demographic questions what kind of OOHC shift we meant. Furthermore another limitation is that our presented data of this pilot study were from 2012 and should be examined in a new research project with a longitudinal study design in consideration of the current health reform in OOHC in Germany and in comparison to rural and urban regions. Moreover, this is a cross-sectional study and thus, we must be cautious to derive causal links from these findings. Significant results might be due to chance and will need to be confirmed in further targeted studies. Moreover, there are no clear statements in the literature concerning the statistical analysis of surveys using Likert scales [47, 48]. Therefore, we handled the Likert scales as an interval which could implicated a potential statistical bias.

Conclusions

The study concludes that our study sample perceived working in OOHC as a general stressor and show low satisfaction with income and working hours. Moreover, less duties in OOHC could increase the overall job satisfaction of GPs and could lead possibly to lower ER-ratio. Our results might support the modification of the current organization of OOHC in the region of Germany studied and could have implications for other regions in Germany. Moreover, it can be recommended that for future health care delivery in OOHC it is important to invest in a continuing professional development. Further research should explore whether the implementation of training programs with the focus on how to deal with the frequently minor ailments of patients in OOHC, how to deal with for example launched triage systems and how to deal with error management could improve the quality of care and could resulted in an improvement of job satisfaction of GPs in OOHC.

Abbreviations

ERI: Effort-reward imbalance; EurOOHnet: European research network for out-of-hours primary health care; GP: General Practitioner; LAU: Local Administrated Units; OECD: Organization for Economic Co-operation and Development; OOHC: Out-Of-Hours Care; SD: Standard deviation

Acknowledgements

The authors would like to thank the physicians for participating in the survey. We also gratefully thank Native Speaker Sarah Berger for reviewing this manuscript.

Authors' contributions

RL, JFM, MS, JS and KG initiated and designed the study. RL and JFM coordinated the study. JFM and KG carried out data analysis. RL and KG wrote the manuscript. All authors (RL, JFM, MS, JS and KG) commented on the draft and approved the final version of the manuscript.

Competing interests
The author KG is an associate editor for BMC Family Practice. The others authors declare that they do not have any competing interests.

Author details
[1]Department of General Practice and Health Services Research, University Hospital Heidelberg, Marsilius-Arcades, Western Tower, Im Neuenheimer Feld 130.3, 69120 Heidelberg, Germany. [2]Headquarter of Control Centre, District Bergstraße, Gräffstrasse 5, 64646 Heppenheim, Germany. [3]Institute of Family Medicine, University Hospital Schleswig-Holstein, Campus Luebeck, Ratzeburger Alle 160, 23538 Luebeck, Germany.

References
1. American College of Physicians. The impending collapse of primary care medicine and its implications for the state of the nation's health care [Internet]. Report January 2006, Available from: https://www.acponline.org/system/files/documents/advocacy/current_policy_papers/assets/dysfunctional_payment.pdf [cited 27 Jun 2016].
2. Leibowitz R, Day S, Dunt D. A systematic review of the effect of different models of after-hours primary medical care services on clinical outcome, medical workload, and patient and GP satisfaction. Fam Pract. 2003;20:311–7.
3. Grol R, Giesen P, van Uden C. After-hours care in the United Kingdom, Denmark, and the Netherlands: new models. Health Aff (Millwood). 2006;25:1733–7.
4. Giesen P, Smits M, Huibers L, Grol R, Wensing M. Quality of after-hours primary care in the Netherlands: a narrative review. Ann Intern Med. 2011;155:108–13.
5. Leutgeb R, Walker N, Remmen R, Klemenc-Ketis Z, Szecsenyi J, Laux G. On a European collaboration to identify organizational models, potential shortcomings and improvement options in out-of-hours primary health care. Eur J Gen Pract. 2014;20:233–7.
6. National Association of Statutory Health Insurance Physicians. [Internet]. Available from: http://www.kbv.de/media/sp/2015_12_31.pdf [cited 12 Apr 2017].
7. Frankenhauser-Mannuß J, Goetz K, Scheuer M, Szecsenyi J, Leutgeb R. Out-of-hours primary care in Germany: general practitioners' views on the current situation. Gesundheitswesen. 2014;76:428–33. German
8. O'Dowd TC, McNamara K, Kelly A, O'Kelly F. Out-of-hours co-operatives: general practitioner satisfaction with governance and working arrangements. Eur J Gen Pract. 2009;12:15–8.
9. van Uden CJ, Nieman FH, Voss GB, Wesseling G, Winkens RA, Crebolder HF. General practitioners' satisfaction with and attitudes to out-of-hours services. BMC Health Serv Res. 2005;5:27.
10. Linzer M, Manwell LB, Williams ES, Bobula JA, Brown RL, Varkey AB, Man B, McMurray JE, Maguire A, Horner-Ibler B, Schwartz MD. Working conditions in primary care: physician reactions and care quality. Ann Intern Med. 2009;151:28–36.
11. Huibers L, Giesen P, Wensing M, Grol R. Out-of-hours care in western countries: assessment of different organizational models. BMC Health Serv Res. 2009;9:105.
12. Margolius D, Bodenheimer T. Redesigning after-hours primary care. Ann Intern Med. 2011;155:131–2.
13. Majeed A. Redesigning after-hours primary care. Ann Intern Med. 2012;156:67–8.
14. Ifediora CO. Assessing the satisfaction levels among doctors who embark on after-hours home visits in Australia. Fam Pract. 2015;33:82–8.
15. Association of Statutory Health Insurance Physicians, Hesse Official regulation of emergency service [Internet]. Frankfurt am Main: Association of Statutory Health InsurancePhysicians, Hesse. 2013. Available from: https://www.kvhessen.de/fuer-unsere-mitglieder/services-und-dienste/aerztlicher-bereitschaftsdienst/ [cited 12 Apr 2017]
16. Scheuer M. Personal communication from the executive emergency doctor of the researched district. [cited 1 Mar 2014].
17. EUROSTAT. Statistics explained [Internet]. Available from: http://ec.europa.eu/eurostat/statistics-explained/index.php/Urban-rural_typology [cited 12 Apr 2017]
18. Warr PJ, Cook J, Wall T. Scales for the measurement of some work attitudes and aspects of psychosocial well-being. J Occup Psychol. 1979;52:129–48.
19. Goetz K, Campbell SM, Steinhäuser J, Broge B, Wilms S, Szecsenyi J. Evaluation of job satisfaction of practice staff and general practitioners: an exploratory study. BMC Fam Pract. 2011;12:137.
20. Siegrist J, Starke D, Chandola T, Godin I, Marmot M, Niedhammer I, Peter R. The measurement of effort-reward imbalance at work: European comparisons. Soc Sci Med. 2004;58:1483–99.
21. Siegrist J, Dragano N, Nyberg ST, Lunau T, Alfredsson L, Erbel R, Fahlén G, Goldberg M, Jöckel KH, Knutsson A, Leineweber C, Magnusson Hanson LL, Nordin M, Rugulies R, Schupp J, Singh-Manoux A, Theorell T, Wagner GG, Westerlund H, Zins M, Heikkilä K, Fransson EI, Kivimäki M. Validating abbreviated measures of effort-reward imbalance at work in European cohort studies: the IPD-work consortium. Int Arch Occup Environ Health. 2014;87:249–56.
22. Loerbroks A, Weigl M, Li J, Angerer P. Effort-reward imbalance and perceived quality of patient care: a cross sectional study among physicians in Germany. BMC Public Health. 2016;16:342.
23. Database of the Association of Statutory Health Insurance Physicians. Available from: http://gesundheitsdaten.kbv.de/cms/html/16392.php [cited 29 March 2018].
24. Ifediora C. Associations of stress and burnout among Australian-based doctors involved in after-hours home visits. Australas Med J. 2015;8:345–56.
25. Bodenheimer T, Pham HH. Primary care: current problems and proposed solutions. Health Aff (Millwood). 2010;29:799–805.
26. Koch K, Miksch A, Schürmann C, Joos S, Sawicki PT. The German health care system in international comparison: the primary care physicians' perspective. Dtsch Arztebl int. 2011;108:255–61.
27. Konrad TR, Link CL, Shackelton RJ, Marceau LD, von dem Knesebeck O, Siegrist J, Arber S, Adams A, McKinlay JB. It's about time: physicians' perceptions of time constraints in primary care medical practice in three national healthcare systems. Med Care. 2010;48:95–100.
28. Huibers L, Moth G, Bondevik GT, Kersnik J, Huber CA, Christensen MB, Leutgeb R, Casado AM, Remmen R, Wensing M. Diagnostic scope in out-of-hours primary care services in eight European countries: an observational study. BMC Fam Pract. 2011;12:30.
29. Smits M, Keizer E, Huibers L, Giesen P. GPs' experiences with out-of-hours GP cooperatives: a survey study from the Netherlands. Eur J Gen Pract. 2014;20:196–201.
30. Campbell JL, Clay JH. Out-of-hours care: do we? Br J Gen Pract. 2010;60:155–7.
31. Chmiel C, Huber CA, Rosemann T, Zoller M, Eichler K, Sidler P, Senn O. Walk-ins seeking treatment at an emergency department or general practitioner out-of-hours service: a cross-sectional comparison. BMC Health Serv Res. 2011;11:94.
32. Kjaer NK, Vedsted M, Høpner J. A new comprehensive model for continuous professional development. Eur J Gen Pract. 2017;23:20–6.
33. Leutgeb R, Engeser P, Berger S, Szecsenyi J, Laux G. Out of hours care in Germany - high utilization by adult patients with minor ailments? BMC Fam Pract. 2017;18:42.
34. Huibers L, Philips H, Giesen P, Remmen R, Christensen MB, Bondevik GT. EurOOHnet-the European research network for out-of-hours primary health care. Eur J Gen Pract. 2014;20:229–32.
35. Smits M, Keizer E, Giesen P, Deilkås EC, Hofoss D, Bondevik GT. The psychometric properties of the 'safety attitudes questionnaire' in out-of-hours primary care services in the Netherlands. PLoS One. 2017;12:e0172390.
36. Bondevik GT, Hofoss D, Hansen EH, Deilkås EC. The safety attitudes questionnaire - ambulatory version: psychometric properties of the Norwegian translated version for the primary care setting. BMC Health Serv Res. 2014;14:139.
37. Klemenc-Ketis Z, Maletic M, Stropnik V, Deilkås ET, Hofoss D, Bondevik GT. The safety attitudes questionnaire - ambulatory version: psychometric properties of the Slovenian version for the out-of-hours primary care setting. BMC Health Serv Res. 2017;17:36.
38. Voltmer E, Rosta J, Siegrist J, Aasland OG. Job stress and job satisfaction of physicians in private practice: comparison of German and Norwegian physicians. Int Arch Occup Environ Health. 2012;85:819–28.
39. Ohlander J, Weigl M, Petru R, Angerer P, Radon K. Working conditions and effort-reward imbalance of German physicians in Sweden respective Germany: a comparative study. Int Arch Occup Environ Health. 2015;88:511–9.
40. Elovainio M, Salo P, Jokela M, Heponiemi T, Linna A, Virtanen M, Oksanen T, Kivimäki M, Vahtera J. Psychosocial factors and well-being among Finnish GPs and specialists: a 10-year follow-up. Occup Environ Med. 2013;70:246–51.
41. Tsutsumi A, Kawanami S, Horie S. Effort-reward imbalance and depression among private practice physicians. Int Arch Occup Environ Health. 2012;85:153–61.

42. Ifediora CO. Burnout among after-hours home visit doctors in Australia. BMC Fam Pract. 2016;17:2.
43. Goetz K, Musselmann B, Szecsenyi J, Joos S. The influence of workload and health behavior on job satisfaction of general practitioners. Fam Med. 2013; 45:95–101.
44. Voltmer E, Spahn C. Social support and physician's health. Z Psychosom Med Psychother 2009; 55:51–69. German.
45. Barry HE, Campbell JL, Asprey A, Richards SH. The use of patient experience survey data by out-of-ours primary care services: a qualitative interview study. BMJ Qual Saf. 2015; https://doi.org/10.1136/bmjqs-2015-003963.
46. Kelley K, Clark B, Brown V, Sitzia J. Good practice in the conduct and reporting of survey research. Int J Qual Health Care. 2003;15:261–6.
47. Norman G. Likert scales, levels of measurement and the "laws" of statistics. Adv Health Sci Educ Theory Pract. 2010;15:625–362.
48. Carifio J, Perla R. Resolving the 50-year debate around using and misusing Likert scales. Med Educ. 2008;42:1150–2.

15

Using a modified nominal group technique to develop general practice

Elisabeth Søndergaard[*] ⓘ, Ruth K. Ertmann, Susanne Reventlow and Kirsten Lykke

Abstract

Background: There are few areas of health care where sufficient research-based evidence exists and primary health care is no exception. In the absence of such evidence, the development of assisted support must be based on the opinions and experience of professionals with knowledge of the relevant field. The purpose of this research project is to explore how the nominal group technique can be used to establish consensus by analysing how it supported the development of structured, knowledge-based, electronic health records for preventive child health examinations in Danish general practice.

Methods: We convened an expert panel of five general practitioners with a special interest in the preventive child health examinations. We introduced the panel to the nominal group technique, a well-established, structured, multistep, facilitated, group meeting technique used to generate consensus. The panel used the technique to agree on the key clinical and socioeconomic themes to include in new electronic records for the seven preventive child health examinations in Denmark. The panel met three times over a four-month period between 2013 and 2014 and their meetings lasted between two-and-a-half and five hours.

Results: 1) The structured and stepwise process of the nominal group technique supported our expert panel's focus as well as their equal opportunities to speak. 2) The method's flexibility enabled participants to work as a group and in pairs to discuss and refine thematic classifications. 3) Serial meetings supported continual evaluation, critical reflection, and knowledge searches, enabling our panel to produce a template that could be adapted for all seven preventive child health examinations.

Conclusion: The nominal group technique proved to be a useful method for reaching consensus by identifying key quality markers for use in daily clinical practice. Our study focused on the development of content and a layout for systematic, knowledge-based, electronic health records. We recommend the method as a suitable working tool for dealing with complex questions in general practice or similar settings, and we present and discuss modifications to the original model.

Keywords: Consensus methods, Nominal group technique, Organisational development, General practice, Primary health care, Qualitative research, Denmark, Electronic health records

Background

General practitioners (GPs) regularly make difficult choices about treatment options. Guidelines are one way of assisting GPs in decision-making and, in an ideal world, guidelines would be based on evidence derived from rigorously conducted empirical studies. In practice, there are few areas of health care where sufficient research-based evidence exists or can even be produced [1], and this is especially so

* Correspondence: elisab@sund.ku.dk
The Research Unit for General Practice and Section of General Practice, Department of Public Health, University of Copenhagen, Copenhagen, Denmark

within primary healthcare [2]. In such situations, the development of assisted support will inevitably be based, largely or in part, on the opinions and experience of clinicians and others with knowledge of the relevant field [3].

Since 2013, a group of Danish GPs has worked on producing systematic and knowledge-based electronic health records for the seven preventive child health examinations (PCHEs) held in general practice.

The Danish National Board of Health provides guidelines for PCHEs, but the recommendations are extensive and cover all aspects of a child's health [4]. There is no structured and systematic process in place to determine which of the comprehensive recommendations is the most important to focus on during the limited time available to carry out the PCHEs, nor is there a nationally aligned process for keeping journal notes. The vision is to make new electronic journal records available to all Danish GPs and the idea is that GPs' use of an electronic health record, with its potential for decision support and easy access to previous findings, will support their work and make it easier to keep an overview of the patient's case history.[1] The development of electronic records therefore holds the potential for a quality development in child healthcare in Denmark.

Given the likely diversity of opinion that any group of people may display when considering a topic, formalised methods, such as consensus techniques, are essential for organising subjective judgments in group work. Consensus techniques have been successfully used by several research groups in their work to develop quality markers in complex clinical areas, such as angina [5], emergency care [6], cancer [7], and also within the field of child healthcare [8–10].

The three most common consensus methods used for medical and health services research are the Delphi method, the consensus development conference, and the nominal group technique (NGT) [11]. The Delphi method is a forecasting method based on several rounds of questionnaires sent to a panel of experts. The anonymous, written responses are aggregated and shared with the group after each round [12]. The consensus development conference brings together practitioners, researchers, and consumers over a period of several days to seek general agreement, or consensus, on the efficacy, safety, and appropriate conditions for the use of various medical and surgical procedures, drugs, and devices [13]. The third method, and the one we selected in the present study, is the NGT.

The NGT is a structured, well-established, multistep, facilitated, group meeting technique used to generate and prioritise responses to a specific question by a group of people who have expert insight into a particular area of interest [2, 11, 14, 15]. It is an organised process that gives participants an equal opportunity to contribute their personal views before inviting them to build on the reflections of others to develop their own thoughts, and finally to reach consensus about the issues raised in the original question [8]. The NGT has been applied on several occasions for projects in general practice [16–19]. It has an advantage in that its format resembles the way Danish GPs are accustomed to collaborating in network groups, where experiences and challenges from everyday working life in practice are shared and discussed [20].

In this study the NGT was used with a twofold purpose. First, it was a way to systematise and develop the content of PCHEs; and second, it was a method to develop the format of electronic health records to be used in PCHEs. These two parallel purposes were strongly interlinked.

To bridge the gap between research and practice, evidence as well as its applicability should be considered when formulating recommendations. It is important that recommendations are compatible with existing norms and values and it is therefore essential that practitioners, in this case the future users of electronic health records, participate in the development of practice [21].

In this paper we explore how the NGT can be used to establish consensus in a complex clinical field by analysing how it supported the development of structured electronic health records for PCHEs in Danish general practice.

Methods

This study applied group discussions based on the NGT method in an adapted serial meeting design. The adapted design complies with the checklist created by Humphrey-Murto et al. to ensure methodological rigour when using consensus group methods, with only one deviation concerning anonymous re-ranking of feedback [22]. In-depth descriptions of the original steps in the NGT method have been reported extensively elsewhere [8, 23].

The project was conceived and designed by KL and RE, who are both experienced GPs specialising in research on children's health. During the meetings, KL was in the facilitator's role and RE participated as a member of the NGT panel. RE participated on the same terms as the other panel members, meaning that e.g. she waited for her turn to speak in the rounds, and her opinion carried no more weight than any of the other participants. More importantly, RE was aware of her double role in the project and its potential downfalls. This demanded a continuous reflection on her position, which we shall return to in the discussion section.

As well as RE, we purposively identified four GPs known for their broad knowledge and expertise in general practice and their specific interest in the PCHEs. We invited them to constitute the expert panel. Verbal informed consent was given before the four recruited GPs freely and informed chose to participate in the project. All five participating GPs worked either in Region Zealand or in the capital area of Copenhagen in Denmark. Prior to the first meeting the GPs were asked to read the report: *Evaluation of the Preventive Child Consultations in General Practice* [4] and before each meeting they were also asked to read the chapters in the Danish National Board of Health's guidelines on PCHEs [24] relevant for that particular meeting's focus. In this way we pursued a systematic method combining evidence and expert opinion.

In addition to background reading, we asked the participating GPs to be extra observant when carrying out PCHEs in the period leading up to the first meeting. We encouraged them to ask parents about their needs and expectations during the PCHEs. Throughout the working period of four months, the expert panel met three times. The meetings lasted five hours, five hours, and two-and-a-half hours respectively, and the four invited participants were offered compensation for their time. All meetings took place at facilities convenient to the practice of two of the participants.

The main aim of NGT is to generate themes and issues, which are discussed and ranked by the group. At the first meeting, KL described the NGT as a method to the panel members who had the opportunity to ask questions. This introduction was a factual description of the method's different steps and did not have any content or comment that would influence participants and the task in hand. After the introduction, KL asked the panel the nominal question: *What do you consider important to prioritise in the preventive child health examination at five weeks, and what do parents think is important, according to your experience and knowledge?* The question was developed based on KL's extensive work with the PCHEs [25–27] and RE's previous experience with developing electronic health records for antenatal care visits in general practice in Denmark. At this stage, the panel was given no guidance on how broad or narrow their focus should be.

The original plan was to work on the first three PCHEs, which take place when a baby is five weeks, five months, and twelve months old; one PCHE per scheduled meeting. However, while working through the steps of the NGT during the first meeting, the group found it necessary to make adjustments and deviations to the original model, outlined by Gallagher et al. [23].

The five hours allocated to develop a health record for the first PCHE were not enough to meet the project's combined objective: exploratory research involving a qualitative understanding of the priorities; and the development of a concrete product in the form of a systematic electronic health record. As a result, it was agreed in plenum that KL and RE should work with the draft produced by the panel between the first and the second meeting. This work solely concerned linguistic and structural aspects and a conscious effort was made to keep the content unchanged. The re-edited draft was then presented to participants at the second meeting, where it was critically evaluated, adjusted, and approved in plenum. In this way, a mutual understanding was secured in a forum in which the participants were both informants and collaborators. This pattern was repeated between the second and third meetings and became the model for working with drafts of the succeeding electronic

health records (Fig. 1). Consensus was defined as having been achieved when there were no further comments or suggestions for corrections from any of the participants. Achieved consensus determined the process. The continual and circular re-evaluation of the drafts enhanced the process and secured communicative validity [28].

The group's experience from working with the content and structure of the first electronic health record was used strategically at the next meeting when the focus shifted to the succeeding PCHE. During the meetings, the atmosphere was jovial and enthusiastic. The participation of KL and RE as the project's initiators did not seem to affect or influence the four invited GPs. All participants took part in the discussions equally and appeared confident in their roles as well as eager to contribute with their individual perspectives on the work.

In addition to working papers from the meeting rounds and the different draft versions of the electronic health records for the first three PCHEs, material for the present article also consisted of field notes produced during one of the meetings by ES, who participated as an observer. Having an observer in the research project enhanced opportunities for noticing aspects of interpersonal communication and group dynamic that are taken for granted or missed by participants due to their immediate obviousness [29]. The observations and field notes permitted an extra level of abstraction in the discussion of the group's use of the NGT, particularly with regard to the steps of the model where the group deviated from the original structure.

Based on the output of the meetings, including descriptive field notes, we conducted a thematic text analysis to identify important areas of new knowledge and to better understand what the modified version of the NGT meant for the validity of the method.

Results

The use of the NGT made it possible to combine idea generation and problem solving as two complementary parts of the same process. This makes the method well suited for development work in general practice with its complex characteristics and demands for applicability. Three main categories of experience were identified and these are described and appraised below. For clarity, the third category is divided into four sub-categories.

Keeping focus and supporting equal opportunities to speak

The structured and stepwise process of the NGT ensured that the energetic expert panel kept focus on the defined purpose, while the repeated table rounds supported opportunities for participants to be equally heard. The method's face-to-face approach integrated non-verbal communication, such as laughter; while the structured

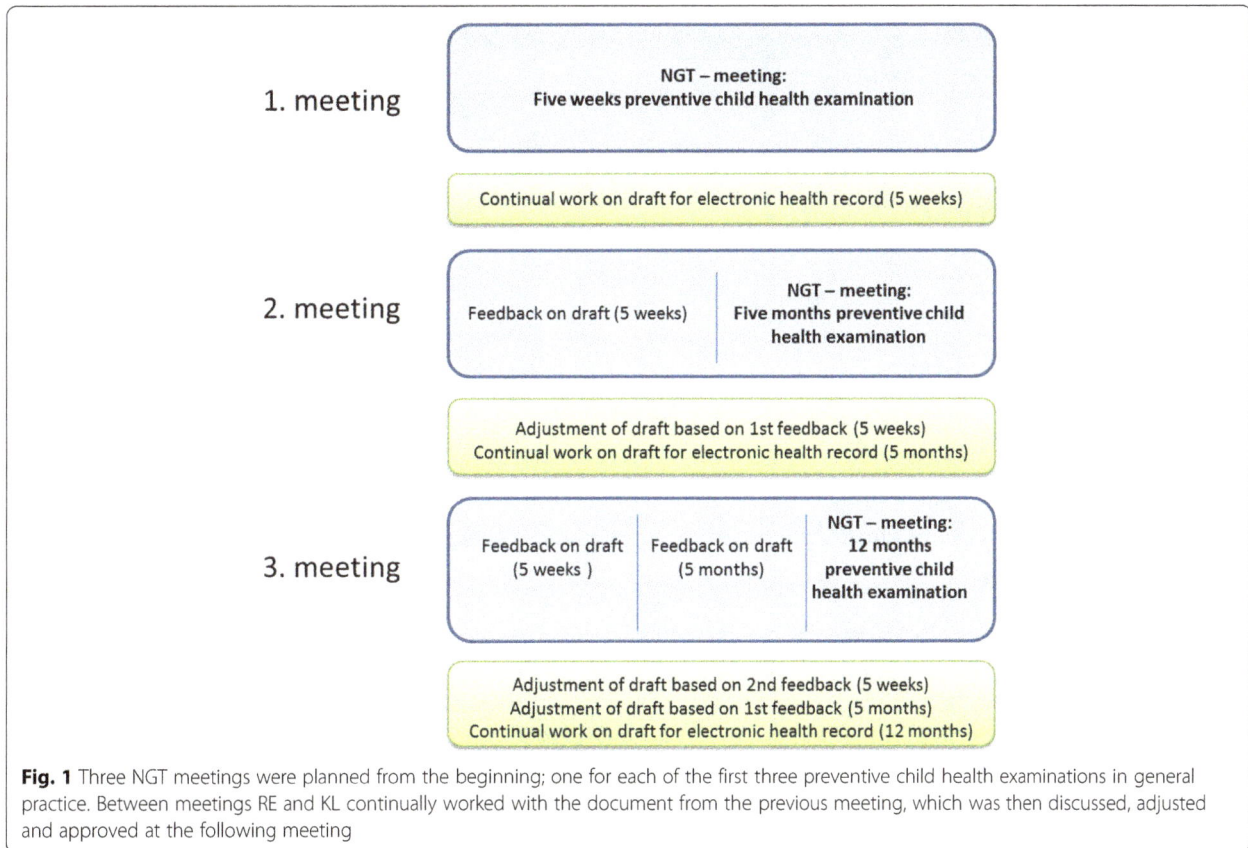

Fig. 1 Three NGT meetings were planned from the beginning; one for each of the first three preventive child health examinations in general practice. Between meetings RE and KL continually worked with the document from the previous meeting, which was then discussed, adjusted and approved at the following meeting

design minimised potential power structures that can appear when participants already know each other, or when one of the panelists is also the initiator of the project, which was our experience on this project.

Generating new perspectives on clinical practice
During steps 4 and 5 (Table 1) the participants became aware of the potential to re-use knowledge previously obtained about the patient (Table 2, column 3). Prior to the seven PCHEs, the Danish preventive healthcare programme has three antenatal care visits and, in principle, all ten visits are conducted by the same GP. Data from antenatal care visits are recorded in the mother's journal, which is not automatically consulted in the PCHEs that follow. The process of the group discussions generated an awareness of the prospective re-use of knowledge gathered during the antenatal care visits, such as the pregnancy's development or the family's socioeconomic situation.

Flexibility of the NGT model
The NGT proved to be a highly flexible model well suited to the complex research question we asked, and conducive to detailed discussion and elucidation of themes and issues.

Discussions and thematic classification in pairs
The panel recognised early in the working process that it would not be favourable to strictly follow the model's original outline. For example, the discussions and clarifications carried out in step 4 (Table 1) revealed that it did not make sense to produce a prioritised list, as the model prescribes. Since all the suggested themes were important, the expert panel found it more relevant to organise them into broader thematic categories and line them up in that way. The work with these categories was carried out first as a group and then the panel divided into pairs to further discuss the categories. This resulted in an outline of the first draft of the electronic health record (Table 2, column 2).

Serial meetings
Serial meetings provided time for continual evaluation and the search for more information.

The original time allocated to work with electronic health records turned out to be too short to produce adequate content and a format for each record. As a consequence, drafts were linguistically and structurally reorganised by KL and RE between meetings (Fig. 1). At the same time, participants had opportunities to test in their practices aspects that had been discussed during the meeting, and to return to the next session with new experience-based knowledge. Participants became aware

Table 1 An outline of the steps in the original NGT model and the deviations and attributions made to the structure during the working process with the development of an electronic health record for the examination of babies at 5 weeks

A case study – working with the preventive child health examination at five weeks

	The original model	Attributions and deviations
Step 1	Introduction	
Step 2	Each individual answers the overall question. Silent generation of ideas in writing.	
Step 3	Table rounds where each participant in turn presents a theme from his/her list. During the presentations, new ideas are generated and rounds continue until all items are listed.	
Step 4	The different themes are discussed and classified. Listing of ideas on flip chart.	The different themes were discussed and organised in categories.
Step 5	Each participant selects 10 of the listed themes in silence. All themes are ranked and given points from 1 to 10. The most important theme receives 10 points.	Working together in pairs the categories were ranged according to the structure of the consultation.
Step 6	Pause, while a prioritised consensus list is produced.	30 min break. No prioritised list produced.
Step 7	The prioritised list is discussed	The thematic categories were presented in plenum and discussed. It was agreed that KL and RE should continue working with the format of the electronic health record in the time until the next meeting.
Step 8	All participants re-evaluate the list. First individually, thereafter in plenum.	Two months' intermission where KL and RE continually worked on a revised version. The newest version of the electronic health record was discussed and adjusted in plenum at the following meeting. 1-month intermission where the electronic health record was further revised. Final discussions in the group during the next meeting.

that some instructions in the guidelines from the National Board of Health were not fully up-to-date; the recommendations for congenital cataract, for example. The serial nature of the meetings meant that such questions of doubt could be checked in the interim and discussed at the next meeting.

Reflections and ethical considerations

The serial character of the meetings and the continual re-evaluation of the drafts (Fig. 1) made room for participants to further reflect between meetings on the topics discussed. During the first meeting, the idea that information collected at the mother's antenatal care visits could automatically be transferred to the child's health record was presented and calmly received in the group. However, at the third meeting an intense discussion arose concerning ethical issues raised by the idea of transferring certain kinds of information to the child's record, e.g. alcohol abuse in the family. The serial application of the method provided time for important critical reflection on themes and, in this case, the ethical challenges around a potential transfer of data.

Adjustable template

Although the group did not succeed at the first meeting in producing a final model for the PCHE at five weeks, the

NGT secured the production of a fruitful draft which was applied as a model for the first and all succeeding PCHEs (See Table 2). The flexibility of the NGT therefore led to the production of a template that could be used and tailored during the development of systematic electronic health records for all seven PCHEs. The template was based on the experience of frontline professionals, the guidelines from the National Board of Health, and best evidence. The findings were practice-near, experience-based, and therefore directly applicable to PCHE work in general practice.

Discussion

Our main findings from working with the NGT relate to its flexibility and modifiability. The flexibility of the method confirmed its suitability for complex research questions, such as ours; while the production of an adjustable template with consensus results made the meetings' outcomes both manageable and tangible. The functionality of the modified serial meeting design provided fruitful time for continued reflection on the results and previous discussions, as well as providing opportunities for relevant checks between meetings where a lack of knowledge or doubts had become apparent. The latter provided openings for systematic development of knowledge.

Table 2 In the first column, all the participants' ideas are shown in the order they appeared during the table rounds and in the short formulations the proposers found adequate

First rounds of the nominal group process	Clarification and categorisation	After linguistic and structural editing by KL and RE
1. Setting the scene: what, why, how – long process.	1. Setting the scene	Information folder
2. The parental experience of pregnancy and birth	At the beginning and at the end of the examination: what, why, how – long process.	(Could we ask the parents a few questions at the same time?)
3. Is there something in particular you would like to discuss?	Vaccinations. What is a preventive child health examination? The goal?	Knowledge previously collected from the antenatal care visits:
4. Has the development from birth until now been satisfying?	Adjust expectations.	The name of the child's father and CPR number. The siblings' names and CPRs.
5. How are things coming along?	Transparency in the examinations.	Relationship status. Chronic diseases among mother or
6. Did anything happen during birth that you experienced as a threat?	Information for parents prior to the consultation.	father. Mother's/father's work title, place of birth.
7. How is the family handling the new family member – network?	To create a feeling of security - future cooperation	Mother's/father's potential threatening social or emotional condition.
8. Follow-up from visiting nurse/ place of birth	2. The parents' experience of pregnancy, birth, and the first weeks with the baby	1. Did the parents have anything particular they wanted to talk with the GP about?
9. The contact between the GP/mother/child/ father	Did anything happen during birth that you experienced as a threat? Has the development	Yes _____ No _____
10. Interaction/Attachment	from birth until this point been satisfying? How are things coming along? Baby blues? (Mother,	2. Follow-up on information transferred from the antenatal care visits, has anything changed?
11. The parents' experience of the parenting role	child, father, the family).	Yes _____ No _____
12. Recognise – Issues with the parents that make me wonder whether this is a vulnerable family	3. Is there something in particular you would like to discuss?	3. The parents' experience of pregnancy and birth
13. Support the parents' belief in their own capabilities	The parents' needs.	3.1 Follow-up on pregnancy. Certain experiences/worries?
14. The objective examination	4. How is the family handling the new family member?	Yes _____ No _____
15. The child's rhythm – sleep patterns, food, crying, bowel function	Hard work – siblings – feeling tired – network.	3.2 Follow-up on birth Certain experiences/worries?
16. The parents own childhood	The parents' experience of the parenting role, making ends meet, frustration. Attachment.	Yes _____ No _____
17. Preventions themes – smoking, falls, and sleeping positions.	Parental leave – is co-parent at home – childcare	3.3 Is contact with a visiting nurse established?
18. Transparency in the examination	5. Follow-up from visiting nurse/ place of birth	Does the visiting nurse have any wishes for themes that should be discussed at the PCHE?
19. Conclusion, transparency and follow-up	Have they attended the relevant examinations? Have they received answers	Yes _____ No_____
20. Advice and guidelines concerning a sick child	from tests?	3.4 Has the child had a PKU-test?
21. Information for parents prior to the consultation	6. Recognise – Issues with the parents that make me wonder whether this is a	Yes _____ No _____
22. Parental leave – is co-parent at home? child care, economy	vulnerable family	Hearing screening test:
23. To create a feeling of security - future cooperation	Economy, resources, education, work. The parents' experiences. Family structure: single, half-half,	Yes _____ No _____
24. Family structure	donor, adopted, etc.	Remarks: _____
25. Support the parents in their care for their child.	7. Objective examination.	4. Parents' experience of the first weeks
	Contact between GP/ mother/child/father interaction.	4.1 How are things coming along? (Mother, father, sibling, family, handling new tasks).
	8. The child's rhythm	4.2 Are mother and child gaining a common rhythm?
	Sleep patterns, food, crying, bowel function, well-being.	Yes _____ No _____
	The GP's evaluation and communication of what is considered as normal.	(Sleep, meals, bowel functions, can the child be comforted when crying? Do mother and father
	9. The parents' own childhood	feel they can cope?).
	Previous/ongoing family trauma. Preconditions for attachments.	4.3 Breast-feeding
	10. Prevention themes	Yes _____ No _____
	Smoking, falls, sleeping positions. Vaccinations.	Partly_____
	Advice and guidelines concerning a sick child.	5. Objective examination
	11. Conclusion	(Specified in 16 items/points following the guidelines from The National Board of Health).
	Reciprocity.	6. Discussed birth control
	Support the parents' belief in their own capabilities	Yes, themes:___ No _____
	Follow-up, appointments.	7. Conclusion
	Transparency	An overall estimation of the child's wellbeing and the family's resources and risks.
		8. Follow-up
		Yes _____ No _____
		E.g. an extra consultation at the GP or a reference to a specialist/or the social system.

In the second column, all the ideas have been elaborated by the original proposer and the group has, both jointly and in pairs, organised the many ideas into categories. The third column shows the final version of both content and structure of the systematic health record. This was completed after discussion and editing at the third and last meeting. This proposal has subsequently been edited into an electronic format which is not shown in this article

Some of our results concur with findings from previous projects working with the NGT and the model's flexibility has been recognised by other studies that also successfully modified the original NGT design and experienced an improvement [5–10]. One study had difficulty with the ranking in step 5 (Table 1) [8], which we also report in our findings. They ended up voting when consensus could not be reached through ranking, while the present study chose to divide the panel into pairs to work with the themes, before returning once more to discussion in plenum. In line with our findings, other studies have also found that the original NGT structure, with one meeting allocated to reach final recommendations, was not sufficient for an in-depth elaboration of themes [8, 30]. The serial character of the meetings in this study is comparable to the Delphi method [12, 15] where consensus is obtained through evaluation of written documents that are sent back and forth among participants a number of times until consensus is reached. Therefore, in the present study we incorporated strength from the Delphi method into the modified version of the NGT.

Experiences emerged during the working processes that, to our knowledge, have not previously been reported by other studies. A central feature of using the NGT is that a question is investigated extensively from a broad spectrum of viewpoints and thereby creates awareness of overlaps, knowledge-sharing, gaps in knowledge, or unproductive working patterns. In this project, our participants became aware of the possibility of using existing knowledge about their patients, but also about the potential ethical downside of such a practice. By documenting all proposals and ideas, the NGT model ensures that no insights are lost through the potential uncertainty of some participants, while at the same time tangible products in the form of written documents are produced.

Implication of findings for future research
Related to the specific research project
It is anticipated that the possibility of using electronic health records as a support when carrying out PCHEs in the future will systematise and develop both the structure and the content of the PCHEs in general practice. However, experience and intuition are fundamental and effective elements of everyday working life in general practice, not least when it comes to diagnosing children [27, 31, 32]. It is therefore crucial that the electronic health records do not compromise this practice, which is why the use of the records will be a supportive option and not a mandatory practice. Lippert et al. have pointed to a need for further discussion about the relationship between situatedness and standardisation in primary care and for further empirical investigations of the possible consequences of standardisation processes [33]. DanChild, of which the present study is a part, has a combined vision to investigate GPs' responses to electronic health records as well as to develop child health through cohort research. While the NGT as a method encourages consensus and practice-near solutions, it is important to emphasise that the success of the electronic health records is dependent on a continued and reciprocal collaboration with general practice [34, 35].

Related to the applicability of the modified method
The modifications we made to the NGT were feasible and did not lose the method's advantageous structure.

We believe this was because the participants and the facilitator shared a common professional background as GPs, limiting the perspectives to one professional grouping. Participants had been asked to read relevant chapters in the Danish National Board of Health's guidelines on PCHEs as well as a thematically relevant report, further enhancing a mutual starting point. However, we did not check whether or not they had read the documents. We felt that this would unnecessarily highlight the fact that one of the participants, RE, was also one of the project's initiators. Therefore we cannot guarantee that all participants had a common starting point for discussion. Finally, the project had a well-defined goal, namely the production of content and a format for electronic health records supporting the PCHEs, and that concrete purpose enabled a softening of the original NGT model's mechanical steps, without the group losing its focus. Based on our experience with the modified NGT all three aspects are crucial for future researchers implementing similar changes to the original NGT model.

Strengths and limitations of the study
By asking highly professionally engaged GPs with a specific interest in the PCHEs to reach consensus and suggest a way forward for all GPs to follow, our results may be ambiguous for the average practitioner. The project group is aware of this risk and will incorporate it into their continued work with electronic health records by pilot testing the product and by giving individual practitioners flexibility to use the record in their own way.

In this project two of the article's authors participated either as facilitator (KL) or as a member of the panel (RE), and they worked with the drafts between the meetings. Double roles like these are not uncommon in similar projects [8], but still worth critical reflection and consideration. Any data collection, analysis, and conclusion are inextricably entwined with the researcher's presuppositions as well as the positions adopted while collecting the data [36, 37]. According to Skjervheim, researchers can only gain access to social phenomena of interest by recognising themselves as a contributing participant [38]. In this case, RE is an experienced GP with a known research interest in child health, and took part in the panel as an equal to the other participants. RE was, however, aware of her double role in the process and continuously reflected on the effect it might have on the way her suggestions and comments were received by the group, and, ultimately, on how it might have affected consensus. One could discuss if KL's and RE's work between the meetings minimised the democratic process, by giving them more influence than the rest of the group. This risk was reduced as much as possible, by the process of repeatedly evaluating their work in plenum at subsequent meetings. During these evaluations the other participants actively suggested critical corrections and this leads us to believe that the final product meets a satisfactory degree of representativeness. Furthermore, we attempted to minimise bias by enrolling co-authors who were not actively implicated in the data producing process. One of them even participated as an observer at one of the meetings. Finally, the authors recognise that objective knowledge in the form of *true* consensus is a naïve understanding of reality. Following Haraway, it might be more fruitful to think of knowledge as situated within a context [39]. While the point of view within a context has a more limited range than disembodied objectivity, situated points of view are richer in content as they take into account the numerous bits of information constituting the context and the environment of that point of view. For the present project, it means acknowledging the influence KL and RE had on consensus, while at the same time recognising this as a given condition that simultaneously supported the success of the group's progressive work.

Conclusions

To our knowledge, this study is the first to report on Danish GPs using the NGT to identify key areas of focus and to structure quality marker development in general practice. The structured interactive process used in this study supported equal opportunities for experienced professionals to significantly contribute to the development of electronic health records to support PCHEs in Danish general practice. By using the modified NGT, participating GPs actively expressed their views through structured discussions as a group, through working in pairs, and through the process of reaching final consensus. In accordance with previous studies [3] we therefore argue that the original NGT model developed in the late 1960s [5] can be modified advantageously and used to explore developmental work and changes in general practice. Due to the integration of experienced professionals from the very beginning of the process the results are practice-based and applicable. We are confident that the NGT model can be useful for capturing group perspectives in complex working areas such as general practice, and we recommend the NGT as a working tool in general practice development in the future.

Endnotes

[1]Creating electronic health records is part of DanChild, a research and quality development project, with the goal to develop a new national birth cohort with potential to nest randomised trials in general practice. The cohort will support the development of knowledge about child health which is highly relevant to the work in general practice.

Abbreviations
ES: Elisabeth Søndergaard; Fig.: Figure; GPs: General practitioners; KL: Kirsten Lykke; NGT: The nominal group technique; PCHEs: Preventive child health examinations; RE: Ruth K. Ertmann

Acknowledgements
We would like to thank all the other members of the expert panel; Morten Jakobsen, Johannes Larsen, Majbrit Brouer and Pia Birgitte Koefoed for their engaged participation.

Funding
The work with developing the electronic health records for the preventive child health examinations was funded by Region Zealand.

Authors' contributions
KL and RE conceived and designed the study and RE participated in the panel while KL moderated the meetings. ES collected and interpreted the data and drafted the article. RE, KL, and SR contributed to drafting of the article, critical revisions to the article, and approved the final draft.

Competing interests
The authors declare that they have no competing interests.

References
1. Chassin M. How do we decide whether an investigation or procedure is appropriate? In: Hopkins A, editor. Appropriate investigation and treatment in clinical practice. London: Royal College of Physicians; 1989. p. 21–9.
2. Campbell SM, Braspenning J, Hutchinson A, Marshall MN. Research methods used in developing and applying quality indicators in primary care. BMJ. 2003;326(7393):816–9.
3. Mann T. Clinical guidelines : using clinical guidelines to improve patient care within the NHS. London: Department of Health; 1996.
4. Michelsen S, Kastanje M, Flachs EM, Søndergaard G, Biering-Sørensen S, Madsen M, AMN A. Evaluation of the preventive child consultations in general practice. Copenhagen: Danish National Board of health, Statens Institut for Folkesundhed, Syddansk Universitet; 2011.
5. Campbell SM, Ludt S, Van Lieshout J, Boffin N, Wensing M, Petek D, et al. Quality indicators for the prevention and management of cardiovascular disease in primary care in nine European countries. Eur J cardiovasc Prev Rehabil. 2008;15(5):509–15.
6. Schull MJ, Guttmann A, Leaver CA, Vermeulen M, Hatcher CM, Rowe BH, et al. Prioritizing performance measurement for emergency department care: consensus on evidence-based quality of care indicators. CJEM. 2011; 13(5):300–9. E28–43
7. Malin JL, Asch SM, Kerr EA, McGlynn EA. Evaluating the quality of cancer care: development of cancer quality indicators for a global quality assessment tool. Cancer. 2000;88(3):701–7.

8.   Gill PJ, Hewitson P, Peile E, Harnden A. Prioritizing areas for quality marker development in children in UK general practice: extending the use of the nominal group technique. Fam Pract. 2012;29(5):567–75.

9.   Giannini EH, Ruperto N, Ravelli A, Lovell DJ, Felson DT, Martini A. Preliminary definition of improvement in juvenile arthritis. Arthritis Rheum. 1997;40(7):1202–9.

10. Wang CJ, McGlynn EA, Brook RH, Leonard CH, Piecuch RE, Hsueh SI, et al. Quality-of-care indicators for the neurodevelopmental follow-up of very low birth weight children: results of an expert panel process. Pediatrics. 2006;117(6):2080–92.

11. Jones J, Hunter D. Consensus methods for medical and health services research. BMJ. 1995;311(7001):376–80.

12. Hasson F, Keeney S, McKenna H. Research guidelines for the Delphi survey technique. J Adv Nurs. 2000;32(4):1008–15.

13. Wortman PM, Vinokur A, Sechrest L. Do consensus conferences work? A process evaluation of the NIH consensus development program. J Health Polit Policy Law. 1988;13(3):469–98.

14. Van de Ven AH, Delbecq AL. The nominal group as a research instrument for exploratory health studies. Am J Public Health. 1972;62(3):337–42.

15. Fink A, Kosecoff J, Chassin M, Brook RH. Consensus methods: characteristics and guidelines for use. Am J Public Health. 1984;74(9):979–83.

16. Stolper E, van Leeuwen Y, van Royen P, van de Wiel M, van Bokhoven M, Houben P, et al. Establishing a European research agenda on 'gut feelings' in general practice. A qualitative study using the nominal group technique. Eur J Gen Pract. 2010;16(2):75–9.

17. Shipman C, Gysels M, White P, Worth A, Murray SA, Barclay S, et al. Improving generalist end of life care: national consultation with practitioners, commissioners, academics, and service user groups. BMJ. 2008;337:a1720.

18. Zhao Y, Chen R, Wang B, Wu T, Huang Y, Guo A. General practice on-the-job training in Chinese urban community: a qualitative study on needs and challenges. PLoS One. 2014;9(4):e94301.

19. Laughlin T, Wetmore S, Allen T, Brailovsky C, Crichton T, Bethune C, et al. Defining competency-based evaluation objectives in family medicine: communication skills. Can Fam Physician. 2012;58(4):217–24.

20. Gannik D. Kvalitet i almen praksis: Praktiserende lægers syn på fagets essens, vilkår og udvikling i Viborg Amt. Forskningsenheden for Almen Praksis i København; 2004.

21. Burgers JS, Grol RP, Zaat JO, Spies TH, van der Bij AK, Mokkink HG. Characteristics of effective clinical guidelines for general practice. Br J Gen Pract. 2003;53(486):15–9.

22. Humphrey-Murto S, Varpio L, Gonsalves C, Wood TJ. Using consensus group methods such as Delphi and nominal group in medical education research. Med Teach. 2017;39(1):14–9.

23. Gallagher M, Hares T, Spencer J, Bradshaw C, Webb I. The nominal group technique: a research tool for general practice? Fam Pract. 1993;10(1):76–81.

24. Vejledning om forebyggende sundhedsydelser til børn og unge. National Board of health: Copenhagen, Denmark; 2011.

25. Lykke K, Christensen P, Reventlow S. The consultation as an interpretive dialogue about the child's health needs. Fam Pract. 2011;28(4):430–6.

26. Lykke K, Christensen P, Reventlow S. GPs' strategies in exploring the preschool child's wellbeing in the paediatric consultation. BMC Fam Pract. 2013;14:177.

27. Lykke K, Christensen P, Reventlow S. "this is not normal ... "-signs that make the GP question the child's well-being. Fam Pract. 2008;25(3):146–53.

28. Steinar K. The social construction of validity. Qual Inq. 1995;1(1):19–40.

29. Corbin Dwyer S. The space between: on being an insider-outsider in qualitative research Int J Qual Methods. 2009;8(1):54–63.

30. He G, Huang WY, Wong SH. Understanding neighborhood environment related to Hong Kong Children's physical activity: a qualitative study using nominal group technique. PLoS One. 2014;9(9):e106578.

31. Van den Bruel A, Aertgeerts B, Bruyninckx R, Aerts M, Buntinx F. Signs and symptoms for diagnosis of serious infections in children: a prospective study in primary care. Br J Gen Pract. 2007;57(540):538–46.

32. Van den Bruel A, Haj-Hassan T, Thompson M, Buntinx F, Mant D. Diagnostic value of clinical features at presentation to identify serious infection in children in developed countries: a systematic review. Lancet. 2010;375(9717):834–45.

33. Lippert ML, Reventlow S, Kousgaard MB. The uses and implications of standards in general practice consultations. Health. 2015;21(1):3–20.

34. Dahler-Larsen P. The Evaluation Society Standford: Standford University; 2012.

35. Munro E. The impact of audit on social work practice. Br J Soc Work. 2004;34(8):1075–95.

36. Reventlow S, Tulinius C. The doctor as focus group moderator - shifting roles and negotiating positions in health research. Fam Pract. 2005;22(3):335–40.

37. Malterud K. Qualitative research: standards, challenges, and guidelines. Lancet. 2001;358(9280):483–8.

38. Skjervheim H. Objectivism and the study of man. Oslo: Universitetsforlaget. 1959.

39. Haraway D. Situated knowledges: the science question in feminism and the privilege of partial perspective. Fem Stud. 1988;14(3):575–99.

16

Diabetes care providers' opinions and working methods after four years of experience with a diabetes patient web portal; a survey among health care providers in general practices and an outpatient clinic

Maaike C. M. Ronda[1]* , Lioe-Ting Dijkhorst-Oei[2], Rimke C. Vos[1] and Guy E. H. M. Rutten[1]

Abstract

Background: To gain insight into the opinions and working methods of diabetes care providers after using a diabetes web portal for 4 years in order to understand the role of the provider in patients' web portal use.

Methods: Survey among physicians and nurses from general practices and an outpatient clinic, correlated with data from the common web portal.

Results: One hundred twenty-eight questionnaires were analysed (response rate 56.6%). Responders' mean age was 46.2 ± 9.8 years and 43.8% were physicians. The majority was of opinion that the portal improves patients' diabetes knowledge (90.6%) and quality of care (72.7%). Although uploading glucose diary (93.6%) and patient access to laboratory and clinical notes (91.2 and 71.0%) were considered important, these features were recommended to patients in only 71.8 and 19.5% respectively. 64.8% declared they informed their patients about the portal and 45.3% handed-out the information leaflet and website address. The portal was especially recommended to type 1 diabetes patients (78.3%); those on insulin (84.3%) and patients aged< 65 years (72.4%). Few found it timesaving (21.9%). Diabetes care providers' opinions were not associated with patients' portal use.

Conclusions: Providers are positive about patients web portals but still not recommend or encourage the use to all patients. There seems room for improvement in their working methods.

Keywords: Patient web portal, E-health, Communication, Physician attitudes, Diabetes portal, Diabetes self-management

Background

The burden of diabetes is rapidly increasing worldwide [1]. Patient web portals are of interest in this respect and many studies focused on the use of portals by patients with diabetes [2, 3]. A patient portal is a secure online website that gives a person access to his or her personal medical information derived from the physician's electronic medical record. Portals have shown a range of benefits, such as improved diabetes outcomes, increased patient satisfaction and patient-provider communication, and reduced office visits [4–8]. However, the number of patients that use a portal is low [9–13].

We demonstrated that patients' unawareness of the existence of a portal is an important barrier for starting its use [14]. So the role of the diabetes care provider seems of importance in the use of patient portals. However, healthcare providers are often also unaware of the existence of a patient portal or of its features [15, 16]. They may underestimate the number of patients that are actually interested in using it [15], are hesitant to start a web-based communication [17], or expect problems with the communication or in the relationship with their patients [18–20]. There is fear for patients experiencing problems with the interpretation of a portal's data [18,

* Correspondence: m.c.m.ronda@umcutrecht.nl
[1]Julius Centre for Health Sciences and Primary Care, University Medical Centre Utrecht, STR 6.131, PO Box 85500, 3508 Utrecht, GA, Netherlands
Full list of author information is available at the end of the article

21, 22], pessimism about patients' motivation and ability to maintain a personal health record [16], and fear for an increase in the physician's workload [23–25]. Concerns about reliability, confidentiality, and security of information are other commonly mentioned barriers [20, 24, 26–28]. However, information about the interaction with patients with regard to portal use is lacking and more insight into the daily practice role of the diabetes care provider in this respect seems warranted.

We aimed to gain insight into the opinions and working methods of diabetes care providers after having used for 4 years a diabetes specific electronically medical record in which patients have full access ("web portal"). The following research questions are addressed:

1. What are the opinions of the diabetes care providers about the portal and its functionality?
2. How do they communicate the possibilities of the portal and to which patients?
3. What are the perceived consequences of the portal?
4. Are provider characteristics and opinions associated with the patients' portal use?

Methods

Study setting
"Diamuraal" is a so-called care group, that coordinates the care of patients with diabetes [29, 30]. Within this care group there are 62 primary care practices working (with general practitioners and nurse practitioners) and one outpatient clinic (with internists with subspecialty diabetology or nephrology and specialized diabetes nurses). All practices and providers use the same type of diabetes electronic medical record (EMR). The diabetes EMR is used simultaneously with and besides the general EMR of both the primary and secondary care practices.

The patient web portal
The general EMR has no portal option, but patients can request a login to access their personal diabetes EMR, via a web portal that provides access to information about the consultation, laboratory results, the so-called 'problem list', treatment goals, as well as to general diabetes information and to an overview of all individual diabetes related examinations and consultations that are needed and/or scheduled. Patients can upload glucose levels measured at home, including comments, and are asked for explanations in case of high and low glucose values ("glucose diary"). They can also contact their physician or nurse by secured electronic messaging. In addition, quarterly monitoring office visits can be substituted by self-monitoring; in that case, the diabetes care provider schedules for a patient to complete a standardized check list in his diabetes EMR. The portal is supplementary; all patients receive regular diabetes care according to the Dutch guidelines [31].

Study design and measures
A postal questionnaire was sent to all 228 diabetes care providers working in Diamuraal. It contained questions about their opinions about the portal and its functionality, to which patients they recommend or discourage the portal's use, how they communicate the possibilities of the portal with the patients and how they perceive the consequences of the portal, not only with regard to patient self-management but also for the healthcare provider. Twenty-six questions had to be scored on a 5-point Likert scale, 15 questions on a 3-point Likert scale, eight questions were multiple choice and one was open ended. In addition, six items about provider characteristics were included (see Additional file 1 for an overview). All issues addressed in the questions were proven relevant based on literature [2, 32] and it was pilot tested by 2 general practitioners, an internist and two diabetes nurses from the Diamuraal care group.

Possible respondents received a reminder twice in a 3 week interval; the first by post, the second by telephone. From the central database of Diamuraal, data were collected about the number of patients with access to the patient portal per practice and about the start date of practices joining Diamuraal.

Statistical analysis
Categorical variables were expressed as counts with percentages and continuous variables as means with standard deviation (SD). Continuous variables were checked for normality. The characteristics and opinions of different type of health care providers were compared with chi-square tests for categorical and unpaired t-tests for continuous variables. Items with a 5-point Likert scale were transformed into three answer categories by combining the two highest and the two lowest response categories. Linear regression was used to assess the association between the number of patients with a login request and the time the practice had been using the portal, and Spearman's rho was used to assess the correlation between provider's opinions and the number of patients with a login request per practice. Data were analysed using SPSS for Windows (version 21, SPSS Inc., Chicago, IL, USA).

Results
In total 129 (56.6%) diabetes care providers completed the questionnaire. One questionnaire was excluded because of > 10% missing values, so 128 questionnaires were analysed. Responders were more often female (75% of participants vs 49% of non-responders, $p < 0.001$) and had a higher proportion of patients with access to the

portal in their practices, although the difference was not significant ($17.6 \pm 11.4\%$ versus $7.9 \pm 6.4\%$ ($p = 0.07$).

Respondents' mean age was 46.2 ± 9.8 years (Table 1). On average 157.8 ± 9.1 diabetes patients were treated in a primary care practice (range 52–508); the outpatient clinic treated 2647 diabetes patients. The outpatient clinic had a higher percentage of patients with access to the portal than the primary care practices (52.8% versus 16.9%). The diabetes EMR with portal was used for 5 years by the outpatient clinic compared to on average 3.8 years in primary care. The medical specialties invited had a differential response rate, ranging from 100% (internists and diabetes nurses) to 76.8% (nurse practitioners) and 35.7% (GPs).

Opinions about the portal and its functionality

The two main reasons for respondents to work with the portal was because they felt that it could improve the quality of diabetes care (77/128 providers, 60.2%) and the supposed improvement of communication between the different members of the diabetes team by working with one common medical record (56/128, 43.8%). Most respondents were positive about the use of a patient portal with respect to the quality of care, patient self-care and consult preparation. However, although most respondents (strongly) agreed that the provided diabetes information on the portal could lead to improved self-management, only 20% thought that it would improve self-management in three quarters of their own patients. In general the internists were more sceptical about the portal, but differences between type of health care provider were not significant (Table 2). Most respondents scored the glucose diary (117/125, 93.6%) and the access to laboratory values and treatment goals for the patients (114/125, 91.2%) as (very) important features of the portal. Other features that were scored as (very) important were the possibility to send an e-message (98/124, 79.0%) and the patient's access to clinical notes (88/124, 71.0%). About two out of three (66.9%) respondents scored web-based scheduling consultations (very) important, the same applied to 'insight in the personal care team' (67.7%) and diabetes information (64.8%). Insight into prescribed medication was scored as (very) important by 61.8% of the respondents. Suggestions for improvement of the portal mainly regarded the glucose diary ("difficult to fill in for patients

with insulin-pump therapy"), the option to add self-measured blood pressure levels by the patient (which actually was an existing feature, but apparently not known by most diabetes care providers working with this portal), adding of other non-diabetes related laboratory values or patient characteristics (e.g. history, type of work and current diet), and tailored diabetes and medication information.

How do diabetes care providers communicate the portal, and to which patients?

Most often the face-to-face method was reported as to communicate the use of the portal. Additional types of informing the patient and communication about the portal were less often utilized (Fig. 1). More than half of the respondents reported that they always or regularly encourage their patients to use the portal for adding glucose values as well as for e-messaging. Preparing a consultation and re-reading the information before and after a consultation were least encouraged (Table 3). Respondents answered that they recommend the portal to most of their patients, but especially to patients with type 1 diabetes mellitus, patients on insulin therapy, younger and higher educated patients (Table 4). Diabetes care providers did not differ in this respect (data not shown).

Perceived consequences for the care provider

One third of the diabetes care providers (40/121, 33.1%) declared that the provider's role in the treatment (strongly) improved, whereas two-thirds of the providers (82/121, 67.8%) felt that the involvement of the patient in the treatment (strongly) improved. Other perceived (strong) improvements were the collaboration with the patient (85/121, 70.2%) and the increased knowledge of patients about diabetes mellitus (70/120, 58.3%). The majority of respondents stated that having access to the EMR stimulates self-management and self-correcting behaviour of patients. Most reported that they did not change their way of medical notation and most also stated that the frequency of patient's personal consultations had not changed after the introduction of the portal (Table 5).

Are provider characteristics and opinions associated with the patients' portal use?

The proportion of patients with access to the portal was not related to the number of years the practice had been using the portal (beta 0.32 (95% CI -0.15 – 0.78), $p = 0.17$). Except for the statement that it can lead to improved self-management in general (r_s-.296, $p = 0.03$), the respondents' opinion about each of the six possible effects of the portal as mentioned in Table 2 was not associated with the proportion of patients within the practice that requested a login to the portal (improving the

Table 1 Characteristics of Responders ($N = 128$)

	General Practitioner	Nurse Practitioner	Internist	Diabetes Nurse
Number	45	56	11	16
Gender, male	27 (60,0%)	0 (0%)	6 (54,5%)	0 (0%)
Age, years ± SD	51.4 ± 12.8	43.2 ± 9.9	46.4 ± 10.8	49.5 ± 10.3

Table 2 Opinions about the possible effects of the diabetes web portal. Percentages of respondents

"I (strongly) agree that….."	All providers (N = 128)	General practitioner (n = 45)	Nurse practitioner (n = 56)	Internist (n = 11)	Diabetes nurse (n = 16)	P-value
a patient portal improves the quality of diabetes care	72.7	77.8	67.9	63.6	81.3	0.60
a patient portal can prevent medical mistakes	55.5	60.0	50.0	45.5	68.8	0.33
the diabetes knowledge that patients gain through the portal can lead to improved self-management	90.6	97.7	85.5[a]	81.8	100	0.30
a positive effect of the patient web portal is that patients can prepare themselves to the diabetes consultation	71.1	73.3	67.9	63.6	81.3	0.76
the use of a patient portal can lead to better self-management in three quarters of my patients	20.3	24.4	16.1	9.1	31.3	0.11
in a cardiometabolically well-controlled patient with portal access, one of the quarterly monitoring visits can be substituted by self-monitoring	69.5	68.9	73.2	45.5	75.0	0.10

[a]1 answer missing

quality of diabetes care r_s – .009, $p = 0.95$; preventing medical mistakes r_s.003, $p = 0.99$; patients being more prepared during consultation r_s – .164, $p = 0.22$; improving self-management in own patients r_s – .211, $p = 0.12$; substitute a quarterly control by self-control r_s-.174, $p = 0.20$).

Discussion

The current study explored the opinions of diabetes care providers on the usefulness of an existing web portal and their working methods with regard to the web portal. They feel it could improve the quality of diabetes care and self-management of patients, but do not recommend it to all of their patients. They mostly explain the use of the portal directly with the patient, but they do not provide additional written information nor inquire into the patient's view. The level of active

encouragement of specific portal features is low, even when physicians or nurses feel those features are important. Both nurses and physicians are selective in promoting the portal. The suggestion that web portals may save time for the diabetes care provider seems not justified.

Several previous surveys have indicated that health care providers are reluctant to encourage patients to gain access to all medical notes; sometimes they considered patient health records more as a resource for physicians than a tool for patients [16, 33]. Physicians expected that patients' access to physician notes would result in greater worry among patients and that they anticipated more questions by patients [19], while afterwards these expectations did not become reality [21], and patients felt that access to physician notes led to an improved understanding, a better relationship with their

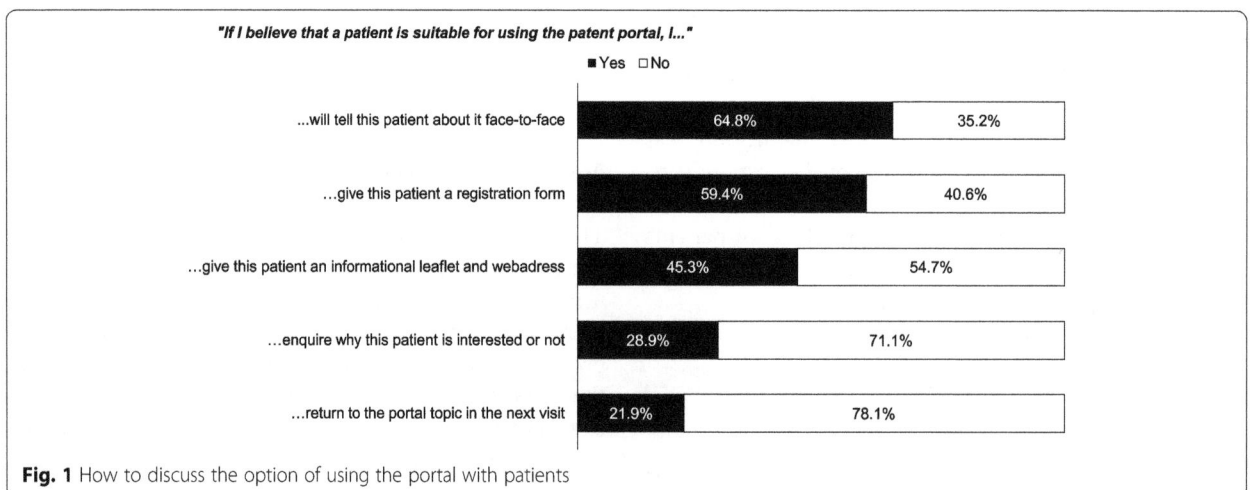

Fig. 1 How to discuss the option of using the portal with patients

Table 3 Encouragement to patients to use certain portal features. Percentages of respondents

"To which extent do you encourage your patient to…"	N	Always or regularly	Sometimes	Rarely or never
send you an electronic message through the portal	122	55.7	15.6	28.7
upload glucose values more often	124	71.8	16.9	11.3
re-read information after a consultation	123	30.1	32.5	37.4
prepare for a consultation by viewing laboratory results and agreed targets	123	19.5	43.1	37.4
inform you when he/she experiences a problem with the portal	123	43.9	26.0	30.1
tell you when the meaning of laboratory values is unclear	123	36.6	27.6	35.8
tell you when medical phrasings used in the health record are unclear	123	39.0	27.6	33.3
turn to you if he/she has questions about self-management	124	47.6	26.6	25.8

provider and improved quality of care and self-care [34]. Such a gap between physicians' expectations on how patients will perceive the use of a web portal and the actual patients 'experience might hinder providers' enthusiasm of discussing a portal with all their patients. Furthermore, health care providers may have insufficient knowledge on the best ways to make use of a web portal as an addition to current diabetes care and they may lack the necessary skills to stimulate patients.

In contrast to what many patients stated about their unawareness of this diabetes portal [14], the majority of the diabetes care providers reported that they informed their patients about the portal, most often face-to face. However, they rarely address it during the next visit, which might have caused the discrepancy between patients' and providers' answers. It is known that general

practitioners rarely assess their diabetic patients' recall or comprehension of new concepts [35]. From the current study we cannot explain why diabetes care providers appreciate for example the portal's glucose diary and patients preparing a consult with the use of the portal, but only encourage the use of these features on a limited scale. With the glucose diary can patients not only upload their glucose levels measured at home, but also must add information to clarify why levels are too high or too low. This is valuable information for the physician who can give the patient subsequent feedback and can also contribute to more self-awareness in patients. Additional training might be necessary to support the providers in discussing the benefits of this with patients, including helping with and checking the patients understanding of the information. Also lack of

Table 4 To what patients do the providers recommend the diabetes portal? Percentages of respondents

	N	Recommend	Neutral	Discourage
Patients with type 1 diabetes mellitus	115	78.3	20.9	0.9
Patients with type 2 diabetes mellitus	125	60.8	39.2	0.0
Patients with good cardiometabolic control	126	65.9	34.1	0.0
Patients with poor cardiometabolic control	126	63.5	27.9	8.6
Patients who do not use diabetes-specific medication	126	28.6	63.5	7.9
Patients who use oral diabetes medication	127	51.2	45.7	3.1
Patients who use insulin	127	84.3	15.7	0.0
Patients without comorbidities	127	55.1	43.3	1.6
Patients with comorbidities	127	52.8	40.2	7.1
Patients without language barriers	126	69.0	30.5	0.0
Patients with language barriers	125	10.2	39.8	47.7
Patients with lower education	126	25.0	48.4	25.0
Patients with higher education	125	73.6	26.4	0.0
Patients < 65 years	127	72.4	27.6	0.0
Patients > 65 years	125	33.6	54.7	9.4

Table 5 Perceived consequences of working with the diabetes patient portal. Percentages of respondents

	N	Yes (%)
"Access to his/her diabetes EMR via a web portal …"	128	
stimulates the self-management and self-correcting behaviour of the patient		75.8
improves communication during consultation with a well prepared patient		44.5
results in saving time		21.9
results in deceased workload		10.9
"I write the medical information…"	128	
as I always did		63.3
in an easier language than before		37.5
with less information than before		7.8
"I think that patients who use the patient portal…"	122	
have an increased frequency of visits		2.5
have an unchanged frequency of visits		80.3
have a decreased frequency of visits		17.2
"How do you feel about patients sending you an e-message?"	128	
(very) positive		65.6
neutral		28.1
(very) negative		6.3
"How many e-messages do you receive per week?"	124	
0 messages		33.1
1–10 messages		59.7
≥ 11 messages		7.3
"Who usually answers the e-message of patients?"	80[a]	
the health care provider answers only the messages of his/her own patients		31.3
the physician (GP or internist) answers all messages		2.5
the nurse (nurse practitioner or diabetes nurse) answers all messages		66.3

[a]All respondents who receive e-messages

time might be a reason for the working methods of the diabetes care providers. They perceived no benefits of the portal in terms of time saving and a decreased workload. Patients' office visit frequency was estimated to have remained similar by most respondents, and this perception is likely to be correct. Other studies led to an increase of both e-messaging and telephone encounters between patients and provider [36, 37], whereas in a study in the USA, patients actually turned to their portals after visits, and portal use did not lead to an increase in primary care visits [38]. We expect that with more experience with the full range of possibilities a patient web portal has to offer, the workload may ultimately decrease as patients will start to use the portal for substitution of care.

Despite the positive attitude of our respondents towards the portal for patient use, only 17.6% of their patients had requested access to the portal. We did not find an association between the opinion of a healthcare provider and the proportion of patients within the practice that requested a login to the portal. These findings suggest that other factors determine whether patients will use the diabetes portal, e.g. insulin use, hypoglycaemic episodes and diabetes knowledge. We did find that diabetes nurses are most optimistic about the portal, while the medical specialists at the same hospital are more sceptical. They both treat the same complex patients who are more likely to request a login [39]. This difference of opinions between type of providers within the same setting might be a reason we did not find an association between positive opinions and proportion of patients within the practice that requested a login. Furthermore, it is also possible that health care providers were more positive about the portal in our questionnaire while in daily use they hold a different opinion and therefore do not recommend it more often. Another possibility is that they are positive but due to e.g. time constraints during consultation do not recommend portal use more actively. We might need to stimulate the providers to play a more active role to increase the number of patients with a login to the portal.

Strengths and limitations of this study

The strength of our study is that we evaluated a web portal that has been in use in daily practice for 4 years. However, several limitations should be considered. First, we have a relatively small surveyed population. Response rates of physician surveys are notoriously low and our rate is comparable to others [40]. One of the researchers works as an internist at the hospital. She had no access to the returned questionnaires, but her position might have influenced the response rate among the diabetes nurses. However, we have no reason to assume that this position influenced the outcomes of the survey. Second, significantly fewer general practitioners responded. However, we found no difference of opinions between general practitioners and internists. Third, the tendency that respondents had a higher percentage of patients with access to the portal than non-respondents might indicate a selection-bias. It is possible that general practitioners who did not return the questionnaire are less positive about using a patient web portal. Finally, our questionnaire was designed based of determinants of patient portal use from literature. It was evaluated by experts but we might have missed information which could have been found if alternative methodologies, such as in-depth interviews, were used. For example, the discrepancy between health care providers' opinions about the portal leading to improvement of self-management and the low number of providers expecting that three quarters of their own patients were able to use the portal to improve their diabetes self-management, might have been the result of the wording ('three quarters') in the questionnaire. It would have been better to phrase it as a more open question.

Implications for clinical practice and further research

Despite positive opinions about the possible effects of a diabetes web portal, diabetes care providers do not offer maximal support and encouragement to patients that are likely necessary to increase the portal use and its possible benefits. They merely discuss the portal with patients face-to-face, hardly provide additional information and hardly check if patients understand how they could benefit from portal use. May be if providers will receive additional training in this respect, the gap between their opinions and their working methods can become smaller. Such training can include teaching care providers how to explore patients' motivation and how to support patients in maintaining their health record and interpreting their data, as well as addressing anticipated problems in electronic communication and the provider-patient relationship. Furthermore, as a result of this study, we are considering adjustments to this web portal to tailor the portal for different categories of patients, for example for patients who use insulin and those who do not.

Acknowledgements
We wish to thank the healthcare providers who returned our questionnaire for their time and participation and Diamuraal for providing data from the central database.

Authors' contribution
G.R. is the principal investigator of this study. M.R collected and analysed the data. M.R. wrote the manuscript which was critically revised by L.D, R.V. and G.R. R.V. additionally analysed data and contributed to the methods and results. All authors read and approved the final manuscript.

Funding
This study was supported by The Diabetes Fund, The Netherlands Organization for Scientific Research in Diabetes (Grant 2010.13.1369) and by the Julius Centre for Health Sciences and Primary Care, University Medical Centre Utrecht.

Competing interests
The authors declare that they have no competing interests.

Author details
[1]Julius Centre for Health Sciences and Primary Care, University Medical Centre Utrecht, STR 6.131, PO Box 85500, 3508 Utrecht, GA, Netherlands. [2]Department of Internal Medicine, Meander Medical Centre, Maatweg 3, 3813 Amersfoort, TZ, Netherlands.

References
1. WHO: Global status report on noncommunicable diseases; 2014.
2. Andreassen HK, Bujnowska-Fedak MM, Chronaki CE, Dumitru RC, Pudule I, Santana S, Voss H, Wynn R. European citizens' use of E-health services: a study of seven countries. BMC Public Health. 2007;7:53.
3. Osborn CY, Mayberry LS, Mulvaney SA, Hess R. Patient web portals to improve diabetes outcomes: a systematic review. Curr Diab Rep. 2010;10(6):422–35.
4. Zhou YYG, Garrido T, Chin HL, Wiesenthal AM, Liang LL. Patient access to an electronic health record with secure messaging: impact on primary care utilization. Am J Manag Care. 2007;13:6.
5. Ralston JD, Hirsch IB, Hoath J, Mullen M, Cheadle A, Goldberg HI. Web-based collaborative care for type 2 diabetes: a pilot randomized trial. Diabetes Care. 2009;32(2):234–9.
6. Holbrook A, Thabane L, Keshavjee K, Dolovich L, Bernstein B, Chan D, Troyan S, Foster G, Gerstein H. Individualized electronic decision support and reminders to improve diabetes care in the community: COMPET5rfcE II randomized trial. CMAJ. 2009;181(1–2):37–44.
7. McCarrier KP, Ralston JD, Hirsch IB, Leweis G, Martin DP, Zimmerman FJ, Goldberg HI. Web-based collaborative care for type 1 diabetes: a pilot randomized trial. Diabetes Technol Ther. 2009;11(4):211–7.
8. Wald JS, Businger A, Gandhi TK, Grant RW, Poon EG, Schnipper JL, Volk LA, Middleton B. Implementing practice-linked pre-visit electronic journals in primary care: patient and physician use and satisfaction. J Am Med Inform Assoc. 2010;17(5):502–6.
9. Greenhalgh T, Hinder S, Stramer K, Bratan T, Russell J. Adoption, non-adoption, and abandonment of a personal electronic health record: case study of HealthSpace. BMJ. 2010;341:c5814.
10. Weppner WG, Ralston JD, Koepsell TD, Grothaus LC, Reid RJ, Jordan L, Larson EB. Use of a shared medical record with secure messaging by older patients with diabetes. Diabetes Care. 2010;33(11):2314–9.
11. Sarkar U, Karter AJ, Liu JY, Adler NE, Nguyen R, Lopez A, Schillinger D. Social disparities in internet patient portal use in diabetes: evidence that the digital divide extends beyond access. J Am Med Inform Assoc. 2011;18(3):318–21.
12. Yamin CK, Emani S, Williams DH, Lipsitz SR, Karson AS, Wald JS, Bates DW. The digital divide in adoption and use of a personal health record. Arch Intern Med. 2011;171(6):568–74.
13. Black H, Gonzalez R, Priolo C, Schapira MM, Sonnad SS, Hanson CW 3rd, Langlotz CP, Howell JT, Apter AJ. True "meaningful use": technology meets both patient and provider needs. Am J Manag Care. 2015;21(5):e329–37.
14. Ronda MC, Dijkhorst-Oei LT, Rutten GE. Reasons and barriers for using a patient portal: survey among patients with diabetes mellitus. J Med Internet Res. 2014;16(11):e263.
15. Fuji KT, Galt KA, Serocca AB. Personal health record use by patients as perceived by ambulatory care physicians in Nebraska and South Dakota: a cross-sectional study. Perspect Health Inf Manag. 2008;5:15.
16. Witry MJ, Doucette WR, Daly JM, Levy BT, Chrischilles EA. Family physician perceptions of personal health records. Perspect Health Inf Manag. 2010;7:1d.
17. Hassol A, Walker JM, Kidder D, Rokita K, Young D, Pierdon S, Deitz D, Kuck S, Ortiz E. Patient experiences and attitudes about access to a patient electronic health care record and linked web messaging. J Am Med Inform Assoc. 2004;11(6):505–13.
23. Miller DP Jr, Latulipe C, Melius KA, Quandt SA, Arcury TA. Primary care Providers' views of patient portals: interview study of perceived benefits and consequences. J Med Internet Res. 2016;18(1):e8.
24. Kittler AF, Carlson GL, Harris C, Lippincott M, Pizziferri L, Volk LA, Jagannath Y, Wald JS, Bates DW. Primary care physician attitudes towards using a secure web-based portal designed to facilitate electronic communication with patients. Inform Prim Care. 2004;12(3):129–38.
25. Keplinger LE, Koopman JK, Mehr DR, Kruse RL, Wakefield DS, Wakefield BJ, Canfield SM. Patient portal implementation: resident and attending physician attitudes. Fam Med. 2013;45(5):335–40.
26. Zwaanswijk M, Verheij RA, Wiesman FJ, Friele RD. Benefits and problems of electronic information exchange as perceived by health care professionals: an interview study. BMC Health Serv Res. 2011;11:256.
27. Bell SK, Mejilla R, Anselmo M, Darer JD, Elmore JG, Leveille S, Ngo L, Ralston JD, Delbanco T, Walker J. When doctors share visit notes with patients: a study of patient and doctor perceptions of documentation errors, safety opportunities and the patient-doctor relationship. BMJ Qual Saf. 2016;26(4):262–70.

28. Kruse CS, Argueta DA, Lopez L, Nair A. Patient and provider attitudes toward the use of patient portals for the management of chronic disease: a systematic review. J Med Internet Res. 2015;17(2):e40.

29. Campmans-Kuijpers MJ, Baan CA, Lemmens LC, Rutten GE. Change in quality management in diabetes care groups and outpatient clinics after feedback and tailored support. Diabetes Care. 2015;38:7.

30. Struijs JN, Baan CA. Integrating care through bundled payments - lessons from the Netherlands. N Engl J Med. 2011;364(11):2.

31. Rutten GEHM, De Grauw WJ, Nijpels G, Houweling ST, Van de Laar FA, Bilo H, Holleman F, Burgers JS, Wiersma TJ, PGH J. NHG-Standaard Diabetes Mellitus type 2 (derde herziening). Huisarts Wet. 2013;56(10):512–25.

32. Weingart SN, Rind D, Tofias Z, Sands DZ. Who uses the patient internet portal? The PatientSite experience. J Am Med Inform Assoc. 2006;13(1):91–5.

33. Grunloh C, Cajander A, Myreteg G. "The record is our work tool!"-Physicians' framing of a patient portal in Sweden. J Med Internet Res. 2016;18(6):e167.

34. Esch T, Mejilla R, Anselmo M, Podtschaske B, Delbanco T, Walker J. Engaging patients through open notes: an evaluation using mixed methods. BMJ Open. 2016;6(1):e010034.

35. Schillinger D, Piette J, Grumbach K, Wang F, Wilson C, Daher C, Leong-Grotz K, Castro C, Bindman AB. Closing the loop: physician communication with diabetic patients who have low health literacy. Arch Intern Med. 2003;163(1):83–90.

36. Liss DT, Reid RJ, Grembowski D, Rutter CM, Ross TR, Fishman PA, Changes in office visit use associated with electronic messaging and telephone encounters among patients with diabetes in the PCMH. Ann Fam Med. 2014;12(4):338–43.

37. Dexter EN, Fields S, Rdesinski RE, Sachdeva B, Yamashita D, Marino M. Patient-provider communication: does electronic messaging reduce incoming telephone calls? J Am Board Fam Med. 2016;29(5):613–9.

38. Leveille SG, Mejilla R, Ngo L, Fossa A, Elmore JG, Darer J, Ralston JD, Delbanco T, Walker J. Do patients who access clinical information on patient internet portals have more primary care visits? Med Care. 2016;54(1):17–23.

39. Ronda MC, Dijkhorst-Oei LT, Rutten GE. Patients' experiences with and attitudes towards a diabetes patient web portal. PLoS One. 2015;10(6):e0129403.

40. Cook JV, Dickinson HO, Eccles MP. Response rates in postal surveys of healthcare professionals between 1996 and 2005: an observational study. BMC Health Serv Res. 2009;9:160.

17

The impact of chronic disease management on primary care doctors in Switzerland: a qualitative study

Olivia Braillard[1*] ⓘD, Anbreen Slama-Chaudhry[1], Catherine Joly[1], Nicolas Perone[2] and David Beran[3]

Abstract

Background: Patient-centeredness and therapeutic relationship are widely explored as a means to address the challenge of chronic disease and multi-morbidity management, however research focusing on the perspective of doctors is still rare. In this study, we aimed to explore the impact of the patient's chronic disease(s) on their healthcare provider.

Methods: A qualitative approach was taken using semi-structured interviews with general practitioners working in outpatient clinics either in individual practices or in a hospital setting in Geneva, Switzerland. Codes were developed through an iterative process and using grounded theory an inductive coding scheme was performed to identify the key themes. Throughout the analysis process the research team reviewed the analysis and refined the coding scheme.

Results: Twenty interviews, 10 in each practice type, allowed for saturation to be reached. The following themes relevant to the impact of managing chronic diseases emerge around the issue of feeling powerless as a doctor; facing the patient's socio-economic context; guidelines versus the reality of the patient; time; and taking on the patient's burden. Primary care practitioners face an emotional burden linked with their powerlessness and work conditions, but also with the empathetic bond with their patients and their circumstances. Doctors seem poorly prepared for this emotional strain. The health system is also not facilitating this with time constraints and guidelines unsuitable for the patient's reality.

Conclusions: Chronic disease and multi-morbidity management is a challenge for healthcare providers. This has its roots in patient characteristics, the overall health system and healthcare providers themselves. Structural changes need to be implemented at different levels: medical education; health systems; adapted guidelines; leading to an overall environment that favors the development of the therapeutic relationship.

Keywords: Primary health care, General practice, Chronic disease, Multimorbidity, Time management, Qualitative research

Background

Chronic diseases are defined by their long duration and slow progression with the current challenge for health systems not only in managing the individual chronic disease, but most notably multi-morbid individuals [1]. Chronic diseases and multi-morbidity lead to both financial and organizational burdens on the health system [2–5]. Patients with multiple chronic diseases face greater healthcare utilization and costs, decreased self-reported health status, depression and reduced functional capacity [1]. In addition the challenge of polypharmacy and managing multiple conditions, including possibly mental health issues, is both a challenge for the individual and healthcare provider(s) [6]. In the United States 84% of total health care costs are related to chronic disease [7] and in the United Kingdom a retrospective cohort study found that 78% of

* Correspondence: Olivia.Braillard@hcuge.ch
[1]Department of Community Medicine, Primary and Emergency Care, Geneva University Hospitals, 1205 Geneva, Switzerland
Full list of author information is available at the end of the article

consultations at primary health care are for people with more than one chronic condition [8].

Very little data exists on the burden of different chronic diseases in Switzerland [9]. In a study of individuals with insurance from a specific company aged 65 or older from all of Switzerland it was found that 76.6% were multi-morbid [10]. Compared to non-multi-morbid individuals these individuals had on average 15.7 consultations versus 4.4 and their associated costs were 5.5 times higher. In Switzerland models for the management of chronic disease are not as well established as in other high income settings[11] with barriers to effectively implement chronic care linked to the organization of the health system, its financing and weaknesses at primary health care level. This means that comprehensive models that have been developed elsewhere may not be implemented in the same way in Switzerland [11, 12].

Given these limitations for primary care doctors in the Swiss health system, and that very little focus and research on the impact of the patient's chronic disease(s) on primary care doctors exists [13], the aim of this study is to explore the impact of the patient's chronic disease(s) on their healthcare provider.

Methods
Context

In Switzerland, due to the federal system, each of the 26 cantons is responsible for the provision of health services, financing of public hospitals as well as subsidizing some of the population's insurance premiums [14]. The Federal government provides the legislative framework which regulates the insurance market, defines the healthcare services covered by the basic insurance package and the way in which these are paid for. One-third of health care spending in Switzerland is from out of pocket payments [14].

Income for primary care doctors' in outpatient settings is dependent on the number of patients they see and the technical acts they perform. The government has delegated to an association of Swiss insurance companies the task of "economically evaluating" doctors by comparing costs generated by each practitioner to an average. Hospital based practitioners do not have the same financial pressure, however time per patient is an issue.

This study took place in Geneva, one of the 26 Swiss cantons [15]. It is characterized by a very diverse population (total 494,000), high density of doctors and the largest university teaching hospital of Switzerland.

Methodological approach

A qualitative approach was taken, with an interview guide created by the team of investigators including three Primary Care specialists (OB, ASC, NP), 1 Public Health Research specialist with a PhD (DB), and a Nurse specialized in Chronic Disease management and Patient Education (CJ). All contributors have experience in qualitative research projects. Discussion topics were related to Chronic Care Model (CCM) [16] and these were used as grand tour questions [17]. The CCM provides a framework for the necessary components to provide integrated chronic disease management. It comprises not only the role of the health system and healthcare provider, but also such elements as policies, the community and patient. For the purpose of this study the CCM was used as a framework to build the interview guide (cf Additional file 1) to guide the interview through the different levels of care (patient, doctor, health system) and the domains that could influence the quality of chronic care (Resources and policies, organization of health care, self-management support, decision support, delivery system design, clinical information systems).

The protocol received ethical approval from the Geneva University Hospitals (HUG) Research Ethics Committee (reference number 14–022). All participants signed a written informed consent form and it was made clear to them they could withdraw from the study at any time. Convenience sampling was used to gain a wide diversity of views. Participants were recruited through an e-mail announcement informing every all primary care practitioners in Geneva (570 in private practices and 40 in the Division of Primary Care Medicine at the HUG) about the study. Selection was done based on those who answered first.

The researcher (CJ) conducting interviews was experienced in interview techniques. She had no professional relation with participants. All participants were made aware of the general objectives of the research which was to explore practitioners' difficulties, needs and resources in the caring for patients with chronic diseases. Interviews were digitally recorded and transcribed verbatim by a person unrelated to the research team and were not returned to the interviewees for comment. Throughout this process, all data were anonymized to guarantee confidentiality using unique codes comprised of SMPR and a number based on the order of interview. These codes are used to present the quotes from interviewees in the results. Interviews took place at participants' workplace (HUG or private practices) between July and August 2014. Only the participant and the interviewer (CJ) were present. Participants received a CHF 50 voucher after completion of interview, in compensation for their time. Interviews were carried out until theoretical saturation was achieved. All interviews were audio recorded and transcribed in French. No field notes were taken. The research and analysis process is presented in Fig. 1.

The interview guide was tested on 2 interviews (excluded from analysis) to check its relevance and clarity. After the 2 test interviews, the guide was refined and a

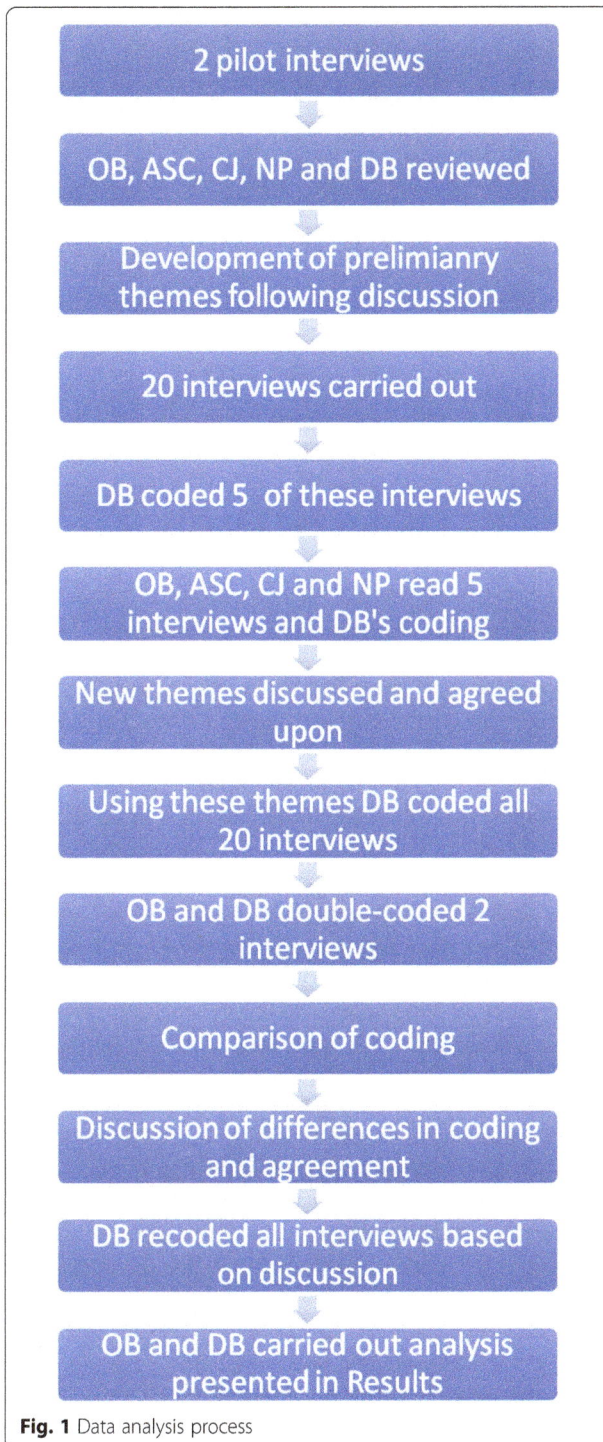

Fig. 1 Data analysis process

visual tool to support the interviews used. (Fig. 2) It was felt that a visual tool was necessary following the 2 test interviews to guide the discussion and allow for an interaction around the key issues between the interviewer and interviewee. The research team read and analyzed 2 test interviews in order to create a coding scheme. These codes were triangulated among the research team to achieve a consensus on their validity for analysis. During the interviews notes and comments were added to Fig. 2 to highlight key issues, remind the interviewer and/or interviewee of some points or as a means to return to certain key issues.

A grounded theory analysis was used. Grounded Theory provides a systematic framework for collecting and analysing qualitative data that is flexible and assists in the creation of theories "grounded in the data collected" [18–21]. An inductive coding scheme was used and analysis was performed using NVIVO 11 for Mac (NVivo qualitative data analysis Software; QSR International Pty Ltd). Analyses were carried out in French, and then translated in English for publication purposes. Five interviews were then analyzed by one member of the team (DB) using this initial coding scheme. Additional codes were added and defined during this process. The research team then reviewed the analysis and refined the coding scheme. Two interviews were double coded (OB and DB) using the second coding scheme and the research team discussed any discrepancy in the analysis. All interviews were then re-coded (DB) using the last coding scheme. Analysis and coding was then discussed and validated by the team. Throughout this process, disagreements and discrepancies were discussed among the researchers until an agreement was validated by the whole team.

Results

Twenty interviews, 10 in each practice type, allowed for saturation to be reached. All participants completed their interviews and there were no repeat interviews. Mean duration of interviews was 51 min (minimum 24 min, maximum 65 min). The characteristics of the interviewees are detailed in Table 1.

The following themes relevant to the impact of managing chronic diseases emerge around the issue of feeling powerless as a doctor; facing the patient's reality; guidelines versus the reality of the patient; time; and taking on the patient's burden.

Feeling powerless as a doctor

Many of those interviewed expressed feeling powerless. SMPR3 states this as "when you are a young doctor, you like to be the savior." SMPR28 describes how for infectious diseases and broken arms doctors can easily find solutions, but that for chronic diseases "it is almost like we give them medicines and we make them sick." SMPR10 and SMPR24 highlight the challenge of patients coming back with recurring complaints that they are unable to provide a solution for.

This powerlessness was also fueled by the perceived patient's view as expressed by SMPR26 "the patient does not

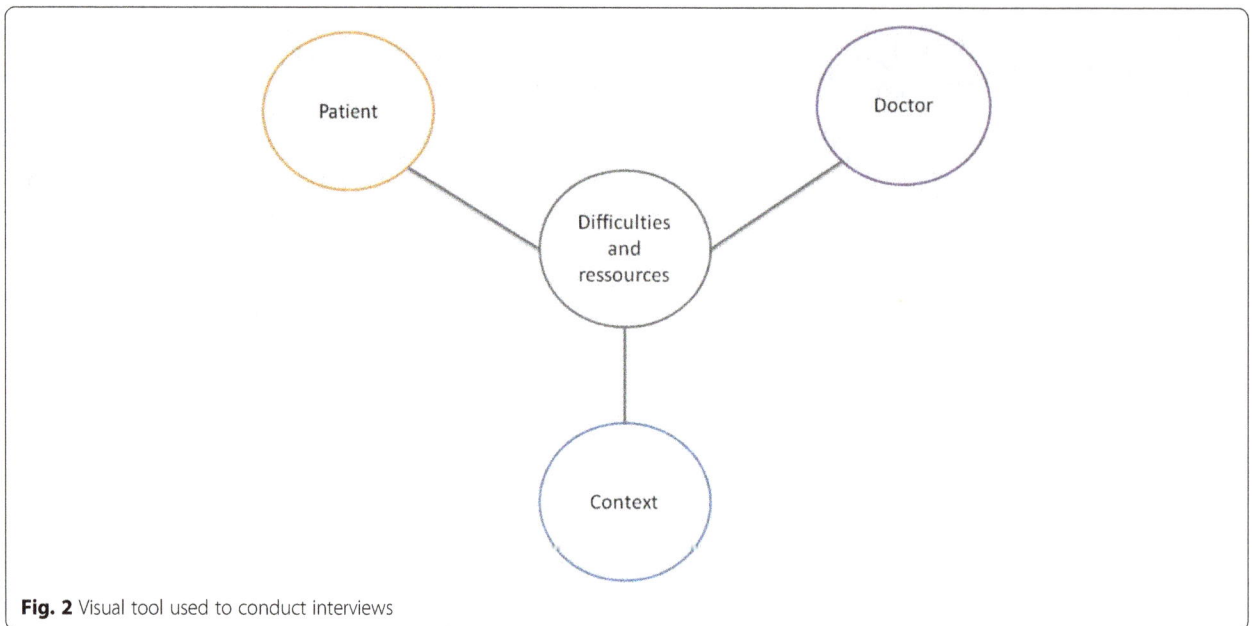

Fig. 2 Visual tool used to conduct interviews

necessarily expect to get better and that is difficult to accept as a doctor". SMPR 10 adds "if we feel that the intervention we are proposing will not change anything our feeling powerless as a doctor increases." This is complemented by SMPR23 saying, "I do not cure them! I just provide treatment!" with SMPR2 highlighting how a transition is needed in the view of being a doctor as a savior and being able to see the limits of what a doctor can do. SMPR3 adds, "With time we are able to relativize a lot and redefine our role as a partner and not a healer."

The patients' reality

Some of this feeling powerless was linked to varying patient characteristics such as social, psychiatric and disease factors. SMPR20 describes this as "the limit of my action in the limits of the context [of the patient] and the difficulty of adapting what I am saying to a reality that I do not know well, therefore the feeling that sometimes I am not in sync with what the patient is living." Different elements comprise the patient's reality, not only including the disease(s) that the doctor is managing, but also their socio-economic characteristics. Patient related factors impacted the management of the patient's chronic disease and could be divided into disease related factors and multi-morbidity and the patient's social context.

Disease related factors and multi-morbidity

With disease related factors, different challenges present themselves at distinctive stages of the disease process. For example, at the time of diagnosis "For some the announcement of having diabetes all of a sudden is an upheaval, we are going to tell them that they need to do various things and I realize that this is a bomb. We put bombs for these patients, but for us it is just diabetes." (SMPR24) This "bomb" at the time of diagnosis is followed by challenges throughout the management of the disease until the last stage of the disease, when the doctor needs to explain "if you are no longer able to

Table 1 Characteristics of interviewees

Code	Practice type	Age	Years of practice
SMPR1	Private practice	52	25
SMPR2	Private practice	59	34
SMPR3	Private practice	55	25
SMPR4	Private practice	53	30
SMPR5	Private practice	65	30
SMPR6	Private practice	67	40
SMPR7	Private practice	58	34
SMPR8	Private practice	42	18
SMPR9	Private practice	67	32
SMPR 10	Private practice	40	21
SMPR 20	Hospital	44	17
SMPR 21	Hospital	53	29
SMPR 22	Hospital	34	7
SMPR 23	Hospital	42	13
SMPR 24	Hospital	35	5
SMPR 25	Hospital	53	27
SMPR 26	Hospital	34	7
SMPR 27	Hospital	39	12
SMPR 28	Hospital	36	10
SMPR 29	Hospital	41	16
	Average Overall (Range)	48 (34–67)	22 (5–40)

breathe it is because you have smoked for 40 years and your body is letting go [...] they have to understand that they are going to die." (SMPR23).

End of life care was identified as a situation with additional challenges (SMPR23), as were chronic disease management in geriatric populations (SMPR23), mental health issues (SMPR7), and specific diseases e.g. HIV/AIDS, diabetes (SMPR7). SMPR24 also describes a vicious cycle in that chronic disease can be disabling for the individual therefore impacting the individual's mental state, which in turn impacts management. As stated by SMPR24, "Somatic chronic diseases often have consequences or come in parallel to difficult psychological situations and it is then difficult to identify what is the cause and consequence." Many doctors in discussing multi-morbidity focused more on psychiatric diseases and addiction (SMPR4, SMPR7, SMPR23, SMPR24 and SMPR25) rather than somatic conditions. SMPR4 portrayed multi-morbidity as "We are juggling many eggs at the same time." This practitioner gave the example of one of their patients having alcohol problems after a bypass surgery and how to manage this added challenge in an individual who already had an eating disorder, problems with their body image, depression and other chronic diseases. The challenge was also how to manage all these issues in parallel (SMPR20).

Patient's social context

A variety of social factors impacting the management of the patient's chronic disease are described by the interviewees. "There are some contexts where as a doctor I take a blood pressure, I use my stethoscope, but that is not the problem! Patients just need to eat, be washed and then access care"(SMPR23). SMPR2, SMPR21, SMPR23, SMPR24 and SMPR25 add to this complexity in mentioning the importance of the patient's surroundings, including: work, life events, family context, financial means, cultural factors, seclusion, and even illiteracy. SMPR25 summarizes this as "the problem is much more non-medical: it is really the surroundings, work, life events that have a bigger impact than us." A specific example is SMPR1 describing how a patient with dyspnea may also be losing his job, having marital trouble and these factors accumulate as elements in their overall suffering.

Doctors seemed ill equipped to manage the patient's social context linked to cultural issues (SMPR5, SMPR7, SMPR20, SMPR21, SMPR23 and SMPR26) and precarious financial situations (SMPR2, SMPR3 and SMPR20). Cultural issues related to barriers in effective communication with the patient and therefore patient's understanding of for example taking medicines. Financial issues were related to the fact that some patients could not access care they needed

(SMPR2), lacked financial means to exercise or afford healthy food (SMPR20), or due to job constraints did not see management of their condition as a priority (SMPR20).

Guidelines versus reality

Guidelines which support evidence-based medicine goals are focused on individual diseases and do not take account the complexity of the patients' reality including socio-economic factors. Therefore, the doctor's efforts to follow guidelines are often a failure. SMPR3 describes a patient who could not check his blood glucose twice a day before and after meals because of his work schedule. This shows that the patients' reality cannot be controlled by the physician. SMPR22 expresses this as "there are things that we can change in the context, and things for which we aren't there. We talk about theory, but once at home..."

This "theory" refers to not being able to follow guidelines due to the nature of the patients disease(s) and other related factors, adding to the doctor's feeling of powerlessness and frustration. Participants described how they are able to put into perspective the importance of guidelines, but that these are limited as guidelines are, "only statistical considerations" (SMPR3), whereas they need to deal with individuals with varying needs.

SMPR20 describes his approach as "trying to find openings where they are, by trying to find strategies which are literally adapted to patient's reality. [It's] useless to talk about changing diet, when the patient eats at a soup kitchen". SMPR24 summarizes it with this statement: "with chronic patients, you need to see further than guidelines, see patient's resources, understand his story, see how he lives with his illness [..]. There are many facets you can't set aside".

Dealing with complexity requires time

Time was a recurrent theme presented by the doctors interviewed. Interviewees described how they struggled with all the tasks they should perform within a limited time frame of a consultation. SMPR28 lists each task he's supposed to do during a single consultation only for diabetes and adds, "And all this in 30 minutes". Therefore, doctors have to prioritize, "in which order and at what time we do things" (SMPR 29), with the risk of "los[ing] track of which exams to do" (SMPR26) or omit something such as stopping a specific medicine no longer required (SMPR 29).

Besides identified specific tasks, many interviewees stated that more time is required to create a therapeutic relationship. For SMPR20, this relationship is "built with the duration and by knowing people" and it is necessary to "enter into patient's life" (SMPR29). SMPR20 summarizes this need for time to build relationship as "if we don't have time, we don't take care of a person but of a disease".

Due to the limit of time imposed by Swiss health system (through its insurance and funding system), many doctors felt frustrated. Several interviewees were quite spirited when discussing this as SMPR2 said, "I can only do my job as a doctor if you allow me more time". SMPR7 had received a warning from an insurance company about the time spent with his patients and stated, "I told them that a society which didn't take time for the bond was a dying one, and that in no way I would agree to reduce the time of my consultations".

Impact of taking on the patient's burden

Many of the doctors interviewed took on their patient's burden with them feeling for their patient and their situation. This had a negative impact in them requiring a lot of energy and a emotional impact. In addition, this also had a positive impact finding motivation and pleasure in some interactions.

Some interviewees stated how consuming it was to take on the patient's burden, and how it made them feel alone. SMPR7 stated "we are bearer of everything [...] psychological, familial issues, the despair, the advancing age". SMPR24 compares some patients as a "very heavy stone to pull", SMPR23 confessed feeling "like pedaling in vain" and being exhausted.

SMPR24 describes the "intensity with the chronic patient that we don't have with any patient [..] it impacts us strongly when in a given day we see patients who feel down because no treatment is working, we still have to continue to accompany them, not to let them down." Due to this bond built on the therapeutic relationship, several interviewees described being affected by their patients' situations (SMPR1, SMPR7, SMPR10, SMPR23 and SMPR24). This is described in different ways, such as "to feel sadness" (SMPR7) about their situation, their issues, or even "to feel what they feel" (SMPR1). All these feelings resulted in energy used to "digest" these emotions (SMPR10).

Interviewees also described positive impact resulting from their work with chronic patients. When SMPR2 talks about a resilient 88-year-old patient with many issues, he relates the pleasure he has to see his fighting spirit, and how it also helps him as a doctor keep motivated. Interviewees described this phenomenon when the patient took their advice (SMPR26), showed resilience facing serious issues (SMPR2, SMPR10), the long-term relationship (SMPR28) or simply through the stories shared by the patients (SMPR2, SMPR10). SMPR10 summarizes, "It's wonderful this relation we can have with people sharing the story of their life, their beliefs [...] It's really touching but in the same time, it also takes energy".

Discussion
Summary

This study describes the complexity from doctors' perspective of managing individuals with chronic diseases. The CCM provided a useful framework for the interview guide as it enabled the investigation of the key element of the doctor/patient interactions. This relationship between patient and healthcare provider is central to this model and essential for the management of chronic diseases. Although wider community and policy issues were not assessed these appeared as barriers to the management of individuals with chronic diseases, such as time limitations on consultations and wider social factors impacting health.

Strengths and limitations

The aim of this study was exploratory in nature therefore a qualitative approach was adopted. As with any qualitative study sampling, data collection, analysis and presentation, as well as contextual bias are limitations [22]. These were mitigated by the experience and diversity of the team involved in this research as well as a clear description of the methods included. To the authors' knowledge this study is unique in its approach and findings and thus serves as a contribution to the literature in understanding the various challenges that primary care doctors face in providing care to patients with chronic diseases.

Comparison with existing literature

Most literature on the issue of primary health care and chronic disease are disease or patient-centered and there are few studies describing doctor's perspective [23–26]. Research shows that 20–40% of primary care doctors are emotionally exhausted due to work-related factors: their income linked to number of patients seen, for especially healthcare providers in private practice, hours of work and stress [27]. A systematic review on primary healthcare provider's perspective on multi-morbidity found that their reaction facing multi-morbidity could reach "something close to despair" [28]. Kenning's study [29] shows the emotional strain experienced by practitioners with the management of complex patients who show little improvement or willingness to engage in their own care. Our study is unique in that it reveals that the emotional burden faced by primary care practitioners is not only linked to their powerlessness and work conditions, but also to the empathetic bond with their patients and their circumstances.

The doctor's feeling of powerlessness is a key finding from this study. Factors such as the training of health professionals, the way guidelines are developed with a disease focus, organization of the health system all contribute to this. From a health system perspective, these components can all be changed. However, patient factors such as disease related factors, multi-morbidity and their social context cannot be modified. It is for the health system and doctor to adapt to these in order to find the appropriate responses. The main challenge identified were the time constraints imposed by the organization of the health system thus preventing the establishment of a therapeutic relationship. The therapeutic relationship is broadly acknowledged as the cornerstone of chronic disease management [29], yet doctors in our study seem poorly prepared for this emotional strain with health system factors also not facilitating this.

Guidelines which should help doctors do not take into account patients' reality and complexity. Parekh and al [30]. in their proposal to improve the management of multi-morbidity include a goal on equipping clinicians. However, this focuses on training, guidelines and identifying best practice and tools. These recommendations fail to address the complexity of the patient, the impact of this on the healthcare provider and the limitations the health system imposes.

Implications for research and practice

Health systems need to drastically change how they support both care for chronic patients and the impact this has on doctors. Wagner et al. [31] point out that each element of the health system, including policies, need to change in order to enable effective care for chronic patients. Most health systems do not provide the propitious environment for patient-centered care or effective teamwork [32]. Although there is some experience in implementing the CCM in practice this is only as part of studies, pilots, or in specific contexts [33]. Financial issues need to be addressed in that time limits on consultations with complex patients are a short-term saving [34]. Resources are also needed to truly have integrated care including inter-professional teams to address the multiple needs of the patients and alleviate the doctor's workload. This should include care coordination as a cornerstone of this effective team and be led by either the primary care practitioner or a trained case manager [35–37]. Prevention must become a top-priority [38] and must be financially rewarded [39]. Well-being and resilience promotion [40, 41] should be a part of medical training to build emotional coping abilities [42]. As management of multi-morbidity involves uncertainty, which is badly tolerated by medical students, and can be a reason not to become a primary care doctor, medical students and young doctors should be taught to cope with this [43]. All of these elements need to be delivered at primary care level and as SMPR28 concludes regarding the primary care specialty: "for nothing else in the world I would do another specialty [...] but it's not easy". Health systems need to find ways to care for their caregivers, such as SMPR28 in order to ensure proper care is provided to chronic and multi-morbid patients.

Conclusion

Chronic disease and multi-morbidity management is a challenge for healthcare providers. This has its roots in patient characteristics, the overall health system and healthcare providers themselves. Structural changes need to be implemented at different levels: medical education; health systems; adapted guidelines; leading to an overall environment that favors the development of the therapeutic relationship. This therapeutic relationship is a cornerstone for properly managing complex patients. To have this requires an investment in terms of time, energy and emotion, but health systems currently do not provide the enabling environment for this. Structural changes need to be implemented at different levels: medical education needs to prepare doctors for this emotional strain; health systems need to find innovative financing mechanisms; consultations need to be adapted and move towards team-based integrated care; and tools such as adapted guidelines need to be developed and used.

Acknowledgements
The authors would like to acknowledge the support of Professor Jean-Michel Gaspoz which allowed them to benefit the "Fonds MIMOSA" grant.
The lead author affirms that the manuscript is an honest, accurate, and transparent account of the study being reported; that no important aspects of the study have been omitted; and that any discrepancies from the study as planned have been explained.

Funding
This study received a grant from the "Fonds MIMOSA", Division of Community Medicine & Primary Care, Faculty of Medicine, Geneva, Switzerland. The funding source had no role in the design of the study and collection, analysis, and interpretation of data and in writing the manuscript.

Authors' contributions
Conceived the idea of the study: ASC. Designed the study: OB, ASC, CJ, NP, DB. Conducted the Interviews: CJ. Coded the data: DB. Mainly conducted data analysis: OB, DB. Participated to data analysis: ASC, CJ, NP. Wrote the manuscript: OB, DB. Critically revised the manuscript for important intellectual content: ASC, NP. Reviewed for final submission: OB, DB. All authors read and approved the final manuscript.

Competing interests
All authors have completed the Unified Competing Interest form (available on request from the corresponding author) and declare no support from any organisation for the submitted work; no financial relationships with any organisations that might have an interest in the submitted work in the previous three years, as well as during this study, no other relationships or activities that could appear to have influenced the submitted work.

Author details
[1]Department of Community Medicine, Primary and Emergency Care, Geneva University Hospitals, 1205 Geneva, Switzerland. [2]Department of Community Health and Care, Geneva University Hospitals, 1205 Geneva, Switzerland. [3]Division of Tropical and Humanitarian Medicine, Geneva University Hospitals and University of Geneva, 1205 Geneva, Switzerland.

References

1. Palladino R, Tayu Lee J, Ashworth M, Triassi M, Millett C. Associations between multimorbidity, healthcare utilisation and health status: evidence from 16 European countries. Age Ageing. 2016;45(3):431–5. PubMed PMID: 27013499. Pubmed Central PMCID: PMC4846796

2. Nolte E, McKee M. Integration and chronic care: a review. In: Nolte E, McKee M, editors. Caring for people woth chronic conditions: a health system perspective. Maidenhead: Open University Press; 2008.

3. McKee M, Nolte E. Responding to the challenge of chronic diseases: ideas from Europe. Clin Med. 2004;4(4):336–42. PubMed PMID: 15372893. Epub 2004/09/18. eng

4. Picco L, Achilla E, Abdin E, Chong SA, Vaingankar JA, McCrone P, et al. Economic burden of multimorbidity among older adults: impact on healthcare and societal costs. BMC Health Serv Res. 2016;16:173. PubMed PMID: 27160080. Pubmed Central PMCID: PMC4862090. Epub 2016/05/11

5. Zulman DM, Pal Chee C, Wagner TH, Yoon J, Cohen DM, Holmes TH, et al. Multimorbidity and healthcare utilisation among high-cost patients in the US veterans affairs health care system. BMJ Open. 2015;5(4):e007771. PubMed PMID: 25882486. Pubmed Central PMCID: PMC4401870. Epub 2015/04/18

6. Wallace E, Salisbury C, Guthrie B, Lewis C, Fahey T, Smith SM. Managing patients with multimorbidity in primary care. BMJ. 2015;350:h176. PubMed PMID: 25616760

7. Moses H 3rd, Matheson DH, Dorsey ER, George BP, Sadoff D, Yoshimura S. The anatomy of health care in the United States. JAMA. 2013;310(18):1947–63. PubMed PMID: 24219951

8. Salisbury C, Johnson L, Purdy S, Valderas JM, Montgomery AA. Epidemiology and impact of multimorbidity in primary care: a retrospective cohort study. Br J Gen Pract. 2011;61(582):e12–21. PubMed PMID: 21401985. Pubmed Central PMCID: PMC3020068

9. Zellweger U, Bopp M, Holzer BM, Djalali S, Kaplan V. Prevalence of chronic medical conditions in Switzerland: exploring estimates validity by comparing complementary data sources. BMC Public Health. 2014;14:1157. PubMed PMID: 25377723. Pubmed Central PMCID: PMC4237788

10. Bahler C, Huber CA, Brungger B, Reich O. Multimorbidity, health care utilization and costs in an elderly community-dwelling population: a claims data based observational study. BMC Health Serv Res. 2015;15:23. PubMed PMID: 25609174. Pubmed Central PMCID: PMC4307623

11. Lauvergeon S, Burnand B, Peytremann-Bridevaux I. Chronic disease management: a qualitative study investigating the barriers, facilitators and incentives perceived by Swiss healthcare stakeholders. BMC Health Serv Res. 2012;12:176. PubMed PMID: 22726820. Pubmed Central PMCID: PMC3483191

12. Peytremann-Bridevaux I, Ebert ST, Senn N. Involvement of family physicians in structured programs for chronic diseases or multi-morbidity in Switzerland. Eur J Intern Med. 2015;26(2):150–1. PubMed PMID: 25638287

13. Campbell C, McGauley G. Doctor-patient relationships in chronic illness: insights from forensic psychiatry. BMJ. 2005;330(7492):667–70. PubMed PMID: 15775003. Pubmed Central PMCID: PMC554923

14. Biller-Andorno N, Zeltner T. Individual responsibility and community solidarity--the Swiss health care system. N Engl J Med. 2015;373(23):2193–7. PubMed PMID: 26630139. Epub 2015/12/03

15. Genève S. Bilan et état de la population du Canton de Genève en 2016. Geneva: République et Canton de Genève; 2016.

16. Wagner EH. Chronic disease management: what will it take to improve care for chronic illness? Eff Clin Pract. 1998;1(1):2–4. PubMed PMID: 10345255

17. Leech BL. Asking questions: techniques for Semistructured interviews. Political Science and Politics. 2002;35(4):665–8.

18. Glaser BG, Holton J. Remodeling Grounded Theory 2004. Available from: http://www.qualitative-research.net/index.php/fqs/article/view/607/1315. [cited 24 August 2018].

19. Charmaz K. Constructing grounded theory. London: Sage; 2007.

20. Corbin J, Straus A. Basics of qualitative research. Thousand Oaks: SAGE Publications; 2008.

21. Braun V, Clarke V. Using thematic analysis in psychology. Qual Res Psychol. 2006;3:77–101.

22. Holloway I. A-Z of qualitative research in healthcare. Chichester: Blackwell Publishing; 2008.

23. McLean G, Gunn J, Wyke S, Guthrie B, Watt GC, Blane DN, et al. The influence of socioeconomic deprivation on multimorbidity at different ages: a cross-sectional study. Br J Gen Pract. 2014;64(624):e440–7. PubMed PMID: 24982497. Pubmed Central PMCID: PMC4073730. Epub 2014/07/02

24. Kurpas D, Bujnowska-Fedak MM, Athanasiadou A, Mroczek B. Factors influencing utilization of primary health Care Services in Patients with chronic respiratory diseases. Adv Exp Med Biol. 2015;866:71–81. PubMed PMID: 26022896. Epub 2015/05/30

25. Sinnige J, Korevaar JC, Westert GP, Spreeuwenberg P, Schellevis FG, Braspenning JC. Multimorbidity patterns in a primary care population aged 55 years and over. Fam Pract. 2015;32(5):505–13. PubMed PMID: 26040310. Pubmed Central PMCID: PMC4576758. Epub 2015/06/05

26. Chetty U, McLean G, Morrison D, Agur K, Guthrie B, Mercer SW. Chronic obstructive pulmonary disease and comorbidities: a large cross-sectional study in primary care. Br J Gen Pract. 2017;67(658):e321–e8. PubMed PMID: 28450344. Pubmed Central PMCID: PMC5409435. Epub 2017/04/30

27. Torppa MA, Kuikka L, Nevalainen M, Pitkala KH. Emotionally exhausting factors in general practitioners' work. Scand J Prim Health Care. 2015;33(3):178–83. PubMed PMID: 26311207. Pubmed Central PMCID: PMC4750721. Epub 2015/08/28

28. Sinnott C, Mc Hugh S, Browne J, Bradley C. GPs' perspectives on the management of patients with multimorbidity: systematic review and synthesis of qualitative research. BMJ Open. 2013;3(9):e003610. PubMed PMID: 24038011. Pubmed Central PMCID: PMC3773648. Epub 2013/09/17

29. Kenning C, Fisher L, Bee P, Bower P, Coventry P. Primary care practitioner and patient understanding of the concepts of multimorbidity and self-management: a qualitative study. SAGE Open Med. 2013;1: 2050312113510001. PubMed PMID: 26770690. Pubmed Central PMCID: PMC4687771. Epub 2013/01/01

30. Parekh AK, Kronick R, Tavenner M. Optimizing health for persons with multiple chronic conditions. JAMA. 2014;312(12):1199–200. PubMed PMID: 25133982

31. Bodenheimer T, Wagner EH, Grumbach K. Improving primary care for patients with chronic illness. JAMA. 2002;288(14):1775–9. PubMed PMID: 12365965. Epub 2002/10/09

32. Rickert J. Patient-Centered Care: What It Means And How To Get There: Health Affairs Blog; 2012. Available from: http://www.healthaffairs.org/do/10.1377/hblog20120124.016506/full/. [cited 7 June 2017].

33. Nuno R, Coleman K, Bengoa R, Sauto R. Integrated care for chronic conditions: the contribution of the ICCC framework. Health Policy. 2012; 105(1):55–64. PubMed PMID: 22071454

34. Bodenheimer T, Wagner EH, Grumbach K. Improving primary care for patients with chronic illness: the chronic care model, part 2. JAMA. 2002; 288(15):1909–14. PubMed PMID: 12377092. Epub 2002/10/17

35. Wagner EH. The role of patient care teams in chronic disease management. BMJ. 2000;320(7234):569–72. PubMed PMID: 10688568. Pubmed Central PMCID: PMC1117605. Epub 2000/02/25

36. Sutherland D, Hayter M. Structured review: evaluating the effectiveness of nurse case managers in improving health outcomes in three major chronic diseases. J Clin Nurs. 2009;18(21):2978–92. PubMed PMID: 19747197. Epub 2009/09/15

37. Hudon C, Chouinard MC, Diadiou F, Lambert M, Bouliane D. Case Management in Primary Care for frequent users of health care services with chronic diseases: a qualitative study of patient and family experience. Ann Fam Med. 2015;13(6):523–8. PubMed PMID: 26553891. Pubmed Central PMCID: PMC4639377. Epub 2015/11/11

38. Fortin M, Chouinard MC, Dubois MF, Belanger M, Almirall J, Bouhali T, et al. Integration of chronic disease prevention and management services into primary care: a pragmatic randomized controlled trial (PR1MaC). CMAJ Open. 2016;4(4):E588–E98. PubMed PMID: 28018871. Pubmed Central PMCID: PMC5173473. Epub 2016/12/27

39. Nolte E, McKee M. Caring for people woth chronic conditions: a health system perspective. Nolte E, McKee M, editors. Maidenhead: Open University Press; 2008.

40. Rahimi B, Baetz M, Bowen R, Balbuena L. Resilience, stress, and coping among Canadian medical students. Can Med Educ J. 2014;5(1):e5–e12. PubMed PMID: 26451221. Pubmed Central PMCID: PMC4563614. Epub 2014/01/01

18

Talking about depression during interactions with GPs: a qualitative study exploring older people's accounts of their depression narratives

Isabel Gordon[1]* [iD], Jonathan Ling[1], Louise Robinson[2], Catherine Hayes[1] and Ann Crosland[1]

Abstract

Background: Older people can struggle with revealing their depression to GPs and verbalising preferences regarding its management. This contributes to problems for GPs in both detecting and managing depression in primary care. The aim of this study was to explore older people's accounts of how they talk about depression and possible symptoms to improve communication about depression when seeing GPs.

Methods: Adopting a qualitative Interpretivist methodological approach, semi-structured interviews were conducted by IG based on the principles of grounded theory and situational analysis. GPs working in north east England recruited patients aged over 65 with depression. Data analysis was carried out with a process of constant comparison, and categories were developed via open and axial coding and situational maps. There were three levels of analysis; the first developed open codes which informed the second level of analysis where the typology was developed from axial codes. The typology derived from second level analysis only is presented here as older people's views are rarely reported in isolation.

Results: From the sixteen interviews with older people, it was evident that there were differences in how they understood and accepted their depression and that this influenced what they shared or withheld in their narratives. A typology showing three categories of older people was identified: those who appeared to talk about their depression freely yet struggled to accept aspects of it (Superficial Accepter), those who consolidated their ideas about depression aloud (Striving to Understand) and those who shared minimal detail about their depression and viewed it as part of them rather than a treatable condition (Unable to Articulate). The central finding was that older people's acceptance and understanding of their depression guided their depression narratives.

Conclusions: This study identified differences between older people in ways they understand, accept and share their depression. Recognising that their depression narratives can change and listening for patterns in what older people share or withhold may help GPs in facilitating communication to better understand the patient when they need to implement alternative approaches to patient management.

Keywords: Primary care, Older people, Depression, Narratives, Communication, Qualitative

* Correspondence: I.Gordon@sunderland.ac.uk
[1]Faculty of Health Sciences and Wellbeing, University of Sunderland, City Campus Chester Road, Sunderland SR1 3SD, UK
Full list of author information is available at the end of the article

Background

In the UK between 4.6 and 9.3% of older adults experience major depression, and an average of 17.1% experience depressive disorders [1]. Of these fewer than one in six will talk to GPs about their symptoms and only half will receive suitable treatment [2] due to poor detection and older people's reluctance to seek help due to isolation or a "nihilistic" attitude [3]. In the UK, primary care is the first point of contact for many older people with health problems, with 22% visiting their GP in a two-week period [4]. Evidence goes some way to explaining why older people can be reluctant to talk to GPs and accept treatment for depression [5–7] yet barriers remain between older people and GPs where the acknowledgement and prioritisation of depression as a legitimate problem requiring medical support prevail [8–14].

Even though older people respond well to probing about their mood by primary care physicians [15] they struggle to reveal depression to GPs [9, 16] or to verbalise their views and preferences relating to the management of their depression [17, 18]. This reluctance conflicts with the value placed on older people talking to GPs about depression whether it is expressing it in terms of situational factors such as loneliness and isolation [12, 13] negotiating how it could be framed as an acceptable concept [11] or establishing justifications for their low mood [10].

Older people's perceptions and beliefs about depression can influence ways they communicate to GPs [9, 10, 13] and they can be unwilling to talk about depression especially when it is normalised in comparison to other health problems [11]. While some older people value talking about depression as a form of help [19] for many it carries a stigma which ultimately is a barrier to seeking help from GPs [9, 10]. Perceptions of depression being a personal responsibility to overcome independently may also deter patients in asking GPs for help, especially when they need help with other physical or social problems [10].

Conceptually older people may not recognize depression as an illness needing treatment [20], rather seeing it as due to circumstances that often accompany old age, such as loneliness [12], and therefore a non-medical problem which is not a GP's responsibility [6, 21] or a moral failing [14].

The use of language and the way GPs and patients talk about depression, in the context of GP practice settings in primary care, has been highlighted as particularly important with older people [8, 13, 15]. For example, those with chronic conditions are likely to frame their depression in the context of their life stories and may describe depression in terms of situations and experiences [10] or loneliness [12]. However, describing depression as a chronic, physical disease which older people find

acceptable and normal in later life rather than a psychiatric brain disease is likely to facilitate communication with GPs [8, 22]. They may also see physical illness as a priority over their depression and that a GPs' capacity to help is limited unless they are suicidal [10] which would deter them from raising depression with GPs. These contrasting rationales for help-seeking indicate complexities and differences underlying how older people validate depression and the impact this has on what they tell GPs.

Evidence shows how depression in later life can slip through the net, where the medical framework used for its detection does not always fit with ways older people frame and talk about it [6, 8, 12, 14, 23] including the complexities of them asking for help with depression in the context of other health or life problems [5, 9–11, 13]. There is little suggestion in the evidence of how GPs can accommodate these factors when older people with depression talk to them. More understanding of the differences and complexities in ways older people conceptualise depression and the impact this has on ways they talk about it would assist GPs in detecting depression according to how older people frame it. The aim of this study was therefore to obtain older people's accounts of how they talk about depression or possible symptoms of depression in order to help improve communication between older patients who have depression and their GPs. Particular focus was on differences in their depression narratives and the factors that influence these.

Methods

Ethical considerations

Ethical approval was obtained from the local NHS National Research Ethics Service (NRES) and from Sunderland and North Tyneside CCGs where practices that recruited participants were located. Approval was also obtained from the University of Sunderland Research Ethics Committee. IG obtained an enhanced disclosure Criminal Records Bureau (CRB) check due to working with a vulnerable group.

Study design

A qualitative study was conducted as part of a PhD. A grounded approach was used; this was informed by the more recent work of Adele Clarke [24] rather than traditional versions by those including Glaser and Strauss [25] that require the researcher to exclude preconceived ideas. Clarke's methods seek to uncover multiplicity, the fluidity of ideas and points of difference rather than commonality; here they were used to facilitate recognition of complex, changing experiences of depression in later life and the range of differences that older people report in their experiences of having depression. Empirical data were generated through in depth semi-structured interviews [26] based on a topic guide developed from the literature. Observational notes were made by IG during interviews to support analysis. No relationships were established with participants prior to the study commencing.

Recruitment and sampling

Letters inviting GP practices to recruit patients were sent via NyReN (Northen and Yorkshire Research Network) to 169 practices along with information about the study explaining reasons for the research and what would happen. GPs working in three practices agreed to recruit patients; at their discretion they identified and sent invitation letters and information to patients over 65 with depression. Data collection, analysis and sampling were carried out iteratively by the lead author.

The first five respondents were interviewed, thereafter a theoretical sample of older people were selected using demographic data which indicated their potential to help explore further or discount ideas being developed. Early interviews (P1–5) indicated a need to gather data from participants who varied in age, gender and socioeconomic status. Accordingly, participants were sought for the second set of interviews (P6–10), which in turn indicated a need for data from those living in deprived inner-city areas and/or who had experienced long term or severe depression. Participants were sought for the third set of interviews as such (P11–16). Selecting patients on the basis of their age and severity/duration of depression was at the discretion of GPs and disclosed by participants at the time of interview if they were willing. The sample size was determined by the number of participants needed to achieve saturation and allow for the production of a full and detailed account of the data.

Interview schedule

The initial topic guide [see Additional file 1] included open ended discussion points and prompts to encourage participants to disclose as much information as they felt comfortable with. This was developed as interviews and analysis progressed, becoming increasingly focused on participants' depression narratives and influences on this, the impact of other people including GPs on their depression narratives, what the differences in their views of depression and its management were, content of their narratives and when and how their views changed, their personal experiences of depression, views of depression and how they felt about seeing GPs for depression. The grounded approach ensured care was taken to use the same vocabulary as the older people as prompts during the interview. After early interviews and analysis (P1–5), a further set of participants were recruited (P6–10) to inform proceeding interviews. This process was repeated with a third set of participants (P11–16) until data saturation. Written consent was obtained prior to data

collection and interviews were transcribed verbatim by IG and an independent transcriber.

Analysis

Transcripts were initially coded and analysed iteratively by IG using the constant comparison method and stepped model of grounded theory [25] where three levels of analysis were undertaken. The constant comparison method informed theoretical sampling of participants where early ideas were tested with subsequent participants and found to either support or disconfirm developing ideas. Coding and interpretations were inspected and discussed by three others in the research team at monthly meetings and for each level of analysis in a process of triangulation [27, 28] to increase validity. Interpretations were available to participants on request but this was not taken up and no feedback was given.

In line with the stepped model of grounded theory three levels of analysis were carried out. Open codes were derived from the data during first level analysis and emergent axial codes noted, grouped together and categorised. This informed the second level of analysis where possible themes were explored further with later participants. These themes were supported with more data were developed into axial codes where a typology of older people with characteristics found in their narratives formed three distinct groups positioned on a continuum.

In the larger PhD study typologies for both older people and GP were developed. Third level analysis brought these two data sets together in a theoretical model [29]. The typology developed from second level analysis of older people's data only is reported here as their views are underrepresented and seldom reported in isolation. Doing this underlines the importance of their voice being heard and allows an in-depth account of ways they communicate about depression.

A series of situational, social and positional maps [24] were used to explore the contextual, background and key influences in the data and enrich interpretations. Observations made during interviews (IG) were also considered in analysis and assisted the development of groups in the typology.

Findings

Interviews were completed with 16 older people at their homes and lasted 1–2 hours; only participants and the researcher were present in all interviews. The sample consisted of 10 women and 6 men with a reported age range of 67–88 years. Data from all participants was included in the analysis plus observational notes made by IG during interviews; no participants refused to participate or dropped out, and there were no repeat interviews. No characteristics about the interviewer (IG) or

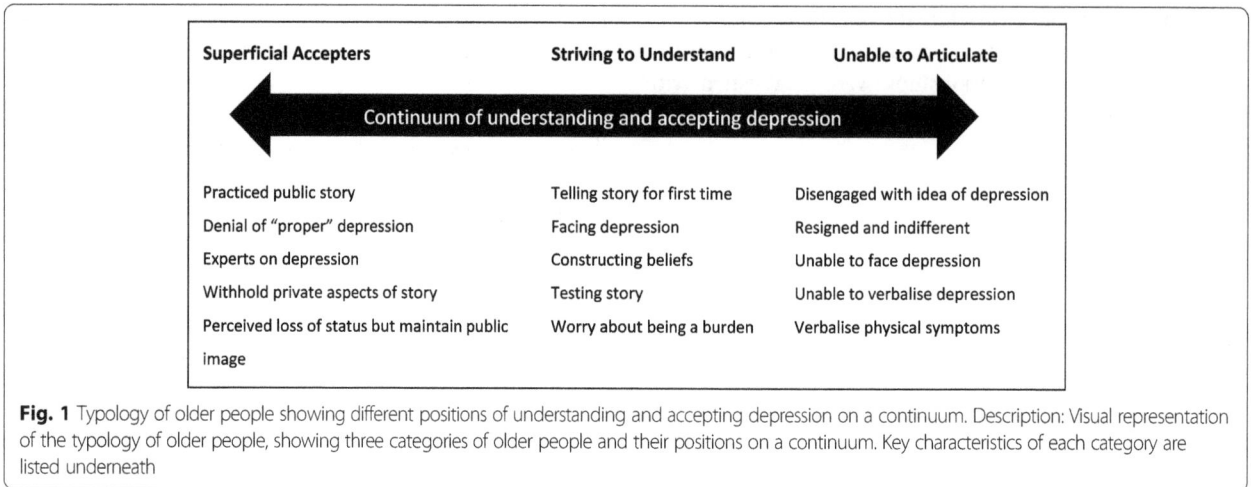

Superficial Accepters	Striving to Understand	Unable to Articulate

Continuum of understanding and accepting depression

Superficial Accepters	Striving to Understand	Unable to Articulate
Practiced public story	Telling story for first time	Disengaged with idea of depression
Denial of "proper" depression	Facing depression	Resigned and indifferent
Experts on depression	Constructing beliefs	Unable to face depression
Withhold private aspects of story	Testing story	Unable to verbalise depression
Perceived loss of status but maintain public image	Worry about being a burden	Verbalise physical symptoms

Fig. 1 Typology of older people showing different positions of understanding and accepting depression on a continuum. Description: Visual representation of the typology of older people, showing three categories of older people and their positions on a continuum. Key characteristics of each category are listed underneath

influences over participants' views were reported. De-scribed here is a summary of axial codes derived from first level analysis of interview data: components of narratives, constructions and experiences of depression, narrative agendas. This leads to the typology consisting of Superficial Accepters, Striving to Understand and Unable to Articulate categories.

Components

All participants recognised their narratives of depression were made up of different components which they shared or withheld from others. The most commonly cited components derived from open codes identified in early analysis of data were: descriptions of what depression feels like, what depression means, explanations for its cause, minimising depression, private and public stories and preferences in what to tell GPs. Differences between the ways older people talked about depression, language they used, what they told and withheld were prominent and began to define categories of the typology.

Constructions and experiences

While all participants described their constructions and experiences of depression they did so to differing degrees of detail using a variety of vocabulary. Not all used the term depression saying it was an inaccurate reflection of the problems they were experiencing and offered their own explanations for it. Some did not see depression as a medical problem or minimised theirs compared to others' who they saw as having "proper" (P3) depression. Others' ideas about their depression did not appear as concrete where they were starting to put their experiences into words or questioned what had happened to them rather than providing explanations or views.

Narrative agendas

Participants appeared to have differing agendas in their narratives of depression; some focused on certain aspects of their story regardless of any interview prompts, others were less focused and seemed to talk through ideas without any obvious direction. The remaining participants' narratives were brief and closed, with conversation about depression minimal. All explained their reasons for telling their story in certain ways; they were motivated by how others saw them, telling their story for the first time, consolidating their ideas or regaining control in some way. Some did not want to talk directly about depression yet their narratives about their life contexts revealed how they saw depression in themselves and the impact it had on what they shared and withheld about depression.

"I want to forget [experiences of depression], I don't want to think about it cos it just brings it all back to me." (P1).

Further data analysis led to the identification of a typology consisting of three distinct categories: Superficial Accepters ($n = 5$), Striving to Understand ($n = 6$) and Unable to Articulate ($n = 8$). These categories were shaped by the way older people spoke about depression in their interviews, the way they reported telling their stories of depression to other people including GPs, information about their depression they shared and withheld in comparison to each other and what they said about their experiences of seeing GPs for depression. Geographical location, affluence, reported severity/duration of depression and participants' ages were not found to be influential over the categories.

The typology indicates variation in participants' understanding and acceptance of depression and in their constructions and narratives at different positions on a continuum (Fig. 1). The continuum is used to emphasise that older people's positions are not fixed, and that flexible, "porous" [24] boundaries are likely to exist between categories. This flexibility accounts for participants who describe change in ways they conceptualise their depression during their life prompting a move between categories, or where participants display characteristics in their storytelling from two categories.

"all of a sudden the ECT [electroconvulsive therapy] had obviously sorted out my head and I said to myself, 'look, this is silly, they are obviously not treating you for cancer they are treating you for mental problems'. Once I realised that then it [the depression] started to sort itself out." (P8).

Analytical maps were used to set out multi factorial relationships identified between open and axial codes, around which analytical memos were developed to form categories of the typology. These were based around components of their stories they shared and withheld, their constructions and experiences of depression, their narrative agendas and perceived indications of change in ways they talked about depression.

Superficial accepters

All participants in this category talked of their depression willingly and it appeared they had accepted it. Further probing revealed denial of having depression where they either compared themselves to others with depression in its "true form" (P5), stated theirs was not a "proper" (P3) illness or commented on others with depression appearing not to see themselves in the same category.

"I would feel a bit down but not to the state that I couldn't get out of the chair like I'd seen in my wife." (P5).

"I never called it as depression I just felt awful, you know, you feel sad, I think sad is the word that I've always used." (P15).

This tendency to deny or minimize their depression conflicted with the open and accepting way they initially talked about it. With probing, some comments revealed insecurities and stigma about having depression, which possibly stemmed from concern about a negative effect on their outward image.

"People don't want to listen to you, or worry about your illness, that's how I feel." (P4).

Many of these participants also revealed a stoical desire to hide their depression from their community or workplace for fear it would influence others' perceptions of them, also indicating they may accept their depression only partially.

"I still did my job alright you know, I didn't have any problems. If I did I didn't let anybody know about them I can tell you... It was a secret. My secret you know, I just got on with my job. Was never off sick." (P14).

They demonstrated an inflexible agenda in their interviews, returning to the same topics regardless of any probing. For example, they gave detailed explanations about why they had depression, ensuring their reasoning and convictions about their depression were understood. This component of their narratives appeared practiced and lacked detail of their feelings or their views, as if they had prepared it for other people.

"I would like to know what's causing it... I have been very successful - I have been a head in four schools, successful as an artist, if I say so myself I am well liked in the village... so there is none of those things. It's just...tiredness." (P9).

Many in this category portrayed themselves as experts on depression by reporting they had greater knowledge of their depression than healthcare staff and/or that their symptoms were not fully understood. In doing this some revealed anger and distrust of healthcare staff, expressing dissatisfaction with many aspects of their treatment or with doctors for putting a label on their depression.

"Have you got any ailment that you always think oh well I know more about that than any of the doctors do? Well it's the same thing .... I've given a lot of thought to it and read [about] it myself and understand exactly what my condition is, but a lot of them don't." (P3).

Participants frequently referenced achievements in their education or careers. They often described facing a loss of status in some way, through career or position in family, and seemed to attach a lot of importance on how they presented themselves to others. Their style of talking about their experiences of depression focused on presenting facts, without giving much detail of how it felt or their views of it; they also tended to be articulate and the public components of their depression narratives were spoken with conviction. Although participants in this category were mostly men this did not appear to influence other characteristics; their willingness to talk about their experiences may simply have been because they were more sociable or better socialised through having a strong support network (as described by women) or a prominent career (as described by men).

Striving to understand

A key characteristic of this category was that many used the interview to talk about their depression for the first time to anybody in such terms, or in any depth outside GP consultations. Some reported their motivation for taking part to be to offload to somebody or to "come clean" (P13). These older people were the most emotionally open of all categories in the typology when describing their thoughts and showing their feelings about depression.

> "I've talked to you more than I've ever talked to anybody [about my depression]." (P15).

Some participants described testing different explanations for their depression aloud or practicing their story, sometimes as a way of reconnecting with other people. In doing this they appeared to be coming to terms with what had happened to them and were trying to clarify and articulate their understanding of depression.

> "I was detached from everybody else, I didn't know why, and I didn't know how then to reconnect and re communicate, it was very difficult." (P10).

Participants' narratives were often long with little need for prompting; they tended to start talking immediately on contact, seemingly determined to tell their story. Their narratives could sound confused when they were remembering chronological events or what had happened to them, and they often appeared lost in their thoughts during interviews.

All participants in this category explored possibilities around their constructions of depression aloud. Though this category's constructions of depression were not as developed as others, they described seeing it as an illness, a weakness of character, a normal feeling in old age and even questioned whether depression existed as a concept at all. They tended to alternate between the labels for depression possibly as they were still establishing their ideas and may not have been certain why they had been diagnosed with depression. Their uncertainty led to numerous contradictions in their narratives, but also prompted changes in their perspectives influenced by consolidating their ideas in the interview. For example, one participant had seldom spoken to anyone about her depression "I've talked to you more than I've ever talked to anybody" (P15) but by the end of the interview she felt older people with depression should "talk to their family if they can and get them to understand; a lot of people don't understand depression." (P15). Similarly,

another interviewee described how he told his GP about his depression initially by talking about his physical symptoms,

> "I didn't tell him [the GP] the details I just said, it started off with me feet and then I got a rash up me back and even in my face." (P13).

By the end of the interview P13 was calling his condition depression and seemed more comfortable talking about it in terms of emotional experiences.

People in this category were clear that the right timing was essential to opening up about their depression. Many described their interviews as a starting point to talk to others about their depression despite uncertainty about being ready or concern about being "a burden" (P13). Others spoke of having to "face up" (P8) to their depression or having ignored it in the past now felt ready to explore it further. Bereaved participants were common in this category, reporting this as a trigger for their depression but needing to pass through a crisis point before they could look back and reflect on their experiences out loud and share this with someone else.

> "She [the counsellor] said what I want you to do is write a letter, put your thoughts on paper, and, you know, I couldn't do that, not at that time I couldn't, I was too upset, like." (P6).

> "I intend to come clean today, because I tend when the family ring me up I'm always alright, even when I'm not, and...I don't want to be a burden." (P13).

This category may not have established what they felt comfortable sharing and so switched between private and public components of their narratives. For participants in this category the opportunity to establish what was private and what they were willing to share in hindsight of depression appeared empowering as their depression narratives grew increasingly confident during interviews. This suggested that confirming their story aloud may have helped regain a sense of control which they typically described having lost when depressed.

> "If I needed to ask them for their support they would be absolutely furious that I hadn't done it [earlier], but my feeling was, I've got to cope with it... It's just silly, but if I told my son that he would have said mum, for heaven's sake..." (P10).

Unable to articulate

Older people in the Unable to Articulate category had difficulty articulating their experiences, understandings or feelings about having depression into words, and appeared disengaged with the idea of it. They accepted they had depression and appeared resigned to it. This category revealed little more than the basic facts about their depression and while they cited a number of traumatic life events, they provided minimal detail of these by closing conversations. They described dealing with depression by blocking out trauma or disconnecting from it, which led them to withhold much of their depression narratives.

"I want to forget, I don't want to think about it cos it just brings it all back to me." (P1).

"My family history is so appalling...it's important that you know. I probably had one of the unhappiest childhoods [I've] ever heard of in my life... father committed suicide, sister committed suicide, mother who attempted suicide on numerous occasions... But that childhood, whether that has any bearing, I don't know." (P9).

Willingness to talk was low among participants in the category but there was variation. All tended to open up more about their daily lives or activities and doing so gave some insight into their constructions of depression, underlining the importance of life narratives for this category. It was common for participants to start talking about an experience of depression then quickly draw the story to a close.

"I sat here for weeks you know, couldn't go out anywhere it affected me so much, but luckily I've got over it." (P2).

Two participants avoided talking about depression completely in interviews but still gave insight into their depression. P12 focused on heartbreak from losing people she loved during her life and this was how she defined her depression. Her narrative was stoical and she came across as detached from her depression, not wanting to talk about it at all. Similarly, P1 avoided talking about her depression, instead talking about pain in her back which seemed to be a way of expressing her feelings about her depression. The most extreme example within this category was P11 who said very little, and then only saying a few words about her life with heavy prompting. She appeared numb to her feelings and not to care about her depression or herself any more. She listed traumatic events that had happened during her life with brief, closed statements and minimal explanation.

There was a feeling within this category that their depression had completely taken them over for a long

time, that they had no hope of things changing and no desire for exploring their own feelings and understanding depression. They described other people (e.g. doctors or family) or the medication to be in control of most aspects of their lives, and when asked how they felt about having depression said.

"Well I've more or less accepted it, I've not got much choice." (P11).

People in this category had relatively fixed views on the reason for their depression (e.g. their personality) indicating they had long accepted the idea of having depression but were less likely to describe pivotal events or decisions to change their narratives than other categories.

They were unlikely to use the label depression, instead not talking about it directly or expressing it through physical symptoms such as *"heartbreak"* (P12) or *"my back"* (P1). P16 described many physical problems including tinnitus and pain on her face, explaining her depression by talking about these; she did not seem able to face her psychological distress or explain it any other way.

Participants in this category reported severe episodes of depression throughout their lifetimes managed in both primary and secondary care. They all described trying a range of medications and treatments appearing resigned and disconnected from these experiences. Their views were passive about how their depression was managed and their descriptions suggested they were used to doctors making decisions without their involvement.

Discussion
Summary of findings
Our findings highlight clear differences in the ways in which older people talk about their depression and provides a typology categorising their approach according to their narratives and how their understanding and acceptance of depression underpins this. This underlines a need for flexibility in the help provided to older people with depression and may provide opportunities for health care professionals to improve communication and understanding of how older people make sense of their depression.

Focus on older people's depression narratives addresses an area known to be a problematic between older people and GPs [9–11, 13]. Older people value talking through their depression over biomedical treatments which may be less acceptable to them [5, 9, 19]. This study offers a framework to support GPs in understanding the complexities of the narratives older people may bring to consultations which tend to focus on their life story [10]. The typology here could also be considered for use outside the GP consultation by non-clinical staff, a factor on which importance is placed elsewhere [9].

This study supports literature suggesting that older people communicate their symptoms in line with their perceptions of depression [6, 23] and that this can deter them from asking for help [8, 13, 19]. It builds on evidence showing a need for patients to gain an understanding of their depression including its cause and what has happened to them [30, 31] so they can explain their experiences to others [32]. Here, older people's acceptance of depression was a key influence for what they told GPs, where varying degrees of acceptance were a reason to tell or withhold parts of their story. Some struggled to recognise depression in themselves, typically denying or attributing it to something else (Superficial Acceptors), others were open to accepting it but needed to make sense of what had happened to them first (Striving to Understand) whereas those who had accepted it appeared to have reached an impasse and saw no way of progressing (Unable to Articulate). The resulting patterns of storytelling may indicate a way for GPs to open a dialogue with older people about help they would find acceptable rather than relying on them reporting symptoms.

Parallels can be found between this study and the work of others dating back as far as the 1950s which promotes the importance of the family doctors' role in building personal relationships and understanding the individual [33–35]. These ideas about patient centredness began to redefine the role of the family doctor to recognize the mind and body as inextricably linked with the patient's individuality at its core.

"to restore the primacy of the person, one needs a medicine that puts the person in all his wholeness in the center of the stage and does not separate the disease from the man, and the man from his environment." ([35], p., 910]).

The findings of this study, particularly that the meaning of depression for older people and the way they communicate about it is built around their life contexts, echo these ideas and suggest they could be revisited by primary care health professionals in consultations with older people.

For McWhinney (1975) this is manifest in achieving a friendship-like relationship with personal knowledge [36], knowing the person both in good and ill health, treating the person before the illness so that the doctor gains understanding of the patients' perceptions of their condition and what it means to them [37]. Evidence in the field often features the perspectives of clinicians and practice staff [11, 13, 14, 37, 38] whereas the focus of this study is solely the patient and their perspectives and

may serve to enhance communication between patients' and physicians so that their personalized life story is recognised. McWhinney proposes that achieving understanding on a personal level between patient and physician can "lead to quicker and more accurate diagnoses and more effective treatment" ([35], p., 910]) even though doctors have less time to listen and patients have higher expectations and make more demands of their physicians [37]. Evidence here which exposes how older patients both make sense of their depression and create meaning may be of value to GPs and other health professionals who spend more time with older patients.

It has been noted that recognising depression and articulating it can be challenging for older people who instead may describe a change in their sense of self in the context of their life stories [10]. Similarly, the life stories of participants in this study were integral to their constructions of depression, where their accounts would give insight into their experience of having depression. Identification of depression in clinical guidance is based on questionnaire scoring systems and identification of symptoms and may rely on the patient's willingness to verbalise these and the extent to which they can articulate their narratives to GPs [39, 40]; this may not be suitable for all patients especially if they struggle to communicate about their depression in a clinical setting. This gold standard approach does not take into account the way older people conceptualise, accept and articulate depression which are the three main factors shown in this study to influence the way they communicate their depression to GPs. Opportunity could be found here for debate or reflection on the one size fits all approach taken in the guidance, which by the very nature of standardization is unavoidable.

This tension between standardisation and personalisation also points to a need for an approach which fits with older people's ways of communicating about depression rather than expectations for them to report clinical symptoms. Confronting this may be daunting for GPs who may have little time to explore patients' narratives in depth [41]. Likewise, their perspectives on managing older people with depression can be characterised by negativity when they have a lack of confidence in their expertise and tend to focus on problems and barriers [13, 37, 38]. They may also view depression as a consequence of patients' life circumstances for which they cannot offer change and for which the treatments they can offer are limited in their effectiveness [42, 43]. The low response rate of 3 practices out of 169 agreeing to take part in the study could be a reflection of these factors. Development of approaches outside the GP consultation that fit with older people's ways of communicating are in their infancy [9] but a lack of available services for older people means a time saving method of doing this that considers the demands of working in general practice could potentially support GPs.

The impact of stigma and assumptions about others' views of depression may also act as a barrier to dialogue between older people and GPs [9, 10, 19]. Feeling a responsibility to avoid burdening other people has been recognised in those with depression [10, 19] where not taking responsibility to look after oneself is perceived by people with depression as a personality flaw or a reason to look down upon others with depression. Reluctance to "be a burden" (P13) prevented older people in this study from sharing their depression with family, friends and GPs and instead internalising it. During interviews the Striving to Understand category were responsive to probing and challenging whilst constructing their ideas, suggesting this stage of depression may be an opportunity to challenge these barriers. With suicide among older people estimated to be the tenth most common cause of death in the older population worldwide by 2020 [44, 45] the need to confront this perception is timely.

Strengths and limitations

The typology is based on participants' accounts of past episodes of depression or coming out of a recent episode so were likely to be recounting views with hindsight. Some described their depression as severe or mild but in the end this did not shape categories in the typology. While not being generalisable the study is potentially transferrable to other similar contexts and settings.

GPs recruited patients at their discretion and it was not known if a formal diagnosis of depression had been made. This method of recruitment was feasible within the research ethics framework as opposed to recruiting participants without a known diagnosis. Participants talked about their condition using a range of vocabulary. We recognise that older people who have not been given a diagnosis may talk about their condition and experiences differently to those who have, as they have not been given a label for their condition. Exploration of the impact of a diagnosis or no diagnosis on ways older people talked about depression was therefore not possible within the study design.

Data collection and analysis was undertaken by the lead author from a non-clinical perspective. This may have been valuable for patients who find it difficult to express their feelings to GPs and for addressing problems between older people and GPs relating to a condition that has become progressively more medicalised among older people who may see it as a non-medical problem.

The approach here is an unusual attempt to explore patients' views with minimal influence or bias from the clinical setting or context, using methods that allow patients to lead the development of ideas in the data. Reporting older people's perspectives in isolation underlines the importance of their voice being heard and allows an in-depth account of ways they communicate about depression.

Implications for practice and research

This study raises the question, what help do older people need for their depression? The findings indicate that older people need flexible support depending on how they conceptualise depression and the extent to which they can articulate their problems and needs. Implications here are for a personalised approach to listening and decoding older people's narratives about depression that recognises the importance of their situational and life contexts.

Future work is needed to develop strategies for GPs to quickly identify appropriate help for older people with depression that better fits with how they frame and talk about it and which also recognises the demands of general practice. Observations of GP consultations to consolidate the typology groups and further exploratory work to confirm acceptable support for each typology category is required. A model showing appropriate support for different categories of older people in the typology may have implications for other clinical and non-clinical practitioners, or others older people talk to, who may be able to listen for patterns in older people's depression narratives and offer support, advise or signpost older people to getting the help they need.

Conclusions

This study provides insight into how older people's constructions of depression manifest in their depression narratives to increase understanding of ways they communicate about depression. It highlights the importance of recognising differences between older people in their understanding, acceptance and willingness to share their stories of depression and suggests the value of these differences as cues to determine appropriate support. The typology presented in this study may help GPs recognise patterns in patients' narratives, their different conceptual positions regarding depression and explore their life contexts to gain more insight into their depression. This personalised approach may assist GPs when they need to try new communication strategies with patients or try to get to the core of what depression means to an individual to provide the best care for them.

Abbreviations

AC: Professor Ann Crosland; CH: Dr.Catherine Hayes; GP: General Practitioner; IG: Dr. Isabel Gordon; JL: Professor Jonathan Ling; LR: Professor Louise Robinson; NHS: National Health Service; PHQ9: Patient Health Questionnaire PHQ9 for depression

Acknowledgements

This project was funded by the University of Sunderland. The views in this article are those of the authors and not necessarily those of the University of Sunderland. Thanks to patients for giving their time and sharing their stories, and Greg Rubin, a co supervisor for the PhD study, for his expertise. JL is a Senior Investigator and Associate Director of Fuse, the Centre for Translational Research in Public Health, a UKCRC Public Health Research Centre of Excellence. Funding for Fuse from the British Heart Foundation, Cancer Research UK, Economic and Social Research Council, Medical Research Council, the National Institute for Health Research, is gratefully acknowledged.

Funding

This study was funded by the University of Sunderland, who had no input into the study design or collection, analysis and interpretation of the data. They did not contribute to writing the manuscript.

Authors' contributions

Drawing on previous experience as a university researcher, IG was responsible for the PhD study conception and design, data collection and analysis and drafting the paper. JL provided guidance and contributed to writing and editing the manuscript. AC was director of studies for the PhD study and provided guidance for the study conception, design, data collection and analysis and contributed to data interpretation. LR is a GP who cares for older patients with depression and has a specialist research interest in patients with dementia. CH taught podogerontology for seven years at the Durham School of Podiatric Medicine and has provided clinical care for older people as a podiatrist. LR and CH were co supervisors for the PhD study, contributing to data interpretation and commented on drafts of the manuscript. All authors read and approved the manuscript.

Competing interests

Authors declare that they have no competing interests.

Author details

[1]Faculty of Health Sciences and Wellbeing, University of Sunderland, City Campus Chester Road, Sunderland SR1 3SD, UK. [2]Newcastle University Institute for Ageing and Institute for Health & Society, Newcastle University, Newcastle upon Tyne NE4 5PL, England.

References

1. Luppa M, Sikrski C, Luck T, Ehrekem L, Konnopka A, Wiese B, Riedel-Heller SG. Age and gender specific prevalence of depression in latest-life – systematic review and meta-analysis. J Affect Disord. 2012;136(36):212–21.
2. Royal College of General Practitioners. Management of Depression in Older People: Why this is Important in Primary Care? Royal College of General Practitioners. In: Fundamental facts about mental health 2016. London: Mental Health Foundation; 2014. https://www.mentalhealth.org.uk/sites/default/files/fundamental-facts-about-mental-health-2016.pdf. Accessed 6 March 2018.
3. Smyth C. Depression in old age is the "next big public health crisis". The Times 8 April 2014. https://www.thetimes.co.uk/article/depression-in-old-age-is-the-next-big-health-crisis-vkb835j05f8. Accessed 17 January 2018.
4. Health and Social Care Information Centre. Health Survey for England, 2005: Health of older people. Health and Social Care Information Centre 2007. http://webarchive.nationalarchives.gov.uk/20170726164150/, https://digital.nhs.uk/catalogue/PUB01184. Accessed 26 Oct 2018.
5. Chew-Graham C, Kovandžić M, Gask L, Burroughs H, Clarke P, Sanderson H, Dowrick C. Why may older people with depression not present to primary care? Messages from secondary analysis of qualitative data. Health Soc Care Community. 2012;20(1):52–60.
6. Bristow K, Edwards S, Funnel E, Fisher L, Gask L, Dowrick C, Chew-Graham C. Help seeking and access to primary care for people from "hard to reach" groups with common mental health problems. Int J Family Med. 2011;2011:1–3.
7. Kessing LV, Hansen HV, Demyttenaere K, Bech P. Depressive and bipolar disorders: patients' attitudes and beliefs towards depression and antidepressants. Psychol Med. 2005;35(8):1205–13.
8. Burroughs HA, Lovell KB, Morley M, Baldwin R, Burns A, Chew-Graham C. Justifiable depression: how primary care professionals and patients view late life depression? A qualitative study Fam Pract. 2006;23(3):369–77.
9. Overend K, Bosanquet K, Bailey D, Foster D, Lewis H, Nutbrown S, Woodhouse R, Gilbody S, Chew-Graham C. Revealing hidden depression in older people: a qualitative study within a randomised controlled trial. BMC Fam Pract. 2015;16:142.
10. Alderson SL, Foy R, Glidewell L, House AO. Patients' understanding of depression associated with chronic illness: a qualitative study. BMC Fam Pract. 2014;15:37.
11. Coventry PA, Hays R, Dickens C, Bundy C, Garrett C, Cherrington A, Chew-Graham C. Talking about depression: a qualitative study of barriers to managing depression in people with long term conditions in primary care. BMC Family Pract. 2011;12:10.
12. Barg FK, Huss-Ashmore R, Wittink MN, Murray GF, Bognor HR, Gallo JJ. A mixed-methods approach to understanding loneliness and depression in older adults. J Gerontol B Psychol Sci Soc Sci. 2006;61(6):S329–39.
13. Murray J, Banerjee S, Byng R, Tylee A, Bhugra D, Macdonald A. Primary care professionals' perceptions of depression in older people: a qualitative study. Soc Sci Med. 2006;63:1363–73.
14. Wittink MN, Barg FK, Gallo JJ. Unwritten rules of talking to doctors about depression: integrating qualitative and quantitative methods. Ann Fam Med. 2006;4(4):302–9.
15. Lawrence V, Murray J, Banerjee S, Turner S, Sangha K, Byng R, Bhugra D, Huxley P, Tylee A, Macdonald A. Concepts and causation of depression: a cross-cultural ctudy of the beliefs of older adults. Gerontol. 2006;46:23–32.
16. Chew-Graham CA, Campion J, Kaiser P, Edwards K. Management of depression in older people: why this is important in primary care. The forum for mental health in. Primary Care. 2011; http://www.psige.org/public/files/NMH_10095_OPMH%20%26%20depression_5.pdf. Accessed 26 Oct 2018.
17. Givens J, Datto C, Ruckdeschel K, Knott K, Zubritsky C, Oslin DW, Nyshadham S, Vanguri P, Barg FK. Older patients' aversion to antidepressants: a qualitative study. J Gen Intern Med. 2006;21:146–51.
18. Gum AM, Areán PA, Hunkeler E, Tang A, Katon W, Hitchcock P, Steffans DC, Dickens J, Unützer J. Depression treatment preferences in older primary care patients. Gerontologist. 2006;46(1):14–22.
19. Kingstone T, Burroughs H, Bartlam B, Ray M, Proctor J, Shepherd T, Bullock P, Chew-Graham CA. Developing a community based psychosocial intervention with older people and third sector workers for anxiety and depression: a qualitative study. BMC Fam Pract. 2017;18:77.
20. Reynolds CF, Charney DS. Unmet needs in the diagnosis and treatment of mood disorders in later life. Biol Psychiatry. 2002;52:145–7.
21. Prior L, Wood F, Lewis G, Pill R. Stigma revisited, disclosure of emotional problems in primary care consultations in Wales. Soc Sci Med. 2003;56:2191–200.
22. van Schaik A, van Marwijk H, Ader H, van Dyck R, de Haan M, Penninx B, van Hout H, Beekman A. Interpersonal psychotherapy for elderly patients in primary care. Ame J Geriatr Psychiatry. 2006;14(9):777–86.
23. Cohen A, Singh SP, Hague J. The primary care guide to severe mental illness. London: The Sainsbury Centre for Mental Health; 2004.
24. Clarke A. Situational analysis: grounded theory after the postmodern turn. London: Sage Publications Ltd; 2005.
25. Glaser BG, Strauss AL. The discovery of grounded theory: strategies for qualitative research. London: Transaction Publishers; 1967. (Fourth paperback printing; 2009)
26. Lincoln YS, Guba EG. Naturalistic enquiry. Beverly Hills, CA: Sage Publications Inc; 1985.
27. Denzin NK. The research act. 2nd ed. Chicago: Aldine; 1978.

28. Flick U. Triangulation in qualitative research. In: Flick U, von Kardoff E, Steike I, editors, Jenner B, translator. A companion to Qualitative Research. London Sage Publications Ltd; 2004.

29. Gordon, I. The perspectives of older people and GPs on depression in later life and its management: the stories they tell and ways they respond to each other. University of Sunderland, February 2013.

30. Lauber C, Falcato L, Nordt C, Rossler W. Lay beliefs about causes of depression. Acta Psychiatr Scand. 2003;108(Suppl 418):96–9.

31. Brown C, Dunbar-Jacob J, Palenchar DR, Kellerher KJ, Breuhlman RD, Sereika S, Thase ME. Primary care patients' personal illness models for depression: a preliminary investigation. Fam Pract. 2001;18(3):314–8.

32. Lewis SE. A search for meaning: making sense of depression. J Ment Health. 1995;4:369–82 McWhinney IR. Family medicine in perspective. N Engl J Med 1975;293(4):176–81. Cited in: Green, L. A. Will people have personal physicians anymore? Dr Ian McWhinney Lecture, 2017. Can Fam Physician 2017;63:910.

33. Green, L. The American Board of Family Medicine Foundation inaugurates the G. Gayle Stephens keystone conference series, Ann Fam Med 2015; 13 (4);391-392. At https://www.ncbi.nlm.nih.gov/pmc/articles/PMC4508190/. Accessed 30 June 2018.

34. Balint M. The doctor, his patient and the illness. Lancet. 1955;1:318.

35. Green LA. Will people have personal physicians anymore? Dr Ian McWhinney lecture. 2017 Can Fam Physician. 2017;63:909–12.

36. Harlow AH Jr. The health care issues of the 1960's, II: the future of the personal physician. Library of Congress catalogue no. 63-21632. New York, NY: group health insurance, Inc; 1964. Cited in: green, L. a. will people have personal physicians anymore? Dr Ian McWhinney lecture, 2017. Can Fam Physician. 2017;63:910.

37. Burroughs HA, Lovell KB, Morley M, et al. Justifiable depression: how do primary care professionals and patients view late life depression? A qualitative study. Fam Pract. 2006;23(3):369–77.

38. Rothera I, Jones R, Gordon C. An examination of the attitude and practice of general practitioners in the diagnosis and treatment of depression in older people. Int J Geriatr Psychiatry. 2002;17(4):354–8.

39. National Institute for Health and Clinical Excellence. Depression in adults: recognition and managment. https://www.nice.org.uk/guidance/cg90. Accessed 26 Oct 2018.

40. Patient Health Questionnaire (PHQ 9). file:///C:/Users/Jim/AppData/Local/Microsoft/Windows/INetCache/IE/A8YWVJ91/DepressionScale.pdf. Accessed 21 March 2018.

41. Oopick P, Aluoja A, Kalda R, Maaroos H. Screening for depression in primary care. Fam Pract. 2006;23:693–8.

42. Chew-Graham CA, May CR, Cole H, Hedley S. The burden of depression in primary care: a qualitative investigation of general practitioners' constructs of depressed people in the inner city. Prim Care Psychiatr. 2000;6(4):137–41.

43. Chew-Graham CA, May CR, Perry MS. Qualitative research and the problem of judgment: lessons from interviewing fellow professionals. Fam Pract. 2002;19(3):285–9.

44. Koponen HJ, Viilo K, Hakko H, Timonen M, Meyer-Rochow VB, Särkioja T, Räsänen P. Rates and previous disease history in old age suicide. Int J Geriatr Psychiatry. 2007;22(1):38–46.

45. Lapierre S, Erlangsen A, Waern M, De Leo D, Oyama H, Scocco P, Gallo J, Szanto K, Conwell Y, Draper B, Quinnett P. International research Group for Suicide among the elderly. A systematic review of elderly suicide prevention programs. Crisis. 2011;32(2):88–9.

19

Effect of administrative information on visit rate of frequent attenders in primary health care: ten-year follow-up study

Anne K. Santalahti[1*], Tero J. Vahlberg[2], Sinikka H. Luutonen[3,4] and Päivi T. Rautava[5,6]

Abstract

Background: Frequent attenders (FAs) use a disproportionately large share of the resources of general practitioners (GPs) working in primary healthcare centres. The aim of this study was to estimate the proportion of FAs among all patients in the primary health care centres of a medium sized city in Finland, and to examine whether providing GPs with administrative information about their frequent attenders (names and numbers of visits per year) can reduce the number of FAs and the frequency of their visits.

Methods: Statistic data on all GP visits ($n = 1.8$ million) to 11 public healthcare centres in one city were collected from the electronic patient records covering the period from 2001 to 2010. A FA-patient was defined as a person who made 10 or more visits to GPs during one year. The baseline situation in 2001 was compared with the situation in 2006 after administrative information had been provided three times to all GPs working in the healthcare centres. Poisson's regression analysis was used, and FA numbers and consultation rates in the years 2002–2005 were compared with the year 2006; figures for 2006 were also compared with those for the follow-up period 2007–2010.

Results: During the years 2001–2006, the proportion of visits of FA-patients fell overall from 9.1 to 8.5%, a decline of 0.6% ($p < 0.0001$). This reduction was equivalent to an annual work load of two GPs in the study center. The proportion of visits of FA patients increased again in the follow-up period (2007–2010), when administrative information was no longer provided.

Conclusion: When GPs are provided with information on the number and names of their FA-patients, the annual rate of FA visits to GPs drops significantly. The method is simple and repeatable. However, without a control group of GPs who have not received such information, it is impossible to assess if the intervention was the only circumstance affecting the reduction in FA consultation rates.

Keywords: Primary care, Frequent attenders, Administrative information, GP's work load

Background

There is no generally accepted definition of a frequent attender (FA). Most studies have used the number of visits per year as the criterion, but the specific number chosen to define a frequent attender varies widely, from 5 visits per year at one end of the range to 20 visits at the other [1–7]. There are studies where FAs are defined as patients who have one-year attendance rates, adjusted for age and gender, above the 90th percentile [8, 9]. In Finnish studies, numerical definitions varying from at 8 to 11 GP visits per year have been generally used [1–4, 10].

The problem of frequent attenders has been studied for more than 60 years. Backett et al. reported in 1954 that 16% of patients made ten or more visits per year to general practitioners (GPs), and that these patients represented 52% of GPs' workload [11]. Frequent consulters are a small proportion of all GPS' patients but account for a disproportionate number of consultations [7]. Vedsted and Christiansen conducted a literature review in 2005, which found that the top 10% of attenders accounted for 30–50% of all GP contacts [12]. It is entirely acceptable to spend a lot of healthcare resources on patients whose

* Correspondence: anne.santalahti@ylojarvi.fi
[1]Turku City Healthcare Center, Turku, Finland
Full list of author information is available at the end of the article

condition demands it, but certain FAs can create unnecessary and unwelcome work and cause frustration for GPs [13].

Research by Heywood et al. (1998) found that FAs received many more prescriptions and were referred to hospital much often that other patients [14]; it is impossible to establish whether these treatment decisions were warranted by the condition of the patients concerned, or whether they represented poor use of healthcare resources. It has been estimated that a decrease of one visit per FA patient per year would decrease the average workload of a GP by 1 % [14]. In Finland, the average frequency of visits to a GP decreased from 1.92 visits to 1.56 visit per inhabitant per year in the period from 2001 to 2010. One FA makes 10 or more visits to a GP per year, so the difference is considerable.

Systematic reviews indicate that FAs often have chronic diseases or other chronic physical or mental problems [4, 12, 15–17], and that they may also have long-lasting somatization and many concomitant disorders [10, 18]. The majority of FAs are elderly females [3, 19, 20]. FAs' socioeconomic status is usually low and they use many social services [12]. Other characteristics are a body mass index over 30, fear of death, low alcohol intake, low satisfaction with healthcare services and irritable bowel syndrome [3].

Studies have been conducted to investigate what kind of interventions might reduce FAs' consultation rates. Research by Bellón et al. showed that intervention with GPs can be effective; in their study, three GPs received 15 h' intervention training which incorporated biopsychosocial, organizational and rational approaches [21]. Jiwa tried to reduce Fas' consultation rates by giving GPs summarized notes on their Fas' medical histories which they could refer to during consultations but this intervention was not successful [22].

The present study was conducted in the city of Turku, which is the sixth largest city in Finland, with 175,000 to 178,000 inhabitants during the years of the study (2001–2010). Turku is an industrial and university city, with an immigrant population of about 8 % and an age distribution similar to most industrialized countries. GPs have a capitation-based contract, where each GP is responsible for about 1500–2700 inhabitants, with a mean of 2312 inhabitants per GP in 2010. Usually, patients first call a nurse, who assesses the type of treatment needed and, if necessary, arranges an appointment with the allocated GP. In this Finnish primary care model, nurses thus control access to GPs to some extent, and as a result FAs do not meet their GPs as often as in many other countries. The duration of GP consultations varies from 10 to 45 min.

The first aim of this study was to establish the total number of FA patients, and how many visits FAs made to the healthcare centres and primary care emergency clinic in Turku in 2001–2010. The second aim was to explore how administrative information provided to each GP about his/her FAs (names and number of visits for each FA in the preceding year) affects frequency of attendance. The hypothesis was that this simple intervention reduces frequent attendance by drawing the attention of GPs to the issue. Thirdly, for the years 2001–2010, we compared the overall workload of the GPs in the study with the workload arising specifically from consultations with FAs. We also asked the GPs to draw up treatment plans for their patients listed as FAs in 2004, and we checked later to see how many plans had in fact been made.

Methods

The research design in this study is a registry-based cohort study. We used the developmental work research method; this model proceeds from evaluation of current action, to model and analysis of novel courses of action, to implementation and final assessment of the new courses of action [23]. In this study, FAs are defined as patients with 10 or more face-to-face visits to a GP during 1 year. The study population was formed by all patients who visited a GP ten times or more per year. The study data were retrieved from the electronic patient record system (Pegasos®) of the city of Turku, where the research was conducted. The electronic patient record system was used by every GP in all of the 11 public healthcare centres in the city and in the primary care emergency clinic during the whole period of 2001–2010. Data were collected on all face-to-face visits to GPs, both in the healthcare centres and the emergency clinic.

In 2002–2005, the chief medical officer of the city of Turku held three short administrative information sessions during regular management meetings with all GPs. In the 2002 session, all the GPs received personalized information about the number of FAs identified in their own patient register for the previous calendar year (2001). The same procedure was repeated in 2003 concerning the data for 2002. In 2005, the list of FAs was updated again according to data covering the year 2004, and the information was passed to GPs as before. In addition, in the 2005 session, the chief medical officer asked the GPs to make treatment plans for the FAs on the 2004 list.

In 2006–2010 the data of the number of FA visits to GPs were collected but in this period, the information was not passed on to GPs. To estimate the impact of providing GPs with administrative information on FAs, we compared the number of FAs and the total number of FA visits in the starting year (2001) with the corresponding figures in 2002–2006. The results are expressed as relative risks (RR) with 95% confidence intervals (95% CI). Then we analyzed the number of FAs and total FA visits in 2007–2010, i.e., over a period when the GPs had not received personalized information about their FAs. Finally, we compared those figures with the ones of 2006. The year 2006 was chosen as the comparison year because the final administrative information session for the GPs had been held in 2005.

The records of all patients listed as FAs in 2004 were checked during the follow-up period to see whether treatment plans had been made for them by their GPS. The number of treatment plans made was recorded.

Information on the number of GPs in 2001–2010, the number of days worked by each GP and the number of individual patients treated per workday was retrieved form the electronic patient record system.

The changes in the number of FA visits as a proportion of all visits to GPs were analyzed using Poisson's regression analysis over the whole period of 2001 to 2010. The natural logarithm of number of all visits to GPs' surgeries was used as an offset parameter in the Poisson model. The results were expressed as risk ratios (RR) with 95% confidence intervals (95% CI). P-values of less than 0.05 were considered statistically significant. Statistical analyses were carried out using the SAS system for Windows, Version 9.2 (SAS Institute Inc. Cary, NC, USA).

Results

All GPs in this study were employed by the city of Turku. They were working in 11 primary healthcare centres in different parts of the city, and in the primary care emergency clinic. The number of full-time tenured GPs increased from 71 in 2001, to 74 in 2006 and 77 in 2010. In 2003, 2005, 2006 and 2008, the number of tenured GPs remained the same as in the previous year. In addition, a large number of locums were employed every year to cover for GPs on annual leave, study leave, and other leaves of absence; these locums were employed for different lengths of time and many worked part-time. Thus, during the years 2001–2010, an average of 135.6

individual GPs per year were employed by the city. Each GP worked 109 days per year on average and treated an average of 1003 individual patients annually.

During the years 2001–2010, a total of 1,816,457 face-to-face visits were made to the GPs, of which 166,059 visits were made by FA patients. The visits of the FA patients accounted for 9.1% (mean value) of all GP visits in primary healthcare. At the same time, FAs represented only 1.8% (mean value) of all patients (Table 1). The average number of individual patients was 73,096 per year, and of FA patients 1327 per year. FAs made on average 16,606 visits per year during the period covered by this study (Table 1).

In 2001, the total number of FA patients was 1415, or 1.9% of all patients who used public healthcare services provided by GPs that year. The number of FAs varied between 1241 and 1415 during the subsequent 9 years (to 2010). The annual mean number of visits to a GP per FA varied between 12.3 and 12.8. The total annual number of FA patient visits went down from 17,627 in 2001, to 15,276 in 2006, although there was a reversal in the downward trend in 2005, when patient visits rose to 16,140 from 15,886 in 2004. FA visits as a proportion of all GP visits varied between 8.5 and 9.8%. Treatment plans were made for 73 of the patients listed as FAs in 2004, i.e. for only 5.9% of all FA patients that year.

At the outset in 2001, FA visits as a proportion of all visits to GPs was 9.1%. The GPs received information on their FAs between 2002 and 2005, and after these interventions, FA visits as a proportion of all visits to GPs decreased significantly in 2003 and even more so in 2006, compared with the situation in 2001. FA visits in 2003 had decreased from 9.1% (2001) to 8.7%, and in 2006 from 9.1% (2001) to 8.5% ($p < 0.0001$ for both comparisons). The number of FA visits was smallest in 2006, when it stood at 15276 visits (Table 1).

During the follow-up period 2007–2010, when there was no administrative information about FAs given to

Table 1 Total number of visits, number of FA visits, and proportion of FAs visits in 2001–2010

Year	Number of all visits	Number of FA visits	Proportion of FA visits of all visits %	Number of patients	Number of FAs	Proportion of FAs of all patients %
2001	194,217	17,627	9.1	75,560	1415	1.9
2002	186,341	16,898	9.1	73,930	1332	1.8
2003	183,184	15,876	8.7	72,302	1292	1.8
2004	180,007	15,886	8.8	71,840	1287	1.8
2005	180,380	16,140	8.9	73,185	1301	1.8
2006	178,987	15,276	8.5	73,208	1241	1.7
2007	179,361	16,620	9.3	72,370	1330	1.8
2008	182,394	17,393	9.5	73,860	1380	1.9
2009	174,486	17,104	9.8	71,968	1338	1.9
2010	177,100	17,239	9.7	72,738	1349	1.8

the GPs, there was a significant ($p < 0.0001$, Table 2) increase in the proportion of FA visits when compared with the proportion of FA visits in 2006.

Between 2001 and 2006, the number of FA visits decreased by 2351 visits. The average number of all patient consultations per GP in 2006 was 1234.4, so this reduction corresponded to the annual workload of 2 GPs. There was a very low response to our request for GPs to draw up treatment plans for their patients listed as FAs in 2004; plans were made for only 73 patients, less than 6% of FAs in that year.

Discussion

In the city where this study was conducted, FAs comprised 1.8% of all patients; this percentage is consistent with other studies which report proportions ranging from 1.7–4.7% [1, 6]. There are studies in which the proportion of FAs was found to be considerably higher - from 10.6% to as much as 15.4% [14, 24]. This can be explained by differences in defining an FA, and differences between healthcare systems. During the first decade of this millennium, the total number of GP consultations decreased in the city in question, and similar decreases happened over the same period elsewhere in Finland, too. Although the reasons for this phenomenon are unclear, it is possible that the overall number of GP consultations has gone down because individual consultations tend to be longer now than before, as patients' problems become more complex and more time-consuming to deal with [25].

In 2002, 2003 and 2005, GPs in the city's primary healthcare system received administrative information about their FA patients: their names and number of GP visits made by each one during the preceding year. This rather simple procedure seemed to reduce the number of FA patients' visits to a GP. Compared with the figure

for 2001 (17,627 FA consultations), the decrease in the annual consultation rate of FA patients was significant in both 2003 and 2006. When the administrative information was no longer provided, the FA consultation rate per year increased again, as seen by comparing the figure for 2006 with the figures for the four subsequent years (2007–2010). A systematic literature review conducted in 2008 concluded that there is no evidence that FAs' utilization of healthcare services can be reduced [26]. The results of our study, however, are more optimistic; the simple procedure of providing administrative information directly to GPs did seem to reduce FAs' consultation rates. In fact, the reduction in the consultation rates of FA patients from 2001 to 2006 corresponds to the annual workload of 2 GPs. This finding is in line with the conclusions of Heywood et al. [14].

The information about FAs was provided once annually in 2002, 2003 and 2005, to all GPs who were working in the city of Turku at the time of the information session, but the fluctuation in the number of individual GPs from year to year, and the low number of full-time GPs might influence the findings. The number of the full-time GPs was unchanged in 2003, 2005, 2006 and 2008. Locums are hardly the explanation for the decrease in FAs' visits in 2003 and 2006. In 2004, on the other hand, the number of full-time GPs changed which may partly explain why there was no reduction in FA patients' visit rates in 2005. Furthermore, no administrative information on FAs was provided in 2004, which may also have contributed to the slight reversal in 2005 in the overall downward trend. During this decade, the number of tenured GPs increased by six, and the number of locums varied. The effects of the fluctuations in the number of full-time GPs and the large number of medical officer locums are not known and cannot be analysed in this study setting.

The administrative information on FA patients was provided in the course of regular team meetings between the GPs and the chief medical officer; thus there was no parallel group of uninformed GPs to act as a control group. The method used was very simple. In the study of Bellón et al., GPs received 15 h' training about the issue of FA-patients, and this intervention, too, yielded a significant reduction in the frequency of FA consultations [21]. Our intervention to GPs was much simpler and considerably less time-consuming, as it took place once a year in the course of normal meeting.

GPs made only few treatment plans to FAs. It is impossible to say whether treatment plans would be helpful in improving the health or reducing the visit rate of FA patients.

The electronic patient record system used in the health care centres involved in this study does not have useful tools for enabling the GPs to monitor their work.

Table 2 Changes in the proportion of FA visits of all visits over the period 2001–2010

Years compared	RR	95% CI		p-value*
2002 with 2001	0.99	0.978	1.03	0.9379
2003 with 2001	0.95	0.93	0.98	< 0.0001
2004 with 2001	0.97	0.95	0.99	0.0104
2005 with 2001	0.99	0.97	1.01	0.1918
2006 with 2001	0.94	0.92	0.96	< 0.0001
2007 with 2006	1.09	1.06	1.11	< 0.0001
2008 with 2006	1.12	1.09	1.14	< 0.0001
2009 with 2006	1.15	1.12	1.17	< 0.0001
2010 with 2006	1.14	1.12	1.17	< 0.0001

Intervention in the form of individualized information to GPs on frequent attendance was provided in 2002, 2003, and 2005. An RR of more than 1.00 signifies that there was an increase in FA visits

RR Relative Risk, CI Confidence Interval

* Statistical significance between years; Poisson's regression analysis

This might be one reason why providing administrative information in face-to-face sessions turned out to be important. For example, the electronic patient record system does not allow for serial numbering of patient contacts during the year; such a feature would enable GPs to recognize instantly the patients making frequent visits.

The strength of the present study is the large amount of data on GP visits during 2001–2010, covering 1,816,457 appointments, including 166,059 appointments with FAs. Also, providing GPs with the administrative information was simple, quick, and easily repeated procedure. A weakness may be the fact that the administrative information provided was not methodologically standardized; it was incorporated into managerial routine. Another weakness was that we had no possibility to use a control group of GPs who had not received information on their FA patients; this methodological drawback arose from the realities of everyday management. The results need to be confirmed by further comparative studies.

Conclusion

Providing administrative information to GPs about their frequently attending patients, including their names and the frequency of their visits, yielded only a modest overall reduction in the number of frequent attenders over the period covered by the study. However, in two of the years (2003 and 2006), there were significant reductions in the total number of visits of FA patients, even though the numbers of FA patients themselves decreased only slightly. It thus seems that this simple intervention can reduce the annual number of visits by FAs to public healthcare centres, rate of frequent attenders was significantly reduced. It seems that such administrative information can reduce the number of annual visits by FA-patients in public healthcare centres, where GPs are working as a team and are led by one chief medical physician. To our knowledge, this is the first study to show that this kind of simple administrative information given by the chief medical officer to the GPs can significantly reduce the consultation rate of frequently attending patients.

Acknowledgements
We thank professor Ivar Sønbø Kristiansen (MD, PhD, MPH Institute of Health Management and Health Economics University of Oslo) and Virpi Rantanen (MD, PhD, adjunct professor in Obstetrics and Gynaecology at the University of Turku) for valuable comments to manuscript. Päivi Ovaskainen, PhD, provided help with literature about information management.

Funding
The study was supported by a government grant for the city of Turku, Healthcare Center in 2009 and 2010.

Authors' contributions
AKS collected the data and performed the drafting of the manuscript. AKS, TJV, SHL and PTR participated in the conception and design of the research, critically revising the manuscript for its intellectual content. AKS, TJV, SHL and PTR have read and approved of the final version.

Ethics approval and consent to participate
Not applicable. According to the Finnish law, register studies do not need Ethics approval, and consent is not required if access to data is provided by a competent authority. The medical record data used in the research has been obtained by the permission of the official authority competent to grant access, who has also evaluated the legality of providing and using the data in accordance with the applicable law. Here the relevant authority has been the City of Turku, Healthcare Center.

Competing interests
The authors declare that they have no competing interests.

Author details
[1]Turku City Healthcare Center, Turku, Finland. [2]Department of Biostatistics, Faculty of Medicine, University of Turku, Turku, Finland. [3]Department of Psychiatry, University of Turku, Turku, Finland. [4]Department of Psychiatry, Turku University Hospital, Turku, Finland. [5]Department of Public Health, Faculty of Medicine, University of Turku, Turku, Finland. [6]Turku Clinical Research Centre, Turku University Hospital, Turku, Finland.

References
1. Jyväsjärvi S. Frequent attenders in primary health care: a cross-sectional study of frequent attenders' psychosocial and family factors, chronic diseases and reasons for encounter in a Finnish health Centre. PhD [dissertation]. Oulu: University of Oulu; 2001.
2. Savonius B. Frequent attendance in healthcare center of Espoo. Finn Med J. 1988;43:1718–20.
3. Koskela T-H. The prognostic risk factors for long term frequent use of the primary health care services. PhD [dissertation]. Kuopio: University of Kuopio; 2008.
4. Karlsson H, Lehtinen V, Joukamaa M. Frequent attenders of Finnish public primary health care: sociodemographic characteristics and physical morbidity. Fam Pract. 1994;11:424–30.
5. Cerney TA, Guy S, Jeffrey G. Frequent attenders in general practice: a retrospective 20-years follow-up study. Br J Gen Pract. 2001;51:567–9.
6. Andersson SO, Mattsson B, Lynoe N. Patients frequently consulting general practitioners at primary healthcare Centre in Sweden – a comparative study. Scand J Soc Med. 1995;23:251–7.
7. Gill D, Sharpe M. Frequent consulters in general practice: a systematic review of studies of prevalence, associations and outcome 1999. J Psychosom Res. 1999;47:115–30.
8. Westhead JN. Frequent attenders in general practice: medical, psychological and social characteristics. J R Coll Gen Pract. 1985;35:337–40.
9. Neal R, Heywood P, Morley S. Frequent attenders' consulting patterns with general practitioners. Br J Gen Pract. 2000;50:972–6.
10. Karlsson H, Joukamaa M, Lahti I, Lehtinen V, Kokki-Saarinen T. Frequent attender profiles: different clinical subgroups among frequent attender patients in primary care. J Psychosom Res. 1997;42:157–66.

11. Backett EM, Heady JA, Evans JCG. Studies of a general practice (II) the doctor's job in an urban area. BMJ. 1954;1:109–15.
12. Vedsted P, Christensen MB. Frequent attenders in general practice care: a literature review with special reference to methodological considerations. Public Health. 2005;119:118–37.
13. Neal R, Dowell A, Heywood P, Morley S. Frequent attenders: who needs treatment? Br J Gen Pract. 1996;46:131–2.
14. Heywood PL, Blackie GC, Cameron IH, Dowell AC. An assessment of the attributes of frequent attenders to general practice. Fam Pract. 1998;15: 198–204.
15. Baez K, Aiarzaguena JM, Grandes G, Pedrero E, Aranguren J, Retolaza A. Understanding patient-initiated frequent attendance in primary care: a case-control study. Br J Gen Pract. 1998;48:1824–7.
16. Foster A, Jordan K, Croft P. Is frequent attendance in primary care disease-specific? Fam Pract. 2006;23:444–52.
17. Jyvasjarvi S, Keinanen-Kiukaanniemi S, Vaisanen E, Larivaara P, Kivela SL. Frequent attenders in a Finnish health Centre: morbidity and reasons for encounter. Scand J Prim Health Care. 1998;16:141–8.
18. Savageau JA, McLoughlin M, Ursan A, Bai Y, Collins M, Cashman SB. Characteristics of frequent attenders at a community health center. J Am Board Fam Med. 2006;19:265–75.
19. Bergh H, Marklund B. Characteristics of frequent attenders in different age and sex groups in primary health care. Scand J Prim Health Care. 2003;21: 171–7.
20. Vedsted P, Fink P, Sorensen HT, Olesen F. Physical, mental and social factors associated with frequent attendance in Danish general practice. A population-based cross-sectional study. Soc Sci Med. 2004;59:813–23.
21. Bellón JA, Rodríguez-Bayón A, de Dios Luna J, Torres-González F. Successful GP intervention with frequent attenders in primary care. Br J Gen Pract. 2008;58:324–30.
22. Jiwa M. Frequent attenders in general practice: an attempt to reduce attendance. Fam Pract. 2000;17:248–51.
23. Engeström Y. Innovative learning in work teams: analyzing cycles of knowledge creation in practice. In: Engeström Y, Miettinen R, Punamäki RL, editors. Perspectives on activity theory. Cambridge: Cambridge University Press; 1998. p. 377–404.
24. Smits F, Brouwer HJ, Riet G, van Weert H. Epidemiology of frequent attenders: a 3-years historic cohort study comparing attendance, morbidity and prescriptions of one-year and persistent frequent attenders. BMC Public Health. 2009;9:36.
25. Ovaskainen PT, Rautava PT, Ojanlatva A, Päkkilä JK, Päivärinta RM. Analysis of primary health care utilisation in South-Western Finland--a tool for management. Health Policy. 2003;66:229–38.
26. Smits FT, Wittkampf KA, Schene AH, Bindels PJ, Van Weert HC. Intervention on frequent attenders in primary care, a systematic literature review. Scand J Prim Health Care. 2008;26:111–6.

20

Correlation between family physician's direct advice and pneumococcal vaccination intention and behavior among the elderly in Japan

Mariko Higuchi[1*], Keiichiro Narumoto[2,3], Takahiro Goto[4] and Machiko Inoue[3,5]

Abstract

Background: Vaccination is an important element of health maintenance in family medicine. The 23-valent pneumococcal polysaccharide vaccine (PPSV23) is highly recommended for the elderly, but its uptake is low in Japan. Primary care system remains under development and preventive services tend to be neglected in the Japanese medical practice. The study aims to investigate the association between family physician's recommendations for PPSV23 during outpatient care and PPSV23 vaccination intention and behavior in the elderly.

Method: We conducted a cross-sectional study with a questionnaire at a family medicine clinic in a rural area in Japan. The participants were over the age of 65 without dementia who had maintained a continuity with the clinic. The questionnaire inquired PPSV23 vaccination status, family physician's advice for PPSV23, socio-demographics, and the constructs in the Health Belief Model. We defined those who had had vaccination intention and behavior as "PPSV23 vaccinated group" and those who had no vaccination and uncertainty about being or no intention to be vaccinated in the future as "PPSV23 unvaccinated group." We used chi-square test for correlation between physician's advice and PPSV23 vaccination/intention, univariate and multivariate logistic regression analysis for factors related to the vaccination/intention, and descriptive analysis for reasons for reluctance to the vaccination.

Results: We analyzed 209 valid responses. There were 142 participants in the PPSV23 vaccinated group and 67 in the PPSV23 unvaccinated group. The PPSV23 vaccination group was more likely to have had their physician's advice (80.2% vs 21.3%, $p < 0.001$). Multivariate logistic regression analysis showed a significant association between PPSV23 vaccination and their physician's recommendation (OR 8.50, 95%CI 2.8–26.0), awareness of PPSV23 (OR 8.52, 95%CI 2.1–35.0), and the perceived effectiveness of PPSV23 (OR 4.10, 95%CI 1.2–13.9). The reasons for reluctance to get vaccinated included lack of understanding of PPSV23, lack of physician's recommendations, and concerns about side effects of PPSV23.

Conclusion: Family physician's recommendation was positively correlated with PPSV23 vaccination intention and behavior in the elderly. This reinforces the importance of providing preventive services during time-constrained outpatient care, even in medical systems where it is undervalued.

Keywords: Family practice, Preventive medicine, 23-valent pneumococcal polysaccharide vaccine, Physician's advice

* Correspondence: myokota-dky@umin.ac.jp
[1] The Department of Internal Medicine, Tsukuba Central Hospital, 1589-3 Kashiwadachou, Ushiku, Ibaraki 300-1211, Japan
Full list of author information is available at the end of the article

Background

Preventive care is an important element in family medicine. However, it tends to be undervalued, as curative medicine is mainstream in Japanese medical practice [1]. Some Japanese primary care physicians experience difficulties practicing preventive medicine in their busy outpatient care because of restricted hours of consultation, perceived difficulties encouraging behavior changes in patients, and the lack of seeing the effectiveness of preventive medicine [2]. In addition, under the current medical billing system, providing preventive services are not adequately paid. Hospital-employed physicians typically need to handle outpatient care in parallel with inpatient management. Therefore, outpatient practice becomes a large burden as they already spend a significant amount of time working on a variety of tasks for inpatient care [3]. These factors restrict the practice of preventive medicine in Japan.

Vaccination is one of the most important parts of health maintenance. The 23-valent pneumococcal polysaccharide vaccine (PPSV23) is recommended for the elderly since it lowers the risks of invasive pneumococcal disease [4] and pneumococcal pneumonia. [5] Pneumonia holds 3rd place for cause of death in the elderly [6], and streptococcus pneumoniae is the most dominant causative bacteria, accounting for 17 to 28% in cases of pneumonia in adults [7–9]. In Japan, the PPSV23 has proven to be effective in reducing the incidence of pneumonia in general as well as pneumococcal pneumonia specifically [10]. However, receiving the PPSV23 vaccine was voluntary until October 1, 2014, when the vaccine was added to the list of routine vaccinations, therefore the uptake of the PPSV23 vaccination was extremely low at just 17.5% in March, 2012 [11]. While the Centers for Disease Control and Prevention recommend both 13-valent pneumococcal conjugate vaccine (PCV13) and PPSV23 for the elderly over the age of 65 [12], only PPSV23 is currently part of routine vaccinations with public health subsidies available every 5 years after 65 years of age in Japan.

Several facilitators of recommended vaccination have been reported: recommendations from family members or friends [13–15], notifications sent to individuals and homepages for public relations purposes set up by each local municipality [16], having knowledge about the vaccine [13, 17], personal record of vaccination [15], and the perceived severity of diseases such as pneumonia, as well as the safety and perceived effectiveness of the vaccine [15, 17, 18]. On the other hand, barriers against vaccination in existing studies included: lack of knowledge about the vaccine, anxiety about its side effects [13, 19, 20], doubting the effectiveness of the vaccine, lack of interest, the cost of self-pay, as well as difficulties making hospital visits due to lack of time [20].

Because preventive medicine provided with the concept of continuity is important in primary care, family physicians have a crucial role in ensuring health maintenance of their patients. Maintaining a continuous relationship with the same family physician or medical institution was positively correlated with receipt of preventive services [21]. In the previous study in Britain, the advice given by general practitioners had the most significant influence on patient's decisions to get PPSV23 [22].

However, in Japan, there is no research on the influence of advice by family physicians on patient's receiving preventive services, specifically PPSV 23 vaccination. Additionally, no investigation into the other factors affecting PPSV23 vaccination in the elderly exists in the Japanese primary care setting.

The purpose of this study was to investigate (1) the association between family physician's direct advice and PPSV23 vaccination intention and behavior in the elderly, (2) factors related to their PPSV23 vaccination intention and behavior, and (3) reasons for reluctance to receive PPSV23 vaccination.

Methods

This is a cross-sectional study of the elderly who regularly visit a single outpatient healthcare clinic, Kikugawa Family Medicine Center, in Shizuoka prefecture, Japan. The study was approved by the Ethics Committee of Kikugawa General Hospital and permission and approval to the investigation were obtained from the clinic.

Setting

The study was conducted at a family medicine clinic in a rural community with a population of approximately 50,000 people. At the clinic, two certified family physicians and 4 family medicine residents were running a group practice at the time of the investigation. The residents had been educated in preventive care as an important element of family medicine by a certified family physician faculty. Therefore, all the physicians at the clinic shared the common ground of a value of preventive medicine in primary care. However, their actual practice might vary according to multiple factors including outpatient time constraint, the complexity of patient health issues and the extent of establishment of patient-physician relationship. Out of the total of 18,756 patients who came to the clinic in 2013, 9094 (48.5%) were elderly patients over the age of 65. The period between clinic visits, depending on their medical conditions and needs, averaged anywhere from 1 week to 3 months. With national health insurance coverage and patients having free access to almost any kind of medical institution, the average outpatient consultation time per patient is between 3 and 15 min in the clinic, according to the complexity of the health problems of each patient.

Participants

We used the convenience sampling method, approaching and distributing the questionnaire to the patients who came to the clinic from November 1, 2013 until a total 500 responses were collected based on predetermined sampling calculation as mentioned in analysis. Inclusion criteria for those to whom the questionnaire was distributed were (1) over the age of 65 as of September 1, 2013, (2) capable of giving their consent to participate in the study and (3) agreed to the study participation. Written informed consent was obtained from all participants prior to the study. After data collection, we then reviewed their electronic medical record (EMR) to confirm the additional inclusion criteria: (4) having had at least 3 consultations in the clinic from August 1, 2011, when the clinic opened, to September 1, 2013 and (5) having no diagnosis of dementia.

Data collection

Participants received the paper-based questionnaire and were asked to complete it while waiting for their outpatient consultation. With visual impairments or difficulty in interpreting the questions, they could have assistance from family members or the research staff at the clinic.

Data confirmation by EMR

After collecting all responses to the questionnaire, we checked the number of clinic visits from the aforementioned period of time (August, 2011 to September, 2013) to evaluate continuity to the clinic as one of the inclusion criteria. We also reviewed the vaccination records of PPSV23 in EMR to validate the answer of the vaccination status in the questionnaire and any documentation regarding the diagnosis of dementia. We defined diagnosis of dementia if one of the following criteria were met: (1) dementia had been registered on the list of diagnosis, (2) there had been a record of Mini-Mental State Examination (MMSE), scoring less than 24 points, or (3) dementia was on the problem list in the progress note.

We excluded the data if the participants did not meet inclusion criteria. We also excluded if there was discordance between responses about vaccination status in the questionnaire and vaccination records in EMR.

The questionnaire

The questionnaire was comprised of a total of 22 items.

First, the questionnaire asked the participants (1) whether they were aware of PPSV23, (2) whether their family physicians had recommended PPSV23 vaccination for their age, and (3) their PPSV23 vaccination status. For those who had not been vaccinated, the questionnaire asked them to choose one from the following three options about their future vaccination intentions (Additional file 1): "I plan to get vaccinated in the future (future vaccination intention).", "I have decided not to get vaccinated (no intention to future vaccination).", and "I don't know if I will get vaccinated or not (uncertainty about future vaccination)." As for those who had not been vaccinated for PPSV23 and who also showed uncertainty about or no intention to be vaccinated in the future, they were asked to choose a single or multiple reasons for their reluctance from 12 items [14, 18–20].

Secondly, the questionnaire asked for the participant's socio-demographic information, including age, gender, educational background, personal financial situation, smoking habits, their medical history of pneumonia and other respiratory diseases, their family history of pneumonia, awareness of PPSV23 and vaccine-related public subsidies, perceived current health conditions, and constructs used in Health Belief Model (HBM) [23–25], by reference to the factors that influenced people's intention to receive vaccination in the previous studies. The HBM is a conceptual model that is widely used to analyze health behaviors. In line with the context of the study, the participants were asked questions about (1) perceived susceptibility to the common cold, (2) perceived susceptibility to pneumonia, (3) perceived severity of pneumonia, (4) perceived effectiveness of PPSV23, and (5) a sense of economic burden as perceived barriers to receiving PPSV23, using a 5-point Likert scale.

Analysis

We defined the respondents who had a history of PPSV23 vaccination confirmed in EMR or who had not been vaccinated but showed the future vaccination intention ("I plan to get vaccinated in the future."), as the "PPSV23 vaccinated group." On the other hand, we defined the respondents who had no history of PPSV23 vaccination and who showed uncertainty about or no intention to future vaccination ("I have decided not to get vaccinated." or "I don't know if I will get vaccinated or not.") as the "PPSV23 unvaccinated group".

It was calculated that a total of 174 responses were necessary in this study (significant level = 0.05, power = 80%, effect size = 0.3) [26, 27]. Since the participants were elderly people over the age of 65, we assumed the response rate or valid response would be low. Therefore, we decided to distribute the questionnaire to 500 people.

We used chi-square test to analyze the association between family physician's advice and PPSV23 vaccination intention/behavior. We applied univariate logistic regression analysis to examine the factors related to PPSV23 vaccination intention/behavior. For multivariate logistic regression analysis, all factors in univariate analysis associated with PPSV23 vaccination at $p < 0.2$ were included.

The dependent variable was PPSV23 vaccination intention/behavior. Independent variables included family physician's direct advice, participant's demographics (age, gender, educational background, personal financial situation, smoking habits, past medical and family history of pneumonia, awareness of PPSV23 and vaccine-related public subsidies, perceived current health conditions), and constructs adapted from Health Belief Model (HBM). We analyzed the responses on the 5-point Likert scale by separating them into the top two and the lower 3 answers as nominal variables. We conducted descriptive analysis on the PPSV23 unvaccinated group's reasoning for reluctance to be vaccinated. The analysis was carried out with R version 3.2.0. statistical software [28].

Results

In the study, "PPSV23 vaccinated group" included those who had had PPSV23 vaccination intention/behavior at the time of the investigation. Of 500 elder patients to whom we distributed the questionnaires, 456 patients agreed to participate in the study. Of 456 respondents, we excluded 247 responses (40: lack of continuity, 43: dementia, 153: discordance in vaccination status in between the questionnaire and EMR, 11: incomplete responses), resulting in a total of 209 valid responses for analysis (Fig. 1).

A hundred nineteen respondents were confirmed vaccinated with PPSV23, and 90 respondents were not vaccinated. Among the unvaccinated, 23 respondents had

future vaccination intention, therefore by definition, there were 142 respondents in PPSV23 vaccinated group and 67 in PPSV23 unvaccinated group.

Table 1 shows characteristics of the participants including 153 respondents whose reports of PPSV23 vaccination status were discordant in between the questionnaire and EMR, categorized as "uncertain PPSV23 vaccine status group." The average ages of PPSV23 vaccinated, unvaccinated and uncertain vaccine status group were 77.6, 72.7, 74.2, respectively. The PPSV23 vaccinated group were more likely to report poor subjective health (72.6% vs. 63.5%, 64.9%), subjectively rated their financial situations as comfortable (12.9% vs 3.2%, 6.5%), and perceived effectiveness of PPSV23 (75.2% vs. 33.3%, 56.6%). The respondents in the PPSV23 vaccinated group were more likely to report family physician's advice on PPSV23 vaccination (78.9% vs 20.3%, 58.5%). Univariate logistic regression analysis revealed that PPSV23 vaccination intention/behavior was significantly correlated with physician's advice ($p < 0.001$), age ($p < 0.001$), awareness of PPSV23 ($p < 0.001$) and vaccination subsidies ($p < 0.001$), perceived susceptibility to the common cold ($p = 0.016$), perceived seriousness of pneumonia ($p = 0.027$), and perceived the effectiveness of PPSV23 ($p < 0.001$) [Table 2].

Multivariate logistic regression analysis showed physician's advice was significantly associated with PPSV23

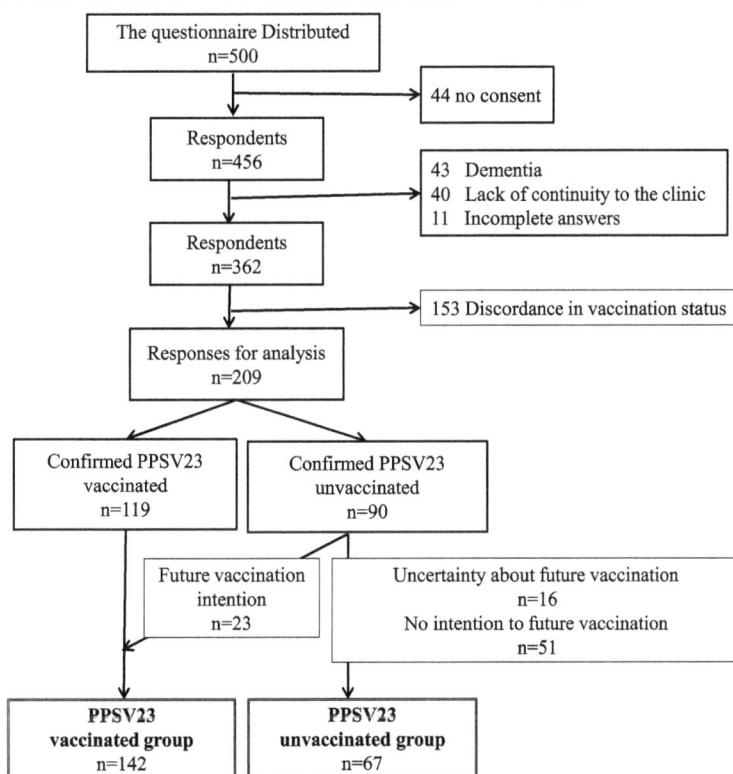

Fig. 1 Selection of participants and definitions of PPSV23 vaccinated and unvaccinated group. It shows the process of selection of the participants and depicts the definitions of PPSV23 vaccinated and unvaccinated group

Table 1 Characteristics of study participants

		PPSV23 vaccinated group (n = 142) n (%) or Mean	PPSV23 unvaccinated group (n = 67) n (%) or Mean	Uncertain PPSV23 vaccine status group (n = 153) n (%) or Mean
Age (±S.E.)		77.6 ± 0.6	72.7 ± 1.0	74.2 ± 0.9
Sex	Male	64 (45.1)	30 (44.8)	71 (46.4)
	Female	78 (54.9)	37 (55.2)	82 (53.6)
Personal medical history of pneumonia	Yes	5 (4.1)	6 (9.4)	8 (10.4)
	No	118 (95.9)	58 (90.6)	69 (89.6)
Personal medical history of respiratory disease	Yes	15 (12.6)	5 (7.8)	4 (5.0)
	No	104 (87.4)	59 (92.2)	76 (95)
Family history of pneumonia	Yes	10 (7.9)	8 (12.7)	10 (11.5)
	No	116 (92.1)	55 (87.3)	77 (88.5)
Regular health check-ups*	Yes	112 (95.7)	59 (98.3)	70 (87.5)
	No	5 (4.3)	1 (1.7)	10 (12.5)
Current smoking habits	Smoker	14 (10.4)	4 (6.3)	7 (7.4)
	Non-smoker	120 (89.6)	60 (93.7)	87 (92.6)
Subjective state of health	Good	37 (27.4)	23 (36.5)	33 (35.1)
	Not good	98 (72.6)	40 (63.5)	61 (64.9)
Subjective sense of economic conditions	Comfortable	17 (12.9)	2 (3.2)	6 (6.5)
	Struggling	115 (87.1)	60 (96.8)	86 (93.5)
Highest level of education completed	Elementary or junior high school	67 (50.4)	32 (51.6)	45 (48.9)
	High school or higher	66 (49.6)	30 (48.4)	47 (51.1)
Living alone or with others	With others	111 (92.5)	54 (87.1)	68 (94.4)
	Alone	9 (7.5)	8 (12.9)	4 (5.6)
Necessity for transportation for clinic visits	Necessary	42 (31.1)	14 (21.9)	31 (33.7)
	Unnecessary	93 (68.9)	50 (78.1)	61 (66.3)
Perceived susceptibility to common colds **	Yes	43 (33.6)	10 (16.4)	27 (31.0)
	No	85 (66.4)	51 (83.6)	69 (69.0)
Perceived susceptibility to pneumonia**	Yes	17 (13.2)	3 (4.8)	18 (20.5)
	No	112 (86.8)	59 (95.2)	70 (79.5)
Perceived severity of pneumonia**	Yes	42 (34.4)	12 (18.8)	34 (40.0)
	No	80 (65.6)	52 (81.2)	51 (60.0)
Perceived effectiveness of PPSV23 **	Yes	91 (75.2)	21 (33.3)	47 (56.6)
	No	30 (24.8)	42 (66.7)	36 (43.4)
Perceived barriers to PPSV23 (sense of economic burden)**	Yes	44 (35.5)	18 (30.5)	27 (35.1)
	No	80 (64.5)	41 (69.5)	50 (64.9)
physician's recommendation	Yes	105 (78.9)	13 (20.3)	38 (58.5)
	No	28 (21.1)	51 (79.7)	27 (41.5)
Awareness of PPSV23	Yes	120 (92.3)	28 (41.8)	69 (76.7)
	No	10 (7.7)	39 (58.2)	21 (23.3)
Awareness of public subsidies	Yes	37 (42.0)	8 (14.3)	18 (34.0)
	No	51 (48.0)	48 (85.7)	35 (66.0)
Difficulty completing the questionnaire	Completed with help.	30 (22.7)	13 (20.6)	13 (14.8)
	Completed without help.	102 (77.3)	50 (79.4)	75 (85.2)

*:Regardless of the frequency of health check-ups, if patients had regular medical check-ups within the last 5 years, the answers were put into the "Yes" category

**:The responses on 5-point Likert scale were separated into the top 2 group and the lower 3 group

The table shows demographic background of the participants and their responses for Health Belief Model related questions. Uncertain PPSV23 vaccine status group was defined by the participants whose reports of PPSV23 vaccination status in the questionnaire and PPSV23 vaccination records in electronic medical record were not consistent vaccination (OR 8.50, 95%CI 2.8–26.0). The other factors that were positively correlated with vaccination were awareness of PPSV23 (OR 8.52, 95%CI 2.1–35.0) and perceived effectiveness of PPSV23 (OR 4.10, 95%CI 1.2–13.9) [Table 3].

There was a significant relationship between the PPSV23 vaccine status and physician's direct advice, awareness of PPSV23, and the perceived effectiveness of PPSV23.

Reasons for not getting vaccinated with PPSV23 included "lack of understanding of PPSV23", "lack of recommendations from their doctors", "lack of interest in PPSV23", "lack of perceived value of the vaccine", and "concerns about the side effects of PPSV23" [Fig. 2].

We conducted sensitivity analysis using different definitions of PPSV23 vaccinated or unvaccinated group. The results from the sensitivity analysis did not differ significantly compared with those from the analysis using the original definition of outcome. First, we carried out an analysis for "confirmed PPSV23 vaccinated (n=119)" and "confirmed PPSV23 unvaccinated (n=90)" groups without intention to get vaccinated taken into consideration for definition of dependent variable. Physician advice was significantly correlated with PPSV23 vaccination in multivariate regression analysis (OR 182,

95%CI 19–1757). Second, since a substantial number of the participants were excluded due to discordance in vaccine status in between the questionnaire and EMR, we analyzed the data based on the definition of PPSV23 vaccine status by either vaccine records in EMR or reports in the questionnaire alone. When the former definition used, a total 362 participants were included in the analysis, where there were 225 (62.2%) and 137 participants in PPSV23 vaccinated and unvaccinated group, respectively. Physician's recommendation remained positively correlated with PPSV23 vaccination (OR 4.73, 95%CI 2.33–9.62) [Tables 4, 5]. When the latter definition used, a total 255 responses in the questionnaire were valid and there were 163 (63.9%) and 92 participants in PPSV23 vaccinated and unvaccinated group, respectively. Physician's recommendation was still positively correlated with PPSV23 vaccination (OR 7.37, 95%CI 2.83–19.22) [Tables 6, 7].

Discussion

The study revealed family physician's direct advice was significantly correlated with PPSV23 vaccination intention/behavior in the elderly in the Japanese primary care setting. To our knowledge, this is the first study in Japan to examine the value of preventive service

Table 2 Univariate logistic regression analysis for factors related to PPSV23 vaccination intention and behavior

	OR	95%CI	p-value
Age	1.09	1.05–1.14	<0.001
Sex	1.01	0.56–1.81	0.968
Personal medical history of pneumonia	0.41	0.12–1.40	0.150
Personal medical history of respiratory disease	1.70	0.59–4.92	0.326
Family history of pneumonia	0.59	0.22–1.58	0.297
Regular health check-ups	0.38	0.04–3.33	0.381
Current smoking habits	1.75	0.55–5.55	0.341
Subjective state of health	0.66	0.35–1.24	0.196
Subjective sense of economic conditions	4.43	0.99–19.84	0.051
Highest level of education completed	0.95	0.52–1.74	0.872
Living alone or with others	1.83	0.67–5.00	0.240
Necessity of transportation to the clinic	1.61	0.80–3.23	0.178
Perceived susceptibility to common colds	2.58	1.19–5.58	0.016
Perceived susceptibility to pneumonia	2.99	0.84–10.60	0.090
Perceived severity of pneumonia	2.27	1.10–4.72	0.027
Perceived effectiveness of PPSV23	6.07	3.11–11.82	<0.001
Perceived barriers to PPSV23 (sense of economic burden)	1.25	0.64–2.44	0.507
Physician's recommendation	14.70	7.03–30.77	<0.001
Awareness of PPSV23	16.70	7.45–37.47	<0.001
Awareness of public subsidies	4.35	1.84–10.28	<0.001
Difficulty in completing the questionnaire	1.13	0.54–2.34	0.741

There were significant relationships between PPSV23 vaccination and the following factors: physician's recommendations, awareness of PPSV23 and public vaccination subsidies, age, perceived susceptibility to common colds, perceived severity of pneumonia, and perceived effectiveness of PPSV23 (p < 0.05)

Table 3 Multivariate logistic regression analysis for factors[*] related to PPSV23 vaccination intention and behavior

	OR	95%CI	p-value
Age	1.05	0.96–1.16	0.269
Personal medical history of pneumonia	0.12	0.01–1.31	0.083
Subjective state of health	0.69	0.20–2.36	0.554
Subjective sense of economic conditions	3.76	0.30–47.84	0.307
The necessity for transportation to the clinic	1.04	0.23–4.67	0.961
Perceived susceptibility to colds	1.17	0.26–5.33	0.836
Perceived susceptibility to pneumonia	7.02	0.50–98.71	0.149
Perceived severity of pneumonia	1.11	0.22–5.53	0.903
Perceived effectiveness of PPSV23	4.10	1.21–13.86	0.023
Physician's recommendations	8.50	2.78–25.99	<0.001
Awareness of PPSV23	8.52	2.07–35.03	0.003
Awareness of public subsidies	1.82	0.51–6.52	0.356

[*]: The independent variables which were associated with PPSV23 at $p < 0.20$ in univariate logistic regression analysis were incorporated to multivariate logistic regression analysis

provided by family physicians during the busy outpatient continuity care.

Among the principles in family medicine, using illness visits as opportunities for preventive medicine [29] is important to achieve comprehensive care. However, the focus in outpatient encounters in primary care is typically more on laboratory tests and treatments with prescriptions rather than providing preventive services due to medical service fees [1, 2]. Therefore, it is questionable whether or not many healthcare providers place a value on preventive medicine during busy outpatient visits. When examining geriatric patients, primary care physicians need to manage not only polypharmacy and multimorbidity but also newly developed acute health issues within constricted outpatient time. Furthermore, it is not uncommon for them to need to address any concern from the patient's caretakers. It is possible that those factors make it challenging for family physicians to practice

preventive medicine. Given the fact that frequency of visiting the clinic is relatively high at 1–2 months intervals in Japan, family physicians might be able to continue to provide preventive services little by little in each visit. However, it has been pointed out that the number of consultations is not necessarily proportional to the providing of preventive healthcare [30]. Under such circumstances, the study results reinforced an important role of family physicians in preventive medicine even during a busy outpatient encounter in the Japanese medical system.

Continuity of care is one of the most important disciplines of family medicine, and family physicians build cumulative knowledge of their patients in the process [31]. It has been suggested that updating immunization records is related to "preference for usual physicians" or "physicians' accumulated knowledge of patients" [32]. In this study, we did not use specific instruments to measure continuity [33]. However, we took a "chronological"

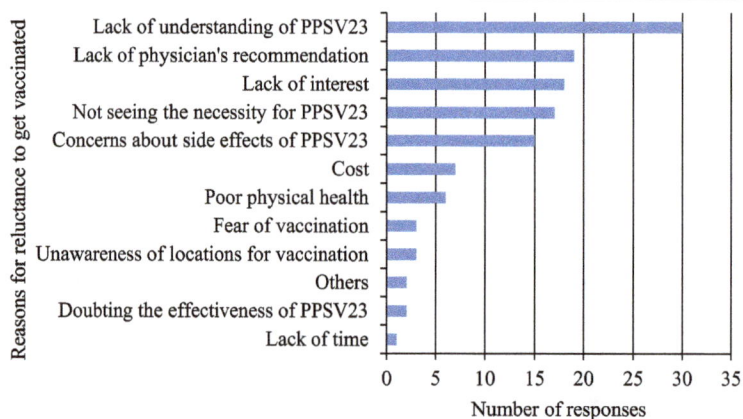

Fig. 2 Reasons for reluctance to get vaccinated in PPSV23 unvaccinated group. It shows the number of responses for each reason for reluctance to get vaccinated in the questionnaire with multiple answers allowed. The question was asked only to the PPSV23 unvaccinated group ($n = 67$)

Table 4 Univariate logistic regression analysis for factors related to PPSV23 vaccination intention and behavior (PPSV23 vaccination status defined by electronic medical record)

	OR	95%CI	p-value
Age	1.01	0.98–1.12	0.234
Sex	1.03	0.57–1.85	0.953
Personal medical history of pneumonia	0.78	0.30–2.02	0.615
Personal medical history of respiratory disease	0.87	0.42–1.79	0.695
Family history of pneumonia	0.46	0.21–1.01	0.053
Regular health check-ups	0.80	0.27–2.39	0.696
Current smoking habits	1.42	0.57–3.52	0.449
Subjective state of health	0.72	0.43–1.20	0.203
Subjective sense of economic conditions	3.11	1.04–9.31	0.043
Highest level of education completed	1.14	0.70–1.86	0.590
Living alone or with others	1.09	0.43–2.74	0.852
Necessity of transportation to the clinic	1.50	0.87–2.59	0.142
Perceived susceptibility to common colds	2.56	1.39–4.69	0.002
Perceived susceptibility to pneumonia	2.73	1.16–6.46	0.021
Perceived severity of pneumonia	1.79	1.03–3.10	0.038
Perceived effectiveness of PPSV23	3.11	1.86–5.22	<0.001
Perceived barriers to PPSV23 (sense of economic burden)	1.27	0.74–2.18	0.388
Physician's recommendation	7.52	4.28–13.23	<0.001
Awareness of PPSV23	4.90	2.76–8.72	<0.001
Awareness of public subsidies	1.47	0.79–2.73	0.227
Difficulty in completing the questionnaire	1.44	0.76–2.73	0.263

The PPSV23 vaccinated and unvaccinated groups were defined by the vaccination records in electronic medical record only, irrespective of the reports of vaccination status in the questionnaire. There were significant relationships between PPSV23 vaccination and the following factors: subjective sense of economic conditions, perceived susceptibility to common colds, perceived susceptibility to pneumonia, perceived severity of pneumonia, perceived effectiveness of PPSV23, physician's direct advice and awareness of PPSV23 ($p < 0.05$)

Table 5 Multivariate logistic regression analysis for factors* related to PPSV23 vaccination intention and behavior (PPSV23 vaccination status defined by electronic medical record)

	OR	95%CI	p-value
Family history of pneumonia	0.35	0.12–1.07	0.066
Subjective sense of economic conditions	3.04	0.76–12.26	0.117
The necessity for transportation to the clinic	1.34	0.61–2.95	0.470
Perceived susceptibility to common colds	2.03	0.81–5.08	0.132
Perceived susceptibility to pneumonia	1.29	0.35–4.77	0.699
Perceived severity of pneumonia	0.96	0.39–2.34	0.924
Perceived effectiveness of PPSV23	2.09	0.98–4.47	0.056
Physician's recommendations	4.73	2.33–9.62	<0.001
Awareness of PPSV23	2.87	1.18–6.96	0.020

*: The independent variables which were associated with PPSV23 at $p < 0.20$ in univariate logistic regression analysis were incorporated to multivariate logistic regression analysis
The PPSV23 vaccinated and unvaccinated groups were defined by the vaccination records in electronic medical record only, irrespective of the questionnaire responses. There were significant relationships between PPSV23 vaccination and physician's direct advice ($p < 0.001$) and awareness of PPSV23 ($p = 0.02$)

continuity into account [34], and it is one of the strengths of our study that, in that context, family physician's advice was associated with the recommended vaccination intention/behavior for the elderly.

"Perceived effectiveness of PPSV23" as facilitators of vaccination and "lack of interest in PPSV23" or "concerns about the side effects of PPSV23" as the reasons for reluctance to get vaccinated were regarded as patient's perceptions of the vaccine, which could indicate the importance of providing preventive services in line with "contexts" in patient-centered clinical methods [35]. The study investigated the presence or absence of "family physician's direct recommendations," and did not explore doctor-patient communications which could influence the patient's decisions to get vaccinated. Since the lack of interpersonal communication skills between physicians and their patients was shown to be the primary obstacle in providing preventive medicine [36], further research in this area will be needed.

The study has some limitations. First, due to the nature of a cross-sectional study, a causal relationship between physician's advice and PPSV23 vaccination

Table 6 Univariate logistic regression analysis for factors related to PPSV23 vaccination intention and behavior (PPSV23 vaccination status defined by questionnaire)

	OR	95%CI	p-value
Age	1.05	0.96–1.17	0.312
Sex	1.07	0.63–2.01	0.972
Personal medical history of pneumonia	0.33	0.12–0.95	0.039
Personal medical history of respiratory disease	1.21	0.56–2.61	0.634
Family history of pneumonia	1.06	0.44–2.51	0.902
Regular health check-ups	1.14	0.35–3.73	0.823
Current smoking habits	1.29	0.51–3.30	0.592
Subjective state of health	0.71	0.41–1.25	0.235
Subjective sense of economic conditions	2.82	0.92–8.62	0.069
Highest level of education completed	0.98	0.58–1.67	0.949
Living alone or with others	1.88	0.73–4.84	0.190
Necessity of transportation to the clinic	1.45	0.80–2.64	0.224
Perceived susceptibility to common colds	1.67	0.90–3.09	0.105
Perceived susceptibility to pneumonia	1.38	0.60–3.17	0.447
Perceived severity of pneumonia	1.47	0.82–2.66	0.197
Perceived effectiveness of PPSV23	4.46	2.49–7.99	<0.001
Perceived barriers to PPSV23 (sense of economic burden)	1.03	0.57–1.83	0.929
Physician's recommendation	7.82	4.29–14.27	<0.001
Awareness of PPSV23	14.32	6.67–30.75	<0.001
Awareness of public subsidies	4.81	2.27–10.16	<0.001
Difficulty in completing the questionnaire	1.11	0.57–2.15	0.756

The PPSV23 vaccinated and unvaccinated groups were defined by the questionnaire responses only, irrespective of the vaccination records in electronic medical record. There were significant positive relationships between PPSV23 vaccination and the following factors: perceived effectiveness of PPSV23, physician's recommendations, and awareness of PPSV23 and public subsidies, while an inverse relationship was observed between PPSV23 vaccination and personal medical history of pneumonia (p < 0.05)

Table 7 Multivariate logistic regression analysis for factors[*] related to PPSV23 vaccination intention and behavior (PPSV23 vaccination was defined by questionnaire responses only)

	OR	95%CI	p-value
Personal medical history of pneumonia	0.27	0.04–1.81	0.179
Subjective sense of economic conditions	3.63	0.38–34.95	0.265
Living alone or with others	1.60	0.28–9.02	0.595
Perceived susceptibility to colds	0.73	0.24–2.23	0.583
Perceived severity of pneumonia	1.24	0.35–4.42	0.744
Perceived effectiveness of PPSV23	2.90	1.03–8.15	0.044
Physician's recommendations	7.37	2.83–19.22	<0.001
Awareness of PPSV23	8.74	2.23–34.31	<0.001
Awareness of public subsidies	1.97	0.68–5.71	0.214

[*]: The independent variables which were associated with PPSV23 at p < 0.20 in univariate logistic regression analysis were incorporated to multivariate logistic regression analysis
The PPSV23 vaccinated and unvaccinated groups were defined by the questionnaire responses only, irrespective of the vaccination records in electronic medical record. There was a significant relationship between PPSV23 vaccination and perceived effectiveness of PPSV23 (p < 0.05), physician's direct advice (p < 0.001) and awareness of PPSV23 (p < 0.05)

cannot be fully understood. Second, there is a possibility that some answer content in the questionnaire might lack accuracy. However, we did conduct the analysis after excluding the data with discordance in vaccination status by reviewing EMR. Third, the relationship between physician's direct advice and PPSV23 vaccination intention/behavior may be over- or underestimated due to a potential effect of clustering of the physician [37] because a history of interacting with the same physician, or the patient-physician correspondence in the practice, for the participants was not evaluated in the study. In addition, the participants in the study were not a representative sample of Japanese primary care practices and therefore generalizing the inference of the result is limited. Lastly, recall bias could lead to overestimation of the association between physician's direct advice and PPSV23 vaccination intention/behavior.

After we carried out the study, routine PPSV23 vaccination for the elderly over the age of 65 began in October, 2014 and each municipality started a public expenditure subsidy policy for vaccination. Although there have been no nationwide epidemiological studies to examine the

Correlation between family physician's direct advice and pneumococcal vaccination intention...

197

changes in the rates of PPSV23 vaccination as the routine PPSV23 vaccination program was introduced, a piece of research conducted at a community hospital showed introduction of the public expenditure subsidy policy increased by 3.4 times the PPSV23 vaccination rates [38]. Under the current circumstances where availability of a public expenditure subsidy for the vaccination and the country's support of the routine PPSV23 vaccination program could have increased the PPSV23 vaccination rate, it is unknown to what extent the physician's advice influences the vaccination behavior.

Currently, we have seen many reports that the provisions of preventive care have been improved by incorporating multidisciplinary cooperation and system-based thinking from those that relied solely on individual recollection and skills. Examples include the introduction of an office system approach based on the characteristics of each medical facility [29], quality improvement activities in clinics, multidisciplinary groups participating in the decision process of a clinic management policy [39], introduction of the reminder system [40], and the presence of the registry [39]. However, these strategies are not necessarily used in medical facilities in Japan, and therefore have a potential to further improve the provisions of preventive medicine in Japanese primary care.

Conclusion

In a busy family medicine outpatient practice, the family physician's direct advice was positively correlated with PPSV23 vaccination intention/behavior in the elderly. In order to improve the PPSV23 vaccination rate at the individual level, it is essential to provide information on PPSV23 with better understanding of patient's perception of the vaccine, using any illness visit as an opportunity for preventive medicine.

Abbreviations

EMR: Electronic medical record; HBM: Health Belief Model; MMSE: Mini-Mental State Examination; PCV13: 13-valent pneumococcal conjugate vaccine; PPSV23: 23-valent Pneumococcal Polysaccharide Vaccine

Acknowledgements

The authors thank Crabtree BF, PhD, Fetters MD, MD, MPH, MA, Oki Y, MD, PhD、medical staff of Kikugawa family medicine center and all of the participants in the study

Authors' contributions

MH conceptualized the study, conducted data collection and interpreted the data. KN supported developing the study and interpreting the data. TG participated in data analysis. MI supported study development and data analysis. All authors were involved in writing the manuscript and took responsibility for the integrity of the data and accuracy of the analysis. All authors read and approved the final manuscript.

Authors' information

MH was a resident of Shizuoka Family Medicine Residency and KN was assistant professor of the Department of Obstetrics, Gynecology and Family Medicine, Hamamatsu University School of Medicine when conducting the study.
MH, MD
KN, MD, MPH
TG, MPharm
IM, MD, MPH, PhD

Competing interests

The authors declare that they have no competing interests.

Author details

[1]The Department of Internal Medicine, Tsukuba Central Hospital, 1589-3 Kashiwadachou, Ushiku, Ibaraki 300-1211, Japan. [2]The Department of Obstetrics and Gynecology, Kikugawa Municipal General Hospital, 1632 Higashiyokoji, Kikugawa, Shizuoka 439-0022, Japan. [3]Shizuoka Family Medicine Residency Program, 1632 Higashiyokoji, Kikugawa, Shizuoka 439-0022, Japan. [4]Yu Pharmacy, 15-1 Otsudori, Shimada, Shizuoka 427-0056, Japan. [5]The Department of Family and Community Medicine, Hamamatsu University School of Medicine, 1-20-1 Handayama, Higashi-ku, Hamamatsu, Shizuoka 431-3192, Japan.

References

1. What is preventive medicine? http://www.yobouigakukai.com/yobouigaku.html. Yobouigakukai. Accessed 25 Feb 2015.
2. Omura S, Kitamura K, Miyazaki K, Mukaibara K. Why is the practice of preventive medicine in everyday practice difficult? What are the solutions? Japanese J Fam Pract. 2004;11(1):24–9.
3. Research on the results verification of revised medical fees in 2010. Descriptive study on reduction of administrative burdens on physicians. Ministry of Health, Labour and Welfare. https://www.mhlw.go.jp/stf/shingi/2r9852000002djkw-att/2r9852000002djt0.pdf. Accessed 24 July 2017.
4. Moberley S, Holden J, Tatham DP, Andrews RM. Vaccines for preventing pneumococcal infection in adults. Cochrane Database Syst Rev. 2013;1: CD000422.
5. Suzuki M, Dhoubhadel BG, Ishifuji T, Yasunami M, Yaegashi M, Asoh N, et al. Adult Pneumonia Study Group-Japan (APSG-J). Serotype-specific effectiveness of 23-valent pneumococcal polysaccharide vaccine against pneumococcal pneumonia in adults aged 65 years or older: a multi-center, prospective, test-negative design study. Lancet Infect Dis. 2017;17(3):313.
6. Ranking leading causes of deaths, the number of age-specific deaths and age-specific mortality rate (population per 100,000). Ministry of Health, Labour and Welfare. https://www.mhlw.go.jp/toukei/saikin/hw/jinkou/geppo/nengai16/dl/h7.pdf. Accessed 24 July 2017.
7. Shindo Y, Ito R, Kobayashi D, Ando M, Ichikawa M, Shiraki A, et al. Risk factors for drug-resistant pathogens in community-acquired and healthcare-associated pneumonia. Am J Respir Crit Care Med. 2013;188(8):985–95.
8. Ishiguro T, Takayanagi N, Yamaguchi S, Yamakawa H, Nakamoto K, Takaku Y, et al. Etiology and factors contributing to the severity and mortality of community-acquired pneumonia. Intern Med. 2013;52(3):317–24.
9. Morimoto K, Suzuki M, Ishifuji T, Abe M, Hamashige N, Aso K, et al. Epidemiology of adult pneumococcal pneumonia. IASR. 2014;10(35):238–9.
10. Maruyama T, Taguchi O, Niederman MS, Morser J, Kobayashi H, Kobayashi T, et al. Efficacy of 23-valent pneumococcal vaccine in preventing pneumonia and improving survival in nursing home residents: double blind, randomised and placebo controlled trial. BMJ. 2010;340:c1004.
11. Pneumococcal polysaccharide vaccine for adults. Infectious disease information center of the National Institute of infectious diseases.Oishi K. Workshop on Health Crisis Management. 2012.
12. Pneumococcal vaccine recommendations. Centers for Disease Control and Prevention. https://www.cdc.gov/vaccines/vpd/pneumo/hcp/recommendations.html. Accessed 25 July 2017.
13. Takahashi O, Noguchi Y, Rahman M, Shimbo T, Goto M, Matsui K, et al. Influence of family on acceptance of influenza vaccination among Japanese patients. Fam Pract. 2003;20(2):162–6.

14. Ishida T, Kaku S, Kochi S. Questionnaire-based investigation of uterine cervical cancer vaccine usage in our hospital. Gen Dent. 2011;60(1):81–5.

15. Liu S, Xu E, Liu Y, Xu Y, Wang J, Du J, et al. Factors associated with pneumococcal vaccination among an urban elderly population in China. Hum Vaccin Immunother. 2014;10(10):2994–9.

16. Kobayashi H, Nakajima Y, Akasaki M. Factors influencing coverage of human papillomavirus (HPV) vaccination: questionnaire survey of local governments in Nara prefecture about the HPV vaccination program and communication campaigns to promote the program. Prog Med. 2012;32:723–59.

17. Klett-Tammen CJ, Krause G, Seefeld L, Ott JJ. Determinants of tetanus, pneumococcal and influenza vaccination in the elderly: a representative cross-sectional study on knowledge, attitude and practice (KAP). BMC Public Health. 2016;16:121.

18. Iwashita Y, Takemura S. Factors associated with willingness to undergo vaccination against Haemophilus influenzae type b (Hib). Nihon Koshu Eisei Zasshi. 2010;57(5):381–9.

19. Haesebaert J, Lutringer-Magnin D, Kalecinski J, Barone G, Jacquard AC, Régnier V, et al. French women's knowledge of and attitudes towards cervical cancer prevention and the acceptability of HPV vaccination among those with 14-18 year old daughters: a quantitative-qualitative study. BMC Public Health. 2012;12:1034.

20. Izumi M, Manabe E, Yoshioka Y. Relevant factors for undergoing uterine cancer screening and HPV vaccination in female college students. Boseieisei. 2013;54(1):120–9.

21. Doescher MP, Saver BG, Fiscella K, Franks P. Preventive care. Does continuity count? J Gen Intern Med. 2004;19:632–7.

22. Kyaw MH, Nguyen-Van-Tam JS, Pearson JCG. Family doctor advice is the main determinant of peumococcal vaccine uptake. J Epidemiol Community Health. 1999;53(9):589–90.

23. Tohnai S, Hata E. Factors affecting health behavior of the people aged forties: a test of the Health Belief Model. Nihon Koshu Eisei Zasshi. 1994; 41(4):362–9.

24. Janz NK, Maiman LA. The Health Belief Model: a decade later. Health Educ Q. 1984;11(1):1–47.

25. Health Belief Model. University of Twente. https://www.utwente.nl/en/bms/ communication-theories/sorted-by-cluster/Health%20Communication/ Health_Belief_Model/. Accessed 28 Feb 2015.

26. Stephane Champely. Package pwr: Basic Functions for Power Analysis. R package version 1.1.1. https://cran.r-project.org/web/packages/pwr/index. html. Accessed 29 Oct 2012.

27. Cohen J. A power primer. Psychol Bull. 1992;112(1):155–9.

28. R Core Team. R: A language and environment for statistical computing. R Foundation for Statistical Computing, Vienna, Austria. http://www.r-project. org/. 2015.

29. Stange KC, Jaén CR, Flocke SA, Miller WL, Crabtree BF, Zyzanski SJ. The value of a family physician. J Fam Pract. 1998;46:363–8.

30. Flocke SA, Stange KC, Goodwin MA. Patient and visit characteristics associated with opportunistic preventive services delivery. J Fam Pract. 1998;47:202–8.

31. Freeman TR. McWhinney's textbook of family medicine. 4th ed. New York: Oxford University Press; 2016.

32. Flocke SA, Stange KC, Zyzanski SJ. The association of attributes of primary care with the delivery of clinical preventive services. Med Care. 1998;36: AS21–30.

33. Saultz JW. Defining and measuring interpersonal continuity of care. Ann Fam Med. 2003;1:134–43.

34. Hennen BKE. Continuity of care in family practice, Part 1: Dimensions of continuity. J Fam Pract. 1975;2(5):371.

35. Stewart M, Brown JB, Weston W, McWhinney IR, McWilliam CL, Freeman T. Patient-centered medicine: transforming the clinical method. 3rd. USA: CRC press; 2013.

36. Pommerenke F, Dietrich A. Improving and maintaining preventive services. Part 1: applying the patient model. J Fam Pract. 1992;34:86.

37. Austin PC, Tu JV, Alter DA. Comparing hierarchical modeling with traditional logistic regression analysis among patients hospitalized with acute myocardial infarction: should we be analyzing cardiovascular outcomes data differently? Am Heart J. 2003;145:27–35.

38. Sugino Y, Kondo Y, Kato S, Matsuura A, Sanda R, Kimura M, et al. Analysis of yearly changes in the number of adults in our hospital receiving 23-valent pneumococcal vaccine. Toyota Iho. 2016;26:86–89.

39. Hung DY, Rundall TG, Crabtree BF, Tallia AF, Cohen DJ, Halpin HA. Influence of primary care practice and provider attributes on preventive service delivery. Am J Prev Med. 2006;30:413–22.

40. Crawford AG, Sikirica V, Goldfarb N, Popiel RG, Patel M, Wang C, et al. Interactive voice response reminder effects on preventive service utilization. Am J Med Qual. 2005;20:329–36.

21

Patient capacity for self-care in the medical record of patients with chronic conditions: a mixed-methods retrospective study

Kasey R Boehmer[1*] (iD), Maria Kyriacou[2], Emma Behnken[1], Megan Branda[1,3] and Victor M Montori[1]

Abstract

Background: Patients with chronic conditions must mobilize capacity to access and use healthcare and enact self-care. In order for clinicians to create feasible treatment plans with patients, they must appreciate the limits and possibilities of patient capacity. This study seeks to characterize the amount, nature, and comprehensiveness of the information about patient capacity documented in the medical record.

Methods: In this mixed-methods study, we extracted notes about 6 capacity domains from the medical records of 100 patients receiving care from 15 primary care clinicians at a single practice. Using a generalized linear model to account for repeated measures across multiple encounters, we calculated the rate of documented domains per encounter per patient adjusted for appointment type and number. Following quantitative analyses, we purposefully selected records to conduct inductive content analysis.

Results: After adjusting for number of appointments and appointment type, primary care notes contained the most mentions of capacity. Physical capacity was most noted, followed by personal, emotional, social, financial, and environmental. Qualitatively, we found three documentation patterns: patients with broad capacity notes, patients with predominantly physical domain capacity notes, and patients with capacity notes mostly in domains other than physical. Records contained almost no mention of patients' environmental or financial capacity, or of how they coped with capacity limitations. Rarely, did notes ever mention how well patients interacted with their social network or what support they provided to the patient in managing their health.

Conclusion: Medical records scarcely document patient capacity. This may impair the ability of clinicians to determine how patients can handle patient work, at what point patient capacity might become overwhelmed leading to poor adherence and health outcomes, and how best to craft feasible treatment programs that patients can implement with high fidelity.

Keywords: Minimally disruptive medicine, Patient capacity, Electronic medical record, Electronic health record, Treatment burden, Treatment planning, Chronic conditions, Chronic illness, Multimorbidity

Background

Patients with chronic conditions must mobilize their abilities and resources to access and use healthcare and enact self-care [1]. Healthcare demands, in many cases, overwhelm the capacity of patients to implement treatment programs. Furthermore, the work of healthcare competes for the same limited capacity with the work of life (e.g., from commitments to family, community, and employment) [1]. Given that capacity is limited and that people often find more meaning in these life activities than in patient work, [2] patients end up "adhering to something else." To reduce the risk of nonadherence to healthcare, clinicians and patients must create feasible treatment plans that reflect an understanding of the role of competing demands, the overall burden of treatment, and the limited capacity patients can mobilize to routinize self-care.

* Correspondence: Boehmer.Kasey@mayo.edu
[1]Knowledge and Evaluation Research (KER) Unit, Mayo Clinic, 200 First Street SW, Rochester, MN 55901, USA
Full list of author information is available at the end of the article

To fashion personalized treatment programs and support patient self-management, clinicians need to understand the limits and possibilities of each patient's capacity, which includes both their strengths to self-manage [3] as well as potential barriers to self-care [4]. They may have access to basic information about patient capacity in the medical record, but the extent to which information about patient capacity for self-care is available in the medical record is currently unknown. Therefore, the aim of this study was to describe the information about patient capacity extractable from the medical record, identifying its amount, nature, and comprehensiveness.

Methods

This study used a mixed methods explanatory sequential design. This type of design first analyzes quantitative data and then uses those findings to inform the scope of qualitative design and analyses (Fig. 1) [5].

Ethics

All study procedures were approved by the Mayo Clinic Institutional Review Board. Minnesota Research Authorization law allows patients to opt out of chart review for research. Patients who did not opt out were considered for inclusion.

Chart selection

Eligible patients were adults 18 years or older, had at least one chronic condition, and had seen a primary care clinician in the previous six months. We defined a chronic condition as one "that lasts 12 months or more and either limits self-care or independent living or requires ongoing medical intervention." [6] We selected six to eight charts per clinician of the most recent visits with eligible patients from the panels of all 15 primary

care clinicians at a single primary care site, within a larger healthcare system, in the upper Midwest. In total, we pulled 100 charts on June 1, 2015. Because this is a sub-study of a larger project in which patients had to give written informed consent, patients who would not be able to provide such consent if approached, e.g., patients with cognitive impairment, were excluded.

Chart review

We reviewed the chart's latest appointment with the primary care clinician and all appointments in the previous six months, with any healthcare professional in which there was a conversation in which capacity information could be elicited. Visits included any visit in- or out-patient that occurred within the healthcare system, and included primary care, care coordination, behavioral health, and specialty care visits. Visits that were simply procedural, i.e., in-patient or out-patient surgical notes, were excluded. From each chart, we extracted appointment date(s), appointment type (ED, hospitalization, primary care, specialty, or other), number of capacity notes mentioned in each domain, and the word-for-word description of capacity information noted. To extract capacity information from the chart, we used a previously described set of categories for documenting patient capacity [7]: financial, environmental, physical, personal, emotional, and social domains. These domains specifically relate to patients' ability to access and use healthcare and enact self-care, rather than considering more traditional clinical characteristics. For each domain, extractors had a list of possible items that could be included in each, which were determined a priori by consensus. Items documented in the clinical notes which clearly conveyed patient capacity but were not on the list, were discussed by the three extractors and added to

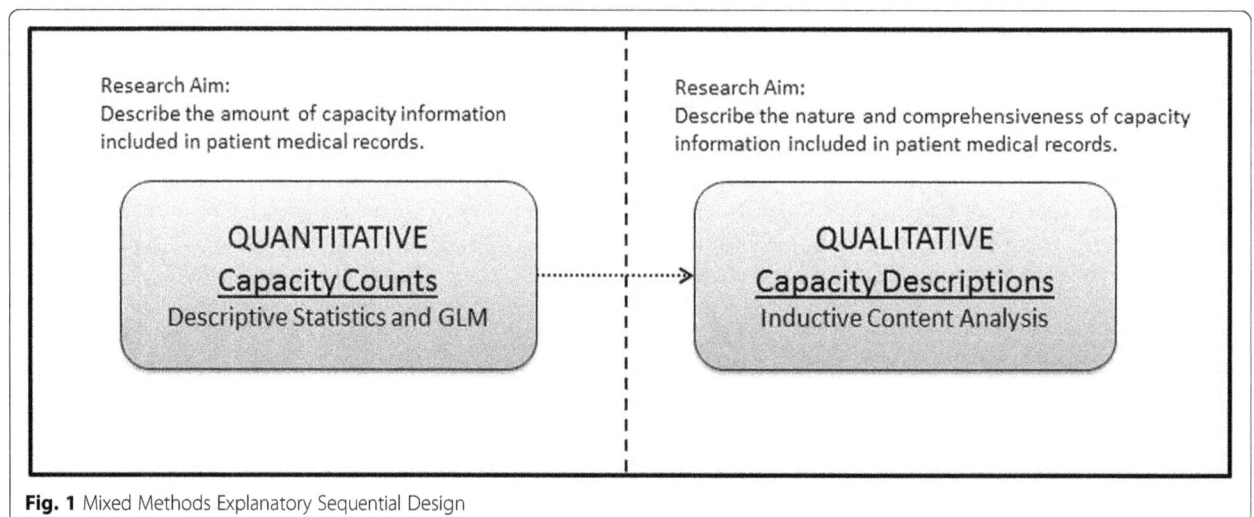

Fig. 1 Mixed Methods Explanatory Sequential Design

the appropriate domain. Table 1 lists the items included in each domain.

KB, EB, and MK reviewed 10 charts in triplicate to ensure reproducible extraction, and met weekly to discuss individual extractions. We determined that after extracting the 10 charts in triplicate, good agreement was established and continued the extraction process individually until all 100 chart reviews were completed. This approach is more consistent with emergent qualitative and mixed methods designs, rather than quantitative a priori designs, which typically establish inter-rater reliability through calculation of intra-cluster correlation coefficients.

Quantitative analysis

In addition to descriptive statistics, we estimated the number of capacity notes per domain per encounter within each appointment type (i.e. all physical capacity notes within primary care appointments was summed then divided by the number of primary care appointments). This rate was then modeled using a generalized linear model to account for repeated measures across multiple encounters. The models were adjusted by appointment type and the following domains had a link of log to account for their distribution (Financial, social, environmental and emotional). The least square means with 95% CI are reported for each capacity domain by appointment type. All quantitative analyses were conducted using SAS software (SAS Institute, version 9.4).

Qualitative analysis

We purposefully selected the charts we would use for qualitative content analysis based upon the quantitative averages. We selected charts that had higher counts of capacity mentioned in any category than their unadjusted mean. We copied the text from each clinical note into NVivo qualitative data analysis software (QSR International Pty Ltd. Version 10, 2014). KB conducted inductive content analysis on all clinical notes [8]. This

process included inductive, line-by-line coding of the entire data set, and we then synthesized these codes to summarize what was learned across all notes.

Results
Quantitative results

Table 2 describes the sample characteristics. The patients included in the sample had a mean age of 49 (19.9) and 52% were female. A diverse range of conditions were included in the sample. Most commonly seen conditions included type 2 diabetes, hypertension, depression, and anxiety, while less common conditions included but were not limited to irritable bowel syndrome, pain conditions, such as fibromyalgia, and asthma. The unadjusted mean of total appointments during the 6-month period was 3.4 (SD 4.0; range 1–20), with 2.1 (SD 1.7; range 1–11) of those, on average, being primary care appointments and 1.3 (SD 2.7; range 0–14) other appointment types.

Table 3 describes the unadjusted mean number of times each capacity domain was documented per patient in a 6 month period. Physical capacity was by far the most mentioned domain followed by personal, emotional, social, financial, and environmental capacity.

Table 4 shows the Least Squares Mean of capacity documentation by domain by appointment type, adjusted for number of appointments and appointment type. Primary care notes provided the most mentions of capacity across most domains, even after adjusting for number of appointments.

Qualitative results

Three patterns, i.e. patient "personas," with above average capacity notes documented emerged: patients with broad capacity notes documented, patients with predominantly physical domain capacity notes documented, and patients with capacity notes documented predominantly in domains other than the physical domain (Fig. 2).

Across all patient personas, we learned little about patients' environmental or financial capacity. For patient personas with high numbers of capacity notes documented across all domains, physical capacity notes were still most prominent, but other notes had fair representation. For patients with high numbers of capacity notes documented predominantly in the physical domain, we were able to get a good understanding of patients' conditions, symptoms, and functional limitations, but not much about their pain and fatigue. In patients with

Table 1 Capacity Domain Information Extracted

Physical	Pain, Fatigue, Disability, Functioning, Conditions, Symptoms, Current physical activity/exercise
Emotional	Anxiety, Depression, Grief, Worry, Stress, Coping
Social	Relationships, Family, Friends, Caregivers (paid/unpaid), Healthcare team, Volunteering, Culture, Safety in Relationships
Personal	Substance use, Smoking, Education, Self-Efficacy, Resilience, Ability to have Conversations/Make Decisions, Clinician Perceptions about Patient, Spirituality
Financial	Job, Sources of Income, Financial Commitments, Financial Difficulty, Medication Costs
Environmental	House, Neighborhood, Community, Anything about Lived Space that Affects Patient Health or Self-Care

Table 2 Sample Characteristics

Age – Mean (SD)	48.7 (19.6)
Gender - % Female	52%
Number of chronic conditions – Mean (range)	3.0 (1–10)

Table 3 Times each capacity domain was mentioned per patient in 6 months of chart records[a]

Capacity Domain	All notes	Primary care notes only	All other notes
Physical	14.0 (21.9), 8 (4, 15), 159	9.5 (10.9), 6 (3, 12), 72	4.6 (12.5), 0 (0, 3.5), 87
Personal	5.7 (6.5), 4 (2, 6), 31	4.0 (3.6), 3 (2, 5), 25	1.8 (4.1), 0 (0, 2), 21
Emotional	3.1 (5.9), 1 (0, 4), 47	2.2 (3.0), 1 (0, 3), 17	0.9 (3.7), 0 (0, 0), 30
Social	2.6 (4.3), 2 (1, 3), 30	1.8 (1.9), 1.0 (0, 3), 12	0.8 (2.9), 0 (0,0), 18
Financial	0.9 (1.5), 1 (0, 1), 11	0.7 (0.8), 1.0 (0, 1), 4	0.3 (0.9), 0 (0,0), 7
Environmental	0.5 (1.0), 0 (0, 1), 6	0.3 (0.6), 0 (0,0), 3	0.2 (0.7), 0 (0, 0), 5

[a]Mean (Standard Deviation), Median (Inter-Quartile Range), Maximum

above average capacity notes documented predominantly in domains other than physical capacity, documentation of emotional capacity problems dominated the record, particularly related to depression and anxiety, as well as occasional documentation of social situations that exacerbated these problems. Across all three personas, financial capacity was barely mentioned, mostly to note employment and the way in which patients earned or received income. Only two charts subjected to content analysis mentioned cost of care or financial difficulty. Personal capacity documentation did not refer to patients' resilience or other personal capacity sources, but rather to patients' ability to understand the plan of care. Social capacity had few mentions per patient, mainly to note the existence of family members or friends. Rarely, did notes ever mention how well patients interacted with their social network or what support these people provided to the patient in managing their health. Across all personas, we also had little information about patients' abilities to cope with capacity limitations.

Discussion

This study highlights the paucity of important capacity information documented in patient medical records. To the extent that lack of documentation reflects lack of awareness of the limits and possibilities of each patient's capacity, medical record silence on capacity impedes clinicians' ability to determine how patients can handle patient work, at what point patient capacity might become overwhelmed leading to poor adherence and health

Table 4 Adjusted times capacity domain mentioned per patient, LSM (CI)*

Capacity Domain	Primary care notes	All other notes	p value
Physical	4.8 (4.2–5.4)	3.1 (2.4–3.7)	<.0001
Personal	2.1 (1.9–2.3)	1.3 (0.9–1.6)	0.0001
Emotional^	1.1 (0.9–1.4)	0.7 (0.4–1.2)	0.08
Social^	1.1 (0.9–1.3)	0.5 (0.3–0.9)	0.02
Financial^	0.41 (0.33–0.50)	0.15 (0.09–0.27)	0.001
Environmental^	0.22 (0.14–0.34)	0.14 (0.06–0.34)	0.37

*CI, 95% confidence interval, LSM, least square means; ^Outcome does not follow a normal distribution therefore a log link is used

outcomes, and how best to craft feasible treatment programs that patients can implement with high fidelity. The medical record is particularly silent when it comes to capacity domains associated with the most disruption by illness and treatments, as uncovered in a previous survey study of patients with chronic disease: emotional capacity, physical capacity, primarily pain and fatigue, and financial capacity [2].

Given the nature of this review, it is impossible to know if the limited mention of capacity domains reflects lack of challenges in patient lives, limited assessment and discussion during clinic visits, or limitations of the documented record. This prompts the need for more in-depth conversation analysis of encounters [9] as well as testing of interventions likely to give light to these issues during consultations [10]. Given the importance of these capacity elements to patients' ability to cope with the burden of treatment and burden of illness, careful assessment of patient capacity is necessary, with sufficient documentation to enable patient-centered team-based care.

The underwhelming documentation of capacity notes in patients with chronic conditions is particularly silent in two areas central to the work of adapting to and managing chronic disease. Both the Burden of Treatment Theory and the Theory of Patient Capacity focus on the importance of patients' social networks in coping with illness and treatment [11, 12]. Furthermore, the Theory of Patient Capacity, as well as previous work in the experience of chronic illness, highlights the importance of patients' biography – their personal story and the extent to which it has been disrupted by their illness [11, 13, 14]. These areas received little to no mention in the notes examined.

The findings of this study cannot be considered fully without discussing its limitations. Key study limitations include: the single-site nature of the study, convenience sampling, the extraction process, and the novelty of the extraction criteria. A single primary care clinic within a large interconnected healthcare system was chosen to undertake this study due to its inclusion as a primary site for recruitment in a subsequent prospective study to test a conversation aid intended to elicit capacity

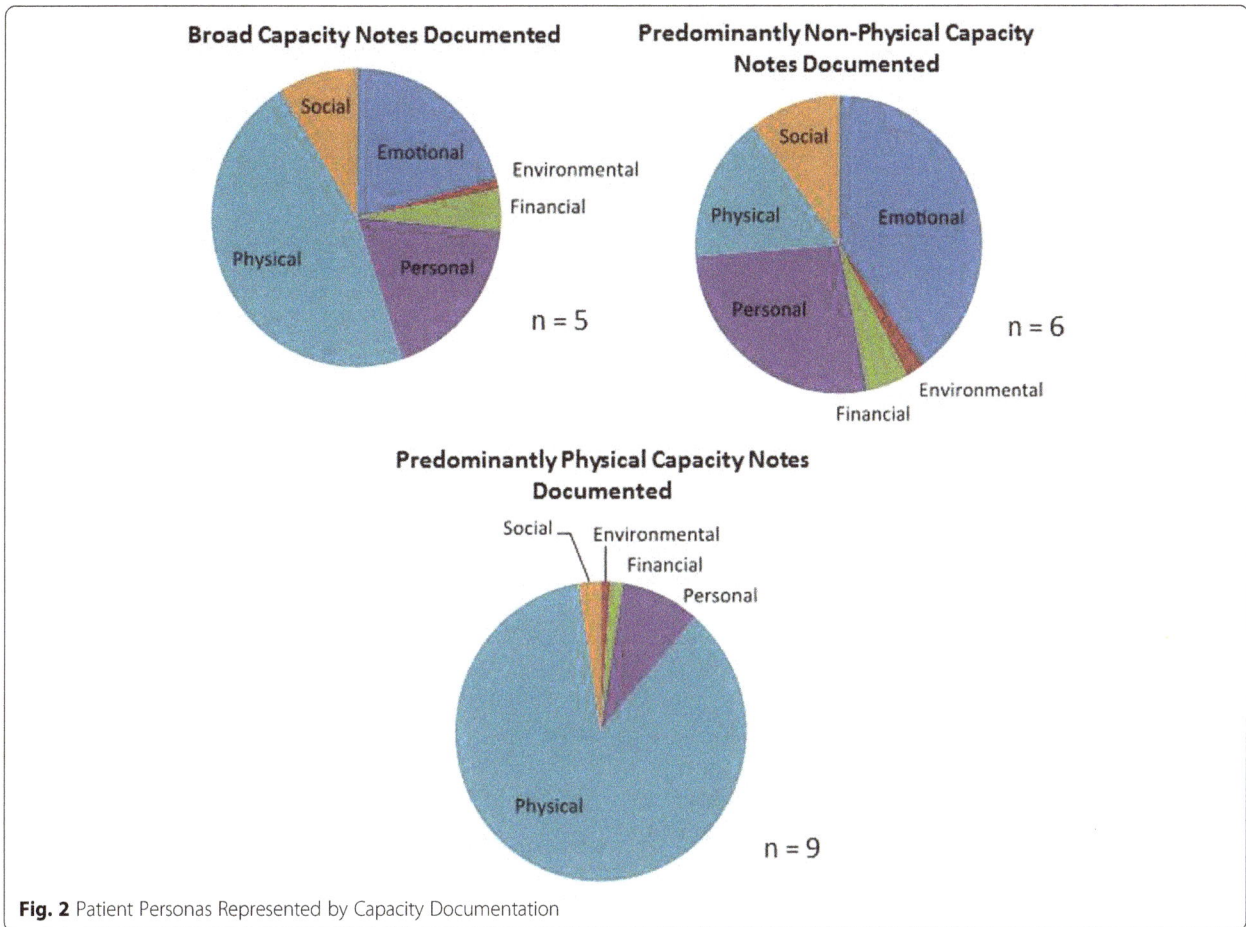

Fig. 2 Patient Personas Represented by Capacity Documentation

information during consultations. While this was a pragmatic choice, it limits the generalizability beyond similar primary care centers in the Midwest and does not necessarily transfer directly to health systems using other medical record systems. Patients included in this study were on clinicians' panels for this individual site. However, we included all notes during the six-month time period regardless of location of care within the health system, and therefore, notes included hospital, specialty, and primary care received at other clinic locations as well. Second, we selected patients consecutively based upon appointment date, a convenience sample and pragmatic choice, but one which could potentially bias results given that it was not random. Next, we took steps to reduce bias as we extracted data from charts, including conducting the first set in triplicate and meeting regularly during the extraction period. While this is typical of the study design used, other more quantitatively-oriented approaches might consider the study stronger if it would have established inter-rater reliability through calculation of intra-cluster correlation coefficients. Finally, the extraction of capacity domains is novel and has not previously been undertaken. Since the time of this analysis, a more robust

Theory of Patient Capacity [11] has been proposed and may warrant similar research using the theory. We have highlighted the key differences in the model used and recent theory in Table 5.

However, despite these limitations, this study has numerous strengths, including its explanatory sequential design. This type of design is the most appropriate for studies in which the research aims seek to explain quantitative findings. Conducting the qualitative analysis after the quantitative analysis is complete allows emergent exploration, where the second phase can be designed to explore the interesting qualitative portions of the data [5]. Therefore, other mixed methods designs, such as a convergent design where qualitative and quantitative analyses are conducted simultaneously would have been weaker for this study's research aims. Furthermore, purely quantitative description of the number of times capacity was mentioned would have been less desirable.

Furthermore, this study is the first to our knowledge that explores capacity descriptions in the medical record and may prompt additional research in other settings. Much of what is captured by documenting patient capacity entails what is often named

Table 5 Overlap and differences between capacity domains used and more recent Theory of Patient Capacity

Theory of Patient Capacity Constructs	Capacity Domains Model Used	Differences
Biography	Personal Emotional	The theory describes the importance of a successful reframing of the patient's biography to include one's condition and self-care. The theory describes that it is not specifically the existence of capacity in these domains, but how they contribute to the overall life of the patient and their ability to pursue their life's hopes, dreams, and purpose.
Resources	Financial Physical	The theory highlights that it is not simply the presence or absence of resources, but that these resources also must be mobilized by patients. Resources captured in the theory are also more encompassing beyond not just financial or physical ones, but include those such as literacy and self-efficacy.
Environment	Environmental	The theory highlights the significant contribution of patients' healthcare environment to their capacity, rather than considering purely home and neighborhood environment characteristics.
Work		This capacity construct is missing from the model used in this manuscript, and it highlights the contribution of experiential learning from patient work that can be accomplished, rather than patient work that is overwhelming, to patients' capacity.
Social	Social	The theory expands upon the social capacity domain by highlighting it is not only the existence of social support in a patient's life, but that patients are able to rely on productive, rather than detrimental, relationships in their social network for emotional and practical support in caring for their conditions.

as social determinants of health. Recently, there have been calls for, expert committee guidance on, conceptual frameworks proposed, and case studies examined of how these social determinants might come to light in and be of importance to the future of medical records [15–17]. Additionally, the practice of geriatrics has been concerned with many of these capacity issue, particularly related to environment, cognition, and physical function in the measurement and documentation of frailty [18, 19]. Ultimately, what our study points to in light of these other bodies of work is that progress is needed for the benefit of patients and the care teams that support them to ensure they are able to fashion care that fits patients' lives.

Conclusion

This study explored the extent to which patient capacity for self-care is documented in the medical record. While mentions of patient capacity appear mostly in primary care notes, the extent is limited, mostly refers to physical capacity concerns (symptoms and functional limitations), with minimal to no mention of the state of other sources of capacity. There is significant room for improving the extent and type of capacity information documented in patient records, and the meaningful conversations and careful assessments with patients these notes should reflect, to improve patient-centered care and to implement minimally disruptive medicine [20].

Funding
No external funding was received for this project.

Authors' contributions
KB conceptualized and oversaw the conduct of the study with mentorship from VM. EB, KB, and MK conducted all data extraction from charts. KB and MB conducted the analyses. KB drafted the manuscript, and all authors provided critical revisions to the manuscript. All authors read and approved the final version of the manuscript.

Competing interests
The authors declare that they have no competing interests.

Author details
[1]Knowledge and Evaluation Research (KER) Unit, Mayo Clinic, 200 First Street SW, Rochester, MN 55901, USA. [2]Phoebe Family Medicine Residency, Albany, GA, USA. [3]Health Sciences Research, Mayo Clinic, Rochester, MN, USA.

References
1. Shippee ND, Shah ND, May CR, Mair FS, Montori VM. Cumulative complexity: a functional, patient-centered model of patient complexity can improve research and practice. J Clin Epidemiol. 2012;65(10):1041–51.
2. Boehmer KR, Shippee ND, Beebe TJ, Montori VM. Pursuing Minimally Disruptive Medicine: Correlation of patient capacity with disruption from illness and healthcare-related demands. *J Clin Epidemiol*. 2016.
3. Monsen KA, Holland DE, Fung-Houger PW, Vanderboom CE. Seeing the whole person: feasibility of using the Omaha system to describe strengths of older adults with chronic illness. Res Theory Nurs Pract. 2014;28(4):299–315.

Patient capacity for self-care in the medical record of patients with chronic conditions: a mixed-methods...

205

4. Bayliss EA, Steiner JF, Fernald DH, Crane LA, Main DS. Descriptions of barriers to self-care by persons with comorbid chronic diseases. Ann Fam Med. 2003;1(1):15–21.

5. Creswell JW, Clark VLP. Designing and conducting mixed methods research. In: SAGE; 2011.

6. AHRQ. AHRQ Announces the Release of the Chronic Conditions Indicator (CCI) for Fiscal Year 2012 (November 2011). 2011; https://www.hcup-us.ahrq.gov/news/announcements/CCI_1111.jsp. Accessed February 2017, 2018.

7. Leppin AL. Montori VM. Extending the Applicability of Clinical Practice Guidelines to Patients with Multiple Chronic Conditions. http://minimallydisruptivemedicine.org/2018/09/28/extending-the-applicability-of-clinical-practice-guidelines-to-patients-with-multiple-chronic-conditions/.

8. Hsieh HF, Shannon SE. Three approaches to qualitative content analysis. Qual Health Res. 2005;15(9):1277–88.

9. Barry CA, Stevenson FA, Britten N, Barber N, Bradley CP. Giving voice to the lifeworld. More humane, more effective medical care? A qualitative study of doctor–patient communication in general practice. Soc Sci Med. 2001;53(4):487–505.

10. Boehmer KR, Hargraves IG, Allen SV, Matthews MR, Maher C, Montori VM. Meaningful conversations in living with and treating chronic conditions: development of the ICAN discussion aid. BMC Health Serv Res. 2016.

11. Boehmer KR, Gionfriddo MR, Rodriguez-Gutierrez R, et al. Patient capacity and constraints in the experience of chronic disease: a qualitative systematic review and thematic synthesis. BMC Fam Pract. 2016;17(1):127.

12. May CR, Eton DT, Boehmer K, et al. Rethinking the patient: using burden of treatment theory to understand the changing dynamics of illness. BMC Health Serv Res. 2014;14:281.

13. Bury M. Chronic illness as biographical disruption. Sociology of health & illness. 1982;4(2):167–82.

14. Charmaz K. The body, identity, and self. Sociol Q. 1995;36(4):657–80.

15. Adler NE, Stead WW. Patients in context—EHR capture of social and behavioral determinants of health. N Engl J Med. 2015;372(8):698–701.

16. DeVoe JE, Bazemore AW, Cottrell EK, et al. Perspectives in primary care: a conceptual framework and path for integrating social determinants of health into primary care practice. Ann Fam Med. 2016;14:104–8.

17. Gottlieb LM, Tirozzi KJ, Manchanda R, Burns AR, Sandel MT. Moving electronic medical records upstream. Am J Prev Med. 48(2):215–8.

18. Clegg A, Bates C, Young J, et al. Development and validation of an electronic frailty index using routine primary care electronic health record data. Age Ageing. 2016;45(3):353–60.

19. Clegg A, Young J, Iliffe S, Rikkert MO, Rockwood K. Frailty in elderly people. Lancet. 381(9868):752–62.

20. May C, Montori VM, Mair FS. We need minimally disruptive medicine. BMJ. 2009;339:b2803.

22

Diabetes mellitus and hyperglycemia control on the risk of colorectal adenomatous polyps

Katarzyna Budzynska[1,3]* (iD), Daniel Passerman[1], Denise White-Perkins[1], Della A. Rees[1], Jinping Xu[2], Lois Lamerato[1] and Susan Schooley[1]

Abstract

Background: Colorectal cancer (CRC) develops from colorectal adenomatous polyps. This study is to determine if diabetes mellitus (DM), its treatment, and hemoglobin A1c (HbA1c) level are associated with increased risk of colorectal adenomatous polyps.

Methods: This was a retrospective cohort study that included patients who had at least one colonoscopy and were continuously enrolled in a single managed care organization during a 10-year period (2002–2012). Of these patients ($N = 11,933$), 1800 were randomly selected for chart review to examine the details of colonoscopy and pathology findings and to confirm the diagnosis of DM. Multivariable logistic regression analyses were performed to assess the associations between DM, its treatment, HbA1c level and adenomatous polyps (our main outcome).

Results: Among the total of 11,933 patients with a mean (standard deviation) age of 56 (± 8.8) years, 2306 (19.3%) had DM and 75 (0.6%) had CRC. Among the 1800 under chart review, 445 (24.7%) had DM, 11 (0.6%) had CRC and 537 (29.8%) had adenomatous polyps. In bivariate analysis, patients with DM had 1.45 odds of developing adenomatous polyps compared to those without DM. This effect was attenuated (odds ratio = 1.25, 95% CI: 0.96–1.62, $p = 0.09$) after adjusting for confounders such as age, gender, race/ethnicity, and body mass index. There was no significant association between type or duration of DM treatment or HbA1c level and adenomatous polyps.

Conclusions: Our study confirmed the known increased risk of adenomatous polyps with advancing age, male gender, Hispanic race/ethnicity and higher body mass index. Although it suggested an association between DM and adenomatous polyps, a statistically significant association was not observed after controlling for other potential confounders. Further studies with a larger sample size are needed to further elucidate this relationship.

Keywords: Adenomatous polyp, Diabetes mellitus, Treatment, Colonoscopy

Background

Colorectal cancer (CRC) develops from colorectal adenomatous polyps. It is estimated that there will be 134,490 new cases of CRC in 2016, 49,190 of those diagnosed will die [1, 2]. Screening colonoscopy prevents development of CRC by removal of precursor adenomatous polyps [3].

Since it takes between 7 and 10 years for the precancerous polyp to develop into a malignant lesion, routine screening colonoscopy has been shown to reduce the incidence of CRC and its subsequent morbidity and mortality [4]. However, despite advances in CRC screening and treatment modalities, CRC continues to be a leading cause of mortality in the United States. This highlights the need for more targeted interventions.

Diabetes mellitus (DM) has been found to be associated with an increased risk of CRC [2]. Several meta-analyses suggested that DM carries an average 30% increased risk

* Correspondence: kbudzyn1@hfhs.org
[1]Department of Family Medicine, Henry Ford Hospital, Detroit, MI, USA
[3]Department of Family Medicine, Henry Ford Health System, 3370 E Jefferson, Detroit, MI 48207, USA
Full list of author information is available at the end of the article

of CRC [5–8]. It has been hypothesized that insulin resistance and the resulting hyperinsulinemia may promote carcinogenesis by directly stimulating colonic cell growth [9, 10]. In addition, insulin is thought to act indirectly by binding to and activating the insulin-like growth factor-1 receptors. Insulin-like growth factor-1 then enhances cell proliferation and inhibits apoptosis [9–12]. Observational studies have shown an increased CRC risk with hyperinsulinemia and elevated insulin-like growth factor-1 levels [13]. This is concerning as the number of Americans with DM has tripled over the last 3 decades [14]. The Centers for Disease Control and Prevention estimates that a total of 29.1 million Americans have DM and 29% of them are undiagnosed [14]. Additionally, it is even more concerning as African American ethnicity is identified as a risk factor for both Diabetes and CRC [15]. African Americans, among other minorities, have a higher prevalence and greater burden of diabetes, and lower screening rates for CRC [16].

Although there are strong data suggesting the association between DM and CRC, the current literature regarding the association between DM and adenomatous polyps, the precursor to CRC, is conflicting and has several limitations [17–20]. Some studies only evaluated a small sample with a short duration of exposure [21, 22] and other studies were conducted outside the United States [6]. In addition, there are only three studies that have evaluated the effect of glycemic control on the risk of adenomatous polyps with conflictual findings [17, 20, 21]. The main goal of this study was to better understand the association between DM and the prevalence of adenomatous polyps in a large managed care organization population. Additionally, the associations between the type of DM treatment (oral medicine vs. insulin), level of glycemic control (i.e., hemoglobin A1c [HbA1c] level), and the prevalence of adenomatous polyps were assessed. The study hypotheses were that: 1) patients with DM have increased prevalence of adenomatous polyps compared to those without DM; 2) higher HbA1c level is associated with higher risk of adenomatous polyps.

Methods

Study population
The initial population was identified by using an administrative database of a single managed care organization (i.e. Health Alliance Plan [HAP]) owned and operated by the Henry Ford Health System (HFHS). HFHS is a large metropolitan health system that spans 3 counties in southeast Michigan, including the city of Detroit. The study inclusion criteria were: 1) adult patients (≥ 18 years); 2) continuously enrolled in HAP for 10 years, who 3) had a colonoscopy during the second half of the 10-year period for either screening or diagnostic purposes. A total of 11,933 eligible patients were identified

within 10 years (January 1, 2002 through December 31, 2012) who received care within the HFHS (Fig. 1). Of them, 1800 patients (the sample population) were randomly selected for medical record review (SPSS software) in 2015. The medical records were then reviewed to determine type of diabetes (type 1 vs type 2) and to identify presence, number, and types of polyp per pathology report (e.g., non-adenomatous polyp, adenomatous polyp, or CRC). The HFHS Institutional Review Board approved this study.

Measurements of main exposure and outcome variables
The main outcome variable was presence of adenomatous polyps. All of the adenomatous polyps were identified by reviewing pathology reports of the colonoscopies. The main independent variable was having the diagnosis of DM within study period (January 1, 2002 to December 31, 2012). DM was categorized further to type 1 or type 2. In the initial total population ($N = 11,933$), a DM diagnosis was based on variables collected in the administrative data using factors employed by the Healthcare Effectiveness Data and Information Set (HEDIS) criteria [23], a long established metric for evaluating care of DM patients. The HEDIS criteria include the use of DM medications as well as DM codes, a methodology that reduces the prevalence of false positive diagnoses compared to the use of diagnostic codes alone [24].

For the sample population ($n = 1800$) that randomly selected for chart review, the diagnosis of DM was determined using information available from the medical record (e.g. fasting plasma glucose ≥126 mg/dl, plasma glucose ≥200 mg/dl at 2 h after a 75 g oral glucose load, HbA1c ≥ 6.5%, presence of medication used to treat DM, presence of insulin antibodies, or office notes indicating a diagnosis of DM).

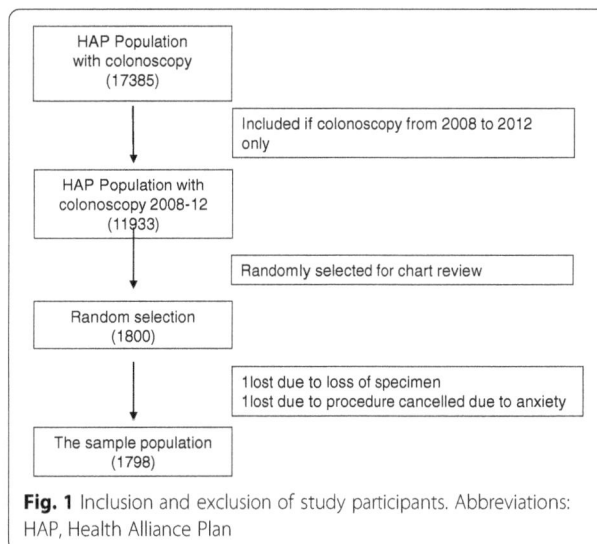

Fig. 1 Inclusion and exclusion of study participants. Abbreviations: HAP, Health Alliance Plan

Covariate assessment

Data on additional covariates were collected from administrative databases of HFHS, including demographic information (age, gender, and race/ethnicity), body mass index (BMI) and HbA1c level. Age was categorized into quintiles ($\leq$ 50, 51–55, 56–60, and >60 years, Table 1). BMI was calculated using height and weight measures and categorized based on World Health Organization criteria (normal BMI < 25, overweight $25 \geq$ BMI < 30 kg/m^2, or obese BMI $\geq$ 30 kg/m^2) [25]. We did not separate underweight patients (BMI < 18.5 kg/m^2) from normal weight patients due to its small percentage. HbA1c was used to represent the level of hyperglycemia control and it was categorized as 4 levels (normal HbA1c < 5.7, pre-DM 5.7–6.4, DM 6.5–7.9, and uncontrolled DM > 7.9) [23]. If more than one value of BMI and HgbA1c level were available in the chart, the median of each variable was used in the model. Type and length of

Table 1 Characteristics of the population and chart review sample

Variables	Population (N = 11,933) N (%)	Chart review sample (N = 1798) N (%)	p value
Age, years, mean (SD)	56.06 (8.77)	56.20 (9.09)	0.468
$\leq$ 50	2036 (17.1)	290 (16.1)	
51~55	4149 (34.8)	628 (34.9)	
56~60	3220 (27.0)	509 (28.3)	
>60	2528 (21.2)	371 (20.6)	
Gender			
Female	6527(54.7)	964 (53.6)	0.317
Male	5406 (45.3)	834 (46.4)	
Ethnicity			
Caucasian	5794 (48.6)	874 (48.6)	0.544
African American	3572 (29.9)	528 (29.4)	
Hispanic	2148 (18.0)	342 (19.0)	
Asian	264 (2.2)	35 (1.9)	
Other/unknown	155 (1.3)	19 (1.1)	
Body mass index, kg/m^2 mean (SD)	31.05 (6.86)	31.05 (7.05)	0.985
< 18.5	34 (0.3)	6 (0.3)	
18.5–24.9	1660 (13.9)	255 (14.2)	
25–29.9	3550 (29.7)	529 (29.4)	
30–39.9	4038 (33.8)	602 (33.5)	
>40	1008 (8.4)	153 (8.5)	
Missing cases	1643 (13.8)	253 (14.1)	
Diabetes			
No	9627 (80.7)	1353 (75.3)	<.0001
Yes	2306 (19.3)	445 (24.7)	

SD standard deviation
P value obtained from chi-square test

medication exposure for oral antidiabetic medications and insulin were determined from filled prescriptions of drugs from HAP database, using the number of months of prescriptions filled prior to the date of colonoscopy, which was categorized as none, < 2 years, and $\geq$ 2 years.

Statistical analyses

Sample characteristics were described using mean and standard deviations for continuous variables and frequencies (numbers and percentages) for categorical variables. Bivariate analysis was used to examine the effect of each of the covariates on prevalence of adenomatous polyps using chi-square test. Multivariable logistic regression models were used to examine the associations between the main exposure variable, DM, and the outcome variable, adenomatous polyps, adjusted for all other covariates. All analyses were performed using SPSS (IBM version of SPSS Statistics 2015).

Results

A total of 11,933 patients met the study eligibility criteria (Fig. 1). Of them, a sample of 1800 patients was randomly selected for medical record review and this is called "the sample population". Two participants were excluded from the sample population analysis: one due to loss of the pathology specimen and one due to the colonoscopy not performed because of patient anxiety of the procedure and poor prep. The demographic characteristics of the sample population (n = 1798) were statistically similar to the total HAP population except that the prevalence of DM diagnosis was greater in the sample population compared to total population (n = 11,933) (Table 1). This is because more patients with DM (25%) were identified by medical record review compared to those identified by HEDIS criteria (19%) in the administrative database of HAP population (p < 0.0001) (Table 1). When we used HEDIS criteria to identify patients with DM in the sample population, we found the prevalence of DM was similar as in the HAP population (P = 0.27, data not shown), which confirms that our randomization was successful. The mean age of the population (n = 1798) was 56.2 ($\pm$ 9.1) years with females comprising 54% of the sample. Eighty-one percent were between ages 50 and 64 years. Forty-nine percent were Caucasian, followed by 30% African-American, 19% Hispanic, 2% Asian and 1% other/unknown. Seventy-one percent of the population was overweight or obese, with a mean BMI of 31.1 kg/m2 ($\pm$ 7.1) (Table 1).

In the bivariate analysis (Table 2), we found significant associations between the presence of adenomatous polyps and older age (p < 0.0001), male gender (p < 0.001), higher BMI (p = 0.004), and a diagnosis of DM (p = 0.001). We found no significant association between presence of adenomatous polyps and race/

Table 2 Characteristics among chart review sample and diabetes mellitus sample by adenomatous polyps

Variables	Adenomatous polyp among chart review sample			
	Total N (%)	No (N = 1261) N (%)	Yes (N = 537) N (%)	P value
Age, years, mean (SD)	56.20 (9.09)	55.39 (9.12)	58.09 (8.75)	< 0.0001
≤ 50	290 (16.1)	233 (80.3)	57 (19.7)	
51~ 55	628 (34.9)	441 (70.2)	187 (29.8)	
56~ 60	509 (28.3)	347 (68.2)	162 (31.8)	
> 60	371 (20.6)	233 (62.8)	138 (37.2)	
Gender				
Female	964 (53.6)	712 (73.9)	252 (26.1)	< 0.0001
Male	834 (46.4)	549 (65.8)	285 (34.2)	
Ethnicity				
Caucasian	874 (48.6)	624 (71.4)	250 (28.6)	0.131
African American	528 (29.4)	380 (72.0)	148 (28.0)	
Hispanic	342 (19.0)	220 (64.3)	122 (35.7)	
Asian	35 (1.9)	24 (68.6)	11 (31.4)	
Other/unknown	19 (1.1)	13 (68.4)	6 (31.6)	
Body mass index, kg/m^2, mean (SD)	31.05 (7.06)	30.70 (7.04)	31.83 (7.03)	0.004
< 18.5	6 (0.3)	6 (100.0)	0 (0.0)	0.013
18.5–24.9	255 (14.2)	196 (76.9)	59 (23.1)	
25–29.9	529 (29.4)	369 (69.8)	160 (30.2)	
30–39.9	855 (47.6)	405 (67.3)	197 (32.7)	
> 40	153 (8.5)	98 (64.1)	55 (35.9)	
Diabetes				
No	1353 (75.3)	976 (72.1)	377 (27.9)	0.001
Yes	445 (24.7)	285 (64.0)	160 (36.0)	
	Adenomatous polyp among patient with Diabetes Mellitus (N = 445)			
Age, years, mean (SD)	58.76 (9.72)	57.54 (9.34)	60.91 (10.03)	0.001
≤ 50	45 (10.1)	35 (77.8)	10 (22.2)	
51~ 55	133 (29.9)	89 (66.9)	44 (33.1)	
56~ 60	128 (28.8)	82 (64.1)	46 (35.9)	
> 60	139 (31.2)	78 (56.1)	61 (43.9)	
Gender				
Female	225(50.6)	155(68.9)	70(31.1)	0.024
Male	220(49.4)	129(58.6)	91(41.4)	
Ethnicity				
Caucasian	169 (38.0)	107 (63.3)	62 (36.7)	0.622
African American	177 (39.8)	119 (67.2)	58 (32.8)	
Hispanic	80 (18.0)	46 (57.5)	34 (42.5)	
Asian	12 (2.7)	7 (58.3)	5 (41.7)	
Other/unknown	7 (1.6)	5 (71.4)	2 (28.6)	

Table 2 Characteristics among chart review sample and diabetes mellitus sample by adenomatous polyps *(Continued)*

Body mass index, kg/m², mean (SD)	34.24 (7.54)	34.28 (7.47)	34.18 (7.67)	0.903
< 18.5	2 (0.4)	1 (50.0)	1 (50.0)	
18.5–24.9	26 (5.8)	15 (57.7)	11 (42.3)	
25–29.9	90 (20.2)	54 (60.0)	36 (40.0)	
30–39.9	205 (46.1)	135 (65.9)	70 (34.1)	
> 40	71 (16.0)	43 (60.6)	28 (39.4)	
Hemoglobin A1c				
< 5.7	15 (3.4)	10 (66.7)	5 (33.3)	0.903
5.7–6.4	126 (28.3)	78 (61.9)	48 (38.1)	
6.5–7.9	214 (48.1)	140 (65.4)	74 (34.6)	
≥ 8.0	71 (16.0)	47 (66.2)	24 (33.8)	
Missing cases	19 (4.3)			
Oral medication exposure				
None	204 (45.8)	130 (63.7)	74 (36.3)	0.916
< 2 years	105 (23.6)	69 (65.7)	36 (34.3)	
≥ 2 years	136 (30.6)	86 (63.2)	50 (36.8)	
Insulin exposure				
None	371 (83.4)	237 (63.9)	134 (36.1)	0.963
< 2 years	24 (5.4)	16 (66.7)	8 (33.3)	
≥ 2 years	50 (11.20	32 (64.0)	18 (36.0)	

SD standard deviation

ethnicity or HbA1c level. Additionally, among patients with DM, only age and gender were found to be associated with adenomatous polyps. Being on insulin or just taking oral DM medications or the length of DM treatment were not associated with adenomatous polyps. There were only seven people with type 1 DM in the subsample, thus no further analysis was done in this group.

In multivariable logistic regression analysis, while the point estimate suggested an increase in odds of adenomatous polyps in patients with DM when compared to those without DM, this association was not statistically significant (*p* = 0.09) after adjusting for age, gender, race/ethnicity, and BMI (Table 3). There was no significant association between HbA1c level and adenomatous polyps when controlling for other factors, such as BMI. In secondary analysis of the subsample that only included patients with DM, neither the type of treatment (insulin vs. oral medications) nor length of treatment (none, < 2 years, or ≥ 2 years) was associated with adenomatous polyps (Table 4).

Discussion

In this retrospective cohort study, we found higher prevalence of colonoscopy-confirmed colorectal adenomatous polyps with older age, male gender, and higher BMI. Although having DM was significantly associated with higher prevalence of adenomatous polyps in the bivariate analysis, the association was attenuated in multivariable logistic regression after controlling for age, gender, BMI, and race/ethnicity. The odds ratio (1.25) was similar in value to that of published data (1.30), but it did not reach statistical significance (*P* = 0.09). In the subsample that included only patients with DM, we did not find any significant associations between HbA1c level, type or duration of DM treatment and prevalence of adenomatous polyps.

Table 3 Multivariable logistic regression predicting adenomatous polyps among chart review sample (*N* = 1798)

	Odds Ratio	95% CI		P value
		Lower	Upper	
Age (ref: ≤50 years)				
51~55	1.97	1.35	2.86	< 0.0001
56~60	2.00	1.36	2.94	< 0.0001
> 60	2.59	1.74	3.86	< 0.0001
Sex (ref: Female)	1.45	1.16	1.81	< 0.0001
Ethnicity (ref: Caucasian)				
African American	0.98	0.76	1.28	0.891
Hispanic	1.44	1.07	1.93	0.016
Asian	1.08	0.48	2.46	0.847
Other/unknown	1.08	0.40	2.94	0.879
Body mass index	1.02	1.00	1.04	0.022
Diabetes (ref: No)	1.25	0.97	1.62	0.091

ref reference group

Diabetes mellitus and hyperglycemia control on the risk of colorectal adenomatous...

211

Table 4 Multivariable logistic regression predicting colorectal adenomatous polyps among diabetes mellitus patients only (N = 445)

	Odds Ratio	95% CI		P value
		Lower	Upper	
Model 1				
Age (ref: ≤50)				
51~55	1.82	0.78	4.25	0.164
56~60	1.92	0.82	4.47	0.132
>60	2.93	1.26	6.85	0.013
Sex (ref: Female)	1.46	0.95	2.24	0.084
Ethnicity (ref: Caucasian)				
African American	0.84	0.52	1.36	0.479
Hispanic	1.25	0.69	2.28	0.463
Asian	1.36	0.33	5.63	0.673
Other/unknown	0.78	0.14	4.37	0.776
Body mass index	1.01	0.98	1.04	0.437
Oral medication exposure (ref: None)				
< 2 years	0.81	0.47	1.39	0.440
≥ 2 years	0.91	0.56	1.49	0.716
Model 2				
Age (ref: ≤50)				
51~55	1.80	0.77	4.18	0.175
56~60	1.88	0.81	4.38	0.145
>60	2.91	1.25	6.78	0.013
Sex (ref: female)	1.44	0.94	2.21	0.093
Ethnicity (ref: Caucasian)				
African American	0.84	0.52	1.36	0.480
Hispanic	1.24	0.68	2.26	0.477
Asian	1.27	0.31	5.23	0.738
Other/unknown	0.75	0.13	4.20	0.741
Body mass index	1.01	0.98	1.04	0.447
Insulin exposure (ref: None)				
< 2 years	1.01	0.40	2.54	0.978
≥ 2 years	1.03	0.53	1.99	0.938
Model 3				
Age (ref: ≤50)				
51~55	1.85	0.73	4.72	0.196
56~60	2.28	0.90	5.77	0.081
>60	3.58	1.42	9.06	0.007
Sex (ref: female)	1.47	0.94	2.30	0.092
Ethnicity (ref: Caucasian)				
African American	0.82	0.49	1.35	0.432
Hispanic	1.24	0.67	2.30	0.497
Asian	1.32	0.32	5.48	0.701
Other/unknown	0.75	0.13	4.27	0.747
Body mass index	1.01	0.98	1.04	0.483

Table 4 Multivariable logistic regression predicting colorectal adenomatous polyps among diabetes mellitus patients only (N = 445) (Continued)

	Odds Ratio	95% CI		P value
		Lower	Upper	
Hemoglobin A1c (ref: < 5.7)				
5.7–6.4	0.91	0.28	3.00	0.880
6.5–7.9	0.99	0.31	3.18	0.992
≥ 8.0	1.03	0.30	3.61	0.962

Model 1 is predicting polyps among diabetic patients on oral medication only; model 2 is predicting polyps among diabetic patients on insulin; and model 3 is predicting polyps among diabetic patients with different levels of Hemoglobin A1c level

The current literature is conflicting regarding the link between DM and colorectal adenomatous polyps. For example, Dash et al. [19], in a nested case-control study (917 cases and 2751 controls) among the Black Women's Health study, found no overall association between DM and risk of adenomatous polyps. In contrast, Suh et al. [6], in a retrospective study of 3505 patients in South Korea reported that patients with DM had a higher proportion of adenomatous polyps. Additionally, Eddi et al. [17], in a case-control study (261 cases and 522 matched controls) in the United States, found an increased risk between DM and colorectal adenomatous polyps. The reason for these contrasting results are not entirely clear but could be related to differences in the study design, population studied, and measurement and control of potential confounders such as BMI, dietary pattern and length of study follow-up. Further prospective cohort studies with a longer follow-up would be needed to clarify these issues.

Current literature is also conflicting regarding the link between glucose level and risk of colorectal adenomatous polyps. We did not find a significant association between HbA1c level and the risk of adenomatous polyps, which is consistent with that reported by multiple investigators [6, 17–19]. In contrast, Siddiqui et al. reported, in a retrospective study with 652 male patients, that diabetic patients with poor glycemic control had a significantly higher prevalence of right-sided adenomatous polyps [19]. This controversy may be a result of the inherent limitation of HbA1c level to reflect the duration or degree of hyperinsulinemia. Though it's a measure of glycemic control in DM patients, HbA1c level cannot be directly translated to the length or extent of hyperinsulinemia. Hyperinsulinemia appears to be a carcinogenic as well as the insulin-like growth factors (IGF) [26, 27]. Further research is needed to investigate this relationship.

The findings of this study confirmed that older age, male gender, and higher BMI were associated with the adenomatous polyps. However, no significant association between type or duration of DM treatment and adenomatous polyp was found as some studies suggested [17, 19]. For example, metformin has been reported to decrease colon adenomatous polyps while insulin therapy may increase them [28–30]. In this study, we could not separate metformin treatment from the use of other oral medications. In addition, the possible protective effect of metformin or the increased risk of insulin on colon adenomatous polyps remains very controversial [17, 19, 21, 26, 31]. While African-American race has been reported as a risk factor for colorectal cancer, data is limited regarding its association with precancerous polyps [32–37]. Our study did not find any significant association between African-American race and adenomatous polyps. Further studies are needed in this area as well.

This study has a number of strengths. It was a large retrospective cohort study of patients continually enrolled in a closed managed care organization for 10 years, with a diverse mix of race/ethnicity. The entire cohort had at least one colonoscopy and the identification of colorectal cancer and adenomatous polyp in the subsample were confirmed by reviewing colonoscopy pathology reports. In addition, the diagnosis of DM was confirmed by chart review, as compared to some of the previous studies where DM was self-reported. This study population that had been continuously enrolled in a closed managed care organization facilitated the inclusion of medication type and duration of DM treatment. Finally, only patients with a colonoscopy done in the second half of the 10-year study period were included in the study minimized the baseline heterogeneity of adenomatous polyp risk in our study population.

Limitations

This study has several limitations. First, as a retrospective cohort study, the study was limited to data reliably found in medical records. Information regarding the possible confounders such as smoking, physical activity, alcohol use, the length of DM and family history of CRC were not available. Second, CRC was not analyzed since there were too few CRC cases in this sample. Third, the study population included only patients who had undergone colonoscopy, which may not be representative of the general population. While our study population was diverse in its mix of race/ethnicity, it cannot be generalized to the entire U.S. population, as this region has overrepresentation of African American race/ethnicity (U.S. census 13% vs and 29% our sample) and underrepresentation of Caucasians (U.S. census 77%, vs. 48% our sample). Finally, the study time frame would exclude any CRC or adenomatous polyp that may have been identified before or after the study period.

Conclusions

Our study findings provide important information and context for future studies focusing on the association between DM and adenomatous polyp and CRC. The relationships between demographics, BMI, DM and its treatment on the development of adenomatous polyps and subsequently CRC are very complex. Up to now, data are inconclusive regarding DM and adenomatous polyp. Determining the effect of these risk factors and their complex interactions with each other on the risk of adenomatous polyp would be invaluable to primary care physicians and public health policy makers. These findings would have potential implications for more targeted CRC screening in individuals with DM, thereby decreasing the incidence rate and mortality from CRC. Considering the high prevalence of type 2 DM in the United States, even a small increase in cancer risk could have considerable consequences at a population level.

Abbreviations

BMI: Body mass index; CRC: Colorectal cancer; DM: Diabetes mellitus; HAP: Health Alliance Plan; HbA1c: Hemoglobin A1c; HEDIS: Healthcare Effectiveness Data and Information Set; HFHS: Henry Ford Health System; Ref: Reference group; SD: Standard deviation

Acknowledgements

We thank the residents Mohamed Eldirani, Nik Gjurashaj, Johnathon Justice, Wajeehullah Muhammad, Priya Murthy, Maliha Nafees, Brittany Okpagu, and Allison Simms for their assistance with the study. We thank Roger Tuttleman and Liying Zhang for their help with the data analysis.

Authors' contributions

KB set up the data protocol, performed chart review, analyzed and interpreted the data and took the lead in the writing process. LL and SS made substantial contribution in the conception and design, data collection, and analysis and interpretation of data. DP, DR and DWP actively participate in writing manuscript and interpreting data. JX made substantial contribution in data analysis, interpretation and writing process. All authors read and approved the final manuscript.

Competing interests

The authors declare that they have no competing interests.

Author details

[1]Department of Family Medicine, Henry Ford Hospital, Detroit, MI, USA. [2]Department of Family Medicine and Public Health Sciences, Wayne State University, Detroit, MI, USA. [3]Department of Family Medicine, Henry Ford Health System, 3370 E Jefferson, Detroit, MI 48207, USA.

References

1. American Cancer Society. Cancer facts and figures 2015. Atlanta: American Cancer Society; 2015.
2. National Cancer Institute. SEER cancer statistics factsheets: colon and rectum cancer. 2015 https://seer.cancer.gov/statfacts/html/colorect.html. Accessed Apr 2015.
3. U. S. Preventive Services Task Force, Bibbins-Domingo K, Grossman DC, Curry SJ, Davidson KW, Epling JW Jr, et al. Screening for colorectal cancer: US preventive services task force recommendation statement. JAMA. 2016; 315:2564–75.
4. Heitman SJ, Ronksley PE, Hilsden RJ, Manns BJ, Rostom A, Hemmelgarn BR. Prevalence of adenomas and colorectal cancer in average risk individuals: a systematic review and meta-analysis. Clin Gastroenterol Hepatol. 2009;7: 1272–8.
5. Deng L, Gui Z, Zhao L, Wang J, Shen L. Diabetes mellitus and the incidence of colorectal cancer: an updated systematic review and meta-analysis. Dig Dis Sci. 2012;57:1576–85.
6. Suh S, Kang M, Kim MY, Chung HS, Kim SK, Hur KY, et al. Korean type 2 diabetes patients have multiple adenomatous polyps compared to non-diabetic controls. J Korean Med Sci. 2011;26:1196–200.
7. Wu L, Yu C, Jiang H, Tang J, Huang HL, Gao J, et al. Diabetes mellitus and the occurrence of colorectal cancer: an updated meta-analysis of cohort studies. Diabetes Technol Ther. 2013;15:419–27.
8. Yuhara H, Steinmaus C, Cohen SE, Corley DA, Tei Y, Buffler PA. Is diabetes mellitus an independent risk factor for colon cancer and rectal cancer? Am J Gastroenterol. 2011;106:1911–21.
9. Giovannucci E. Insulin and colon cancer. Cancer Causes Control. 1995;6:164–79.
10. Giovannucci E. Insulin, insulin-like growth factors and colon cancer: a review of the evidence. J Nutr. 2001;131:3109s–20s.
11. Schoen RE, Weissfeld JL, Kuller LH, Thaete FL, Evans RW, Hayes RB, et al. Insulin-like growth factor-I and insulin are associated with the presence and advancement of adenomatous polyps. Gastroenterology. 2005;129:464–75.
12. Soubry A, Il'yasova D, Sedjo R, Wang F, Byers T, Rosen C, et al. Increase in circulating levels of IGF-1 and IGF-1/IGFBP-3 molar ratio over a decade is associated with colorectal adenomatous polyps. Int J Cancer. 2012;131:512–7.
13. Renehan AG, Zwahlen M, Minder C, O'Dwyer ST, Shalet SM, Egger M. Insulin-like growth factor (IGF)-I, IGF binding protein-3, and cancer risk: systematic review and meta-regression analysis. Lancet. 2004;363:1346–53.
14. Center for Disease Control and Prevention. National diabetes fact sheet: national estimates and general information on diabetes and prediabetes in the United States, 2011. Atlanta: US Department of Health and Human Services, Center for Disease Control and Prevention; 2011.
15. Engelgau MM, Geiss LS, Saaddine JB, Boyle JP, Benjamin SM, Gregg EW, et al. The evolving diabetes burden in the United States. Ann Intern Med. 2004;140:945–50.
16. Doubeni CA, Laiyemo AO, Klabunde CN, Young AC, Field TS, Fletcher RH. Racial and ethnic trends of colorectal cancer screening among Medicare enrollees. Am J Prev Med. 2010;38:184–91.
17. Eddi R, Karki A, Shah A, DeBari VA, DePasquale JR. Association of type 2 diabetes and colon adenomas. J Gastrointest Cancer. 2012;43:87–92.
18. Kim BC, Shin A, Hong CW, Sohn DK, Han KS, Ryu KH, et al. Association of colorectal adenoma with components of metabolic syndrome. Cancer Causes Control. 2012;23:727–35.
19. Dash C, Palmer JR, Boggs DA, Rosenberg L, Adams-Campbell LL. Type 2 diabetes and the risk of colorectal adenomas: black Women's health study. Am J Epidemiol. 2014;179:112–9.
20. Huang X, Fan Y, Zhang H, Wu J, Zhang X, Luo H. Association between serum HbA1c levels and adenomatous polyps in patients with the type 2 diabetes mellitus. Minerva Endocrinol. 2015;40:163–7.
21. Siddiqui AA, Maddur H, Naik S, Cryer B. The association of elevated HbA1c on the behavior of adenomatous polyps in patients with type-II diabetes mellitus. Dig Dis Sci. 2008;53:1042–7.
22. Vu HT, Ufere N, Yan Y, Wang JS, Early DS, Elwing JE. Diabetes mellitus increases risk for colorectal adenomas in younger patients. World J Gastroenterol. 2014;20:6946–52.
23. National Committee for Quality Assurance. Proposed changes to existing measure for HEDIS®1 2015: comprehensive diabetes care (CDC). 2014.

http://www.ncqa.org/Portals/0/HEDISQM/Hedis2015/List_of_HEDIS_2015_Measures.pdf. Accessed 8 Dec 2017.
24. Kasper DL, Braunwald E, Fauci AS, Hauser SL, Longo DL, Jameson JL. Harrison's principles of internal medicine. 16th ed. New York: McGraw-Hill; 2005.
25. James PT, Leach R, Kalamara E, Shayeghi M. The worldwide obesity epidemic. Obes Res. 2001;9:228S–33S.
26. Kath R, Schiel R, Muller UA, Hoffken K. Malignancies in patients with insulin-treated diabetes mellitus. J Cancer Res Clin Oncol. 2000;126:412–7.
27. Rodeck U, Herlyn M, Menssen HD, Furlanetto RW, Koprowsk H. Metastatic but not primary melanoma cell lines grow in vitro independently of exogenous growth factors. Int J Cancer. 1987;40:687–90.
28. Yang YX, Hennessy S, Lewis JD. Insulin therapy and colorectal cancer risk among type 2 diabetes mellitus patients. Gastroenterology. 2004;127:1044–50.
29. Zhang ZJ, Zheng ZJ, Kan H, Song Y, Cui W, Zhao G, et al. Reduced risk of colorectal cancer with metformin therapy in patients with type 2 diabetes: a meta-analysis. Diabetes Care. 2011;34:2323–8.
30. Chung YW, Han DS, Park KH, Eun CS, Yoo KS, Park CK. Insulin therapy and colorectal adenoma risk among patients with type 2 diabetes mellitus: a case-control study in Korea. Dis Colon Rectum. 2008;51:593–7.
31. Schiel R, Muller UA, Braun A, Stein G, Kath R. Risk of malignancies in patients with insulin-treated diabetes mellitus: results of a population-based trial with 10-year follow-up (JEVIN). Eur J Med Res. 2005;10:339–44.
32. Chien C, Morimoto LM, Tom J, Li CI. Differences in colorectal carcinoma stage and survival by race and ethnicity. Cancer. 2005;104:629–39.
33. Jemal A, Siegel R, Ward E, Hao Y, Xu J, Murray T, et al. Cancer statistics, 2008. CA Cancer J Clin. 2008;58:71–96.
34. Mostafa G, Matthews BD, Norton HJ, Kercher KW, Sing RF, Heniford BT. Influence of demographics on colorectal cancer. Am Surg. 2004;70:259–64.
35. Robbins AS, Siegel RL, Jemal A. Racial disparities in stage-specific colorectal cancer mortality rates from 1985 to 2008. J Clin Oncol. 2012;30:401–5.
36. Tawk R, Abner A, Ashford A, Brown CP. Differences in colorectal cancer outcomes by race and insurance. Int J Environ Res Public Health. 2015;13:E48.
37. Wilkins T, Gillies RA, Harbuck S, Garren J, Looney SW, Schade RR. Racial disparities and barriers to colorectal cancer screening in rural areas. J Am Board Fam Med. 2012;25:308–17.

23

The influence of gender concordance between general practitioner and patient on antibiotic prescribing for sore throat symptoms

D. Eggermont[1*†] ⓘ, M. A. M. Smit[1†], G. A. Kwestroo[1†], R. A. Verheij[2], K. Hek[2] and A. E. Kunst[1]

Abstract

Background: Patient gender as well as doctor gender are known to affect doctor-patient interaction during a medical consultation. It is however not known whether an interaction of gender influences antibiotic prescribing. This study examined GP's prescribing behavior of antibiotics at the first presentation of patients with sore throat symptoms in primary care. We investigated whether GP gender, patient gender and gender concordance have an effect on the GP's prescribing behavior of antibiotics in protocolled and non-protocolled diagnoses.

Methods: We analyzed electronic health record data of 11,285 GP practice consultations in the Netherlands in 2013 extracted from the Nivel Primary Care Database. Our primary outcome was the prescription of antibiotics for throat symptoms. Sore throat symptoms were split up in 'protocolled diagnoses' and 'non-protocolled diagnoses'. The association between gender concordance and antibiotic prescription was estimated with multilevel regression models that controlled for patient age and comorbidity.

Results: Antibiotic prescription was found to be lower among female GPs (OR 0.88, CI 95% 0.67–1.09; $p = .265$) and female patients (OR 0.93, 95% 0.84–1.02; $p = .142$), but observed differences were not statistically significant. The difference in prescription rates by gender concordance were small and not statistically significant in non-protocolled consultations (OR 0.92, OR 95% CI: 0.83–1.01; $p = .099$), protocolled consultations (OR 1.00, OR 95% CI: 0.68–1.32; $p = .996$) and all GP practice consultations together (OR 0.92, OR 95% CI: 0.82–1.02; $p = .118$). Within the female GP group, however, gender concordance was associated with reduced prescribing of antibiotics (OR 0.85, OR 95% CI: 0.72–0.99; $p = 0.034$).

Conclusions: In this study, female GPs prescribed antibiotics less often than male GPs, especially in consultation with female patients. This study shows that, in spite of clinical guidelines, gender interaction may influence the prescription of antibiotics with sore throat symptoms.

Keywords: Gender role, Anti-bacterial agents, Drug resistance, Prescriptions, Sore throat, General practitioner

Background

Bacterial resistance is an important topic in today's health policy [1]. Although growing microbacterial resistance is partly a natural process, it can be accelerated with the inappropriate prescription of antibiotics by health care professionals [2]. With this in mind, factors which influence the prescription of antibiotics, other than patient's clinical presentation, became an object of study. Indeed, research suggests the importance of such non-medical factors. General practitioners' (GPs) attitudes such as fear and complacency affect prescribing behavior [3, 4]. Akkerman showed that physicians with more years of practice were more likely to prescribe antibiotics, especially if they felt they had little time per patient [5]. Moreover, GP's perception of patients' expectations concerning medication prescription influences the actual prescribing behavior [6–8]. Overall, these studies imply that doctor-patient interaction

* Correspondence: d.eggermont@amc.uva.nl
†D. Eggermont, Smit MAM and G. A. Kwestroo contributed equally to this work.
¹Department of Public Health, Amsterdam UMC, University of Amsterdam, Meibergdreef 9, Amsterdam 1105, AZ, the Netherlands
Full list of author information is available at the end of the article

has an important influence on antibiotic prescribing behavior.

When focusing on the doctor-patient relationship, the gender of both the doctor and patient are known to influence their interaction [9, 10]. Among others, the GP's gender may determine the communication style, the contents of the consultation, which drugs are indicated and whether they are prescribed [11–13]. In turn, the gender of the patient also affects the interaction between doctor and patient. For example, female patients are more likely to express their emotions during the consultation [14] and had fewer discussions about addictive behavior or heart disease risk [9, 15]. This implies that GPs might make medical decisions which are affected by gender-related considerations and gender stereotypes.

Since both patient's and doctor's gender play a part in the medical process, it is not unlikely that the combination of a patient and doctor of the same gender (compared to dyads of opposite gender) may have additional effects. In interactions between patient and doctor, four gender dyads can be distinguished (male-male, female-female, male-female, female-male) of which two are concordant and two are discordant. It has been found that female-female consultations contain more affective talk and less analytical talk. The opposite occurs in male-male consultations [16]. Moreover, it appears that female concordance leads to communication that is most patient centered [17, 18], which may enhance health outcomes by elevated patients' trust, improved communication and patient satisfaction. Indeed, female gender concordance is associated with more effective treatment of cardiovascular risks [19] and male gender concordance is positively associated with measures on diet, nutrition and exercise counseling [20]. It is however not known whether gender concordance influences prescribing behavior of antibiotics. Possibly, concordance is an additional non-medical factor that affects (inappropriate) antibiotics prescription. Creating awareness of such non-medial factors could result in GPs being less biased, more objective and consistent in their treatments.

Since the 1980's there is an increase in the extent to which primary care practice is influenced by clinical guidelines [21]. For example, some diagnoses are followed by guidelines that leave the physician room to follow a treatment of choice ('non-protocolled' guidelines). Other diagnoses have guidelines in which a 'protocolled' treatment (e.g. antibiotic prescription) is strongly recommended. The power of a clinical guideline is to make sure the patient gets the most effective, evidence-based treatment. A guideline also reduces the variation in treatment for the same diagnoses between GPs.

In this study, we will explore whether the prescription of antibiotics depends on the patients or physicians gender and/or on their gender interaction (concordance). To do this, we will study prescribing behavior concerning patients presenting sore throat symptoms in primary care. This patient group was chosen since the inappropriate prescription of antibiotics is very common in sore throat symptoms [22] and because the majority of antibiotic prescriptions in The Netherlands is issued in primary care [23]. In addition, we will investigate whether gender concordance is less influential in diagnoses corresponding to a strong antibacterial protocol than in diagnoses that leave the GP more room for interpretation and choice.

Methods

The specific objectives of this study were to explore:

1. whether the likelihood that patients will be given a medical prescription depends on the gender of, respectively, the patient and the GP.
2. whether this likelihood depends on the gender concordance between patient and GP, with distinction between male-male and female-female concordance.
3. the role of gender and of gender concordance for prescription policy in non-protocolled guidelines and protocolled guidelines.

Data source

The electronic health records for this study were provided by the Netherlands Institute for Health Services Research (Nivel) Primary Care Database, containing GP practice consultations from 2013. We included general practices that registered information on the function and sex of caregiver. Moreover, the data included information on consultations, prescriptions (coded according to the Anatomical Therapeutical Chemical (ATC) classification) and diagnosis (coded according to the International Classification of Primary Care (ICPC) version 1) [24]. These consultations were handled by health professionals of whom 225, according to information provided by the practice, were known to be trained as GP. Other health professionals were for example physiotherapist, physician assistant, dietician or practice nurse. We used data from 22,412 GP practice consultations concerning patients with sore throat symptoms.

Variables

The electronic health records data contained information on: prescription of antibiotics (did or did not prescribe a medicine with ATC-code J01, which are antibiotics for systemic use), sex of both patient and caregiver, age of patient, function of caregiver (e.g. physiotherapist, physician assistant, dietician, nurse etc.), comorbidity (did or did not suffer from one or more chronic disease according to the GP's medical file) and ICPC-code. The ICPC classification system is used to record diagnosis and/or symptoms. This study focuses on ICPC codes relating to sore throat symptoms (see Table 1). Using the ICPC code, we distinguished between diagnoses based on symptoms versus those based on underlying pathology. ICPC-codes R21 and R22 represent symptoms (e.g. coughing) indicating that at the time of the consultation no real diagnosis (e.g. tonsillitis) was apparent.

We also measured whether the disease was 'protocolled'. For this, the ICPC code R76 (acute tonsillitis/peritonsillar abscess) was regarded as protocolled. The Dutch GP guideline for acute sore throat complaints firmly advises to prescribe antibiotics for this diagnosis [25]. Other ICPC-codes related to sore throat were classified as non-protocolled, i.e. antibiotics are not indicated. To determine the presence of an antibiotic treatment protocol, the GP guideline was analyzed independently by three coders. Intercoder agreement was 100%, as all coders regarded the same ICPC-codes as either 'protocolled' and 'non-protocolled'.

Exclusion criteria

The following exclusion criteria were used to select patients and GP practice consultations for the analyses:

1. This study focuses on the gender interaction between patient and GP in the general practice. Hence, all practice consultations with other health care professionals within the practice (e.g. medical student, physician assistant, dietician, etc.) were excluded.
2. In the communication between a GP and a child, parents are usually involved [26]. Consequently, the

gender interaction between child and GP is complicated by the gender of the parent that is present during the consultation. Therefore, all children (age 0 to 17) were excluded from the study.
3. At first presentation, all treatment options are still possible and patient-doctor interaction may be decisive for prescription. Therefore, we decided to focus on first consultations, which implied that all second and consecutive practice consultations in 2013 for sore throat symptoms were excluded.

Descriptives and demographics

After selecting only the practice consultations handled by a GP, 20511 (91.5%) consultations were available for analysis (see Fig. 1). The second exclusion criterion (only 18+ patients) brought our dataset back from 20,511 to 12,523 (61.1%) consultations. Finally, after applying our last exclusion criterion (only first presentation), 11,285 (55.0%) first consultations, handled by 225 GPs, remained for analysis.

Statistical analyses

Logistic regression was performed to calculate the effect of our main predictors on our outcome variable 'prescription of antibiotics' (dichotomous). In the regression model, our main predictors for antibiotic prescription were patient gender, GP gender and concordance. Patient's age and comorbidity were added as control variables. We also tested whether GP's gender and gender concordance had an interaction effect by creating an interaction term and adding this to the regression model along with its constituting variables. In addition, in further analyses, the regression models were calculated separately for protocolled and non-protocolled prescriptions. In order to explore whether the main predictors have different effects on male and female GP's, the regression models were also calculated separately for male and female GP's consultations.

Due to clustering of observations at the level of GPs and health practices, we applied multi-level models. In a generalized linear mixed model, we entered three different data levels: [1] practice, [2] GP and [3] patient. All analyses were performed with statistical package SPSS versions 22.

Privacy

Dutch law allows the use of electronic health records for research purposes under certain conditions. According to the legislation, neither obtaining informed consent from patients nor approval by a medical ethics committee is obligatory for this type of observational studies containing no directly identifiable data [27]. This study has been approved by the applicable governance bodies of NIVEL Primary Care Database under number NZR-00315.025.

Table 1 Diagnoses for sore throat symptoms

ICPC-code	Diagnoses	Percentage of all consultations ($n = 11,285$)	Protocolled	Symptoms/no diagnosis
R21	Symptoms/complaints throat	19.8%	No	Yes
R22	Symptoms/complaints tonsils	1.0%	No	Yes
R72	Streptococcus/scarlet fever	1.3%	No	No
R74	Acute infection upper airway	67.4%	No	No
R76	Acute tonsillitis/peritonsillar abscess	8.5%	Yes	No
R77	Acute laryngitis/tracheitis	1.9%	No	No

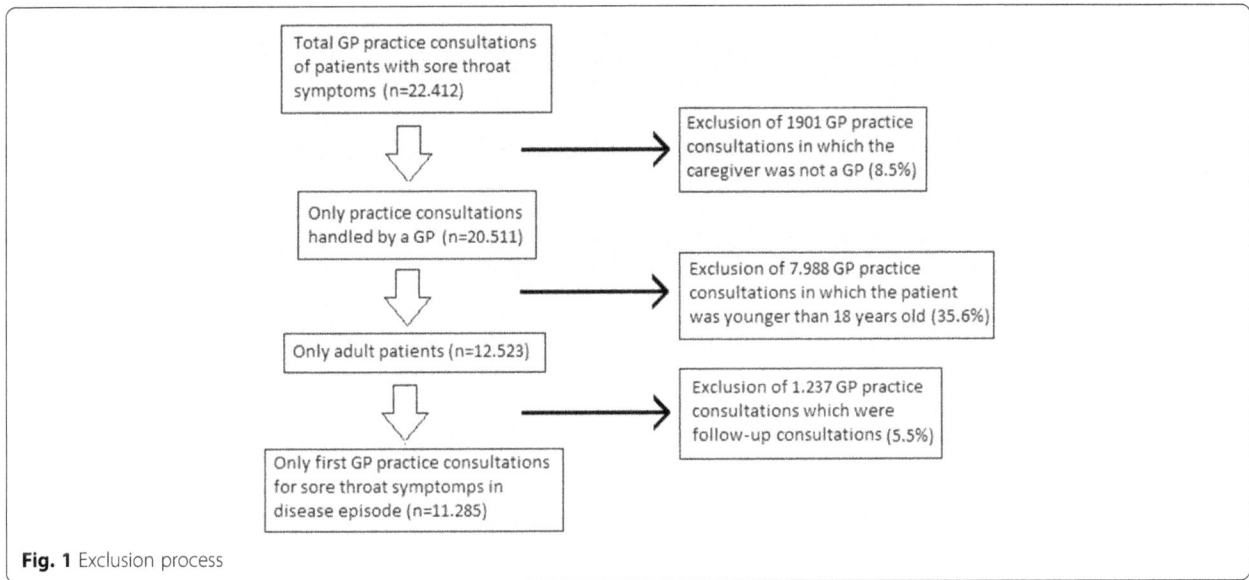

Fig. 1 Exclusion process

Results

Of all GP practice consultations, 52.1% were handled by male GPs. In 39.2% of the consultations the patient was male. Of all cases 27.6% of the patients were prescribed antibiotics. The concordant dyads are represented with 52.8% of the consultations, while 47.2% of the consultations contained discordant couples. For all consultations, 8.5% got assigned an ICPC code labeled as protocolled and 91.5% as non-protocolled.

Table 2 shows that patient age, presence of comorbidity and the amount of consultations without a real diagnosis were similar in consultations with male and female GPs. Male GPs prescribed antibiotics in 29.5% of their consultations. Female GPs did so in 25.7% of their consultations. For female GPs, 64.1% of their consultations were concordant (i.e. with a female patients), while male GPs had same-sex consultations in 42.3% of their consultations. The concordant couples had an antibiotic prescription rate of 26.8% of the consultations, against 28.6% in discordant couples.

Figure 2 shows the percentage of antibiotics prescribed per gender dyad. In accordance with Table 2, it illustrates that female GPs prescribe less antibiotics than male GPs. Female GPs especially prescribe less antibiotics for female patients (24.8% in concordant couples versus 27.3% in discordant couples). In consultations

Table 2 Descriptive of patients seen by male GP vs female GP and concordant vs discordant couples

	Male GP	Female GP	Concordant	Discordant
Sample size	5956	5329	5956	5329
Average age patient (years)	46.7	46.3	46.6	46.4
Comorbidity patient	53.6%	52.5%	53.3%	52.7%
Concordance	42.3%	64.1%	–	–
Symptoms / no diagnosis	20.3%	21.4%	21.5%	20.1%
Protocolled diagnoses	7.9%	9.1%	8.4%	8.6%
Antibiotics prescribed				
All diagnoses	29.5%	25.7%	26.8%	28.6%
-Male GP	–	–	29.6%	29.4%
-Female GP	–	–	24.8%	27.3%
In non-protocolled diagnoses	25.6%	21.5%	22.8%	24.6%
-Male GP	–	–	25.8%	25.5%
-Female GP	–	–	20.7%	23.0%
In protocolled diagnoses	74.1%	67.3%	69.7%	71.7%
-Male GP	–	–	76.9%	72.3%
-Female GP	–	–	65.5%	70.7%

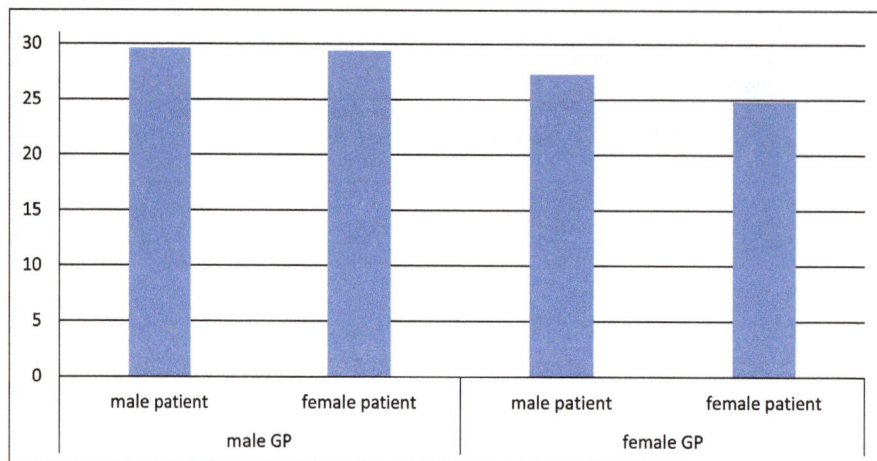

Fig. 2 Percentage of consultations for sore throat symptoms with antibiotic prescription. Female GP's prescribe antibiotics less often than male GP's ($p = .000$). In dyads with a female GP, antibiotics are less often prescribed when there is gender concordance ($p = .044$)

with male GPs, on the other hand, there is no such difference (concordant couples 29.6% versus 29.4% in discordant couples).

Table 3 shows the outcome of the multilevel regression analysis. In the total population, concordance (OR 0.92, OR

Table 3 Predictors for antibiotic prescription after multi-level analysis[a]

	Exp (B)	Lower	Upper	Significance
All GP practice consultations ($n = 11,285$)[b]				
Concordance	0.92	0.83	1.01	$p = .099$
Gender GP	0.88	0.67	1.09	$p = .265$
Gender patient	0.93	0.84	1.02	$p = .142$
Comorbidity	1.09	0.99	1.18	$p = .090$
Age patient	1.00	1.00	1.00	$p = .022$
Non-protocolled ($n = 10,328$)[c]				
Concordance	0.92	0.82	1.02	$p = .118$
Gender GP	0.83	0.58	1.08	$p = .180$
Gender patient	0.96	0.85	1.06	$p = .404$
Comorbidity	1.21	1.01	1.32	$p = .000$
Age patient	1.00	0.99	1.00	$p = .000$
Protocolled ($n = 957$)[d]				
Concordance	1.00	0.68	1.32	$p = .996$
Gender GP	0.65	0.26	1.04	$p = .076$
Gender patient	0.79	0.47	1.10	$p = .184$
Comorbidity	0.92	0.57	1.26	$p = .633$
Age patient	0.98	0.96	0.99	$p = .002$

[a]These findings are based on mulit-level logistic regression analysis
[b]There was no interaction effect of concordance and gender GP ($p = .225$)
[c]There was no interaction effect of concordance and gender GP ($p = .272$)
[d]There was no interaction effect of concordance and gender GP ($p = .145$)

95% CI: 0.83–1.01), female GP (OR 0.88, 95% CI: 0.67–1.09) and female patient (OR 0.93, 95% CI: 0.84–1.02) show lower rates of antibiotic prescription, however not with statistical significance. Similar results were found in both types of prescriptions (protocolled and non-protocolled). Patient age was significantly associated with antibiotics prescription (OR 1.00, 95% CI: 1.00–1.00). This was equally true for protocolled and non-protocolled consultations. Comorbidity was a significant predictor in non-protocolled consultations (OR 1.21, 95% CI: 1.01–1.32), but not in the protocolled consultations (OR 0.92, 95% CI: 0.57–1.26).

Table 4 shows that for female GPs concordance is associated with antibiotic prescription after controlling for comorbidity and patient age. In female concordant consultations less antibiotics were prescribed (OR 0.85, 95% CL: 0.72–0.99). The lower section of Table 4 shows that for male GPs concordance is not associated with antibiotic prescription after controlling for comorbidity and patient age (OR 0.99, 95% CL: 0.86–1.11).

Discussion

Summary of results

In this study, we assessed whether gender concordance between GP and patient was associated with antibiotics prescribing. Gender concordance among females is associated with less prescription of antibiotics, i.e. female GPs appear to issue fewer antibiotics prescriptions to female patients than to male patients. Concordance appears not to have a similar effect in prescribing behavior of male GPs. For both concordant dyads combined, prescription rates were lower than for discordant dyads, but this difference was not statistically significant. Whether the treatment was protocolled did not appear to affect these findings.

Table 4 The model of predictors for antibiotic prescription according to gender of GP[a]

	Practice consultations with female GP (n = 5410)				Practice consultations with male GP (n = 5875)			
	Exp (B)	Lower	Upper	Significance	Exp (B)	Lower	Upper	Significance
Concordance	0.85	0.72	0.99	p = .034	0.99	0.86	1.11	p = .827
Comorbidity	1.16	1.02	1.31	p = .028	1.02	0.89	1.16	p = .731
Age patient	1.00	1.00	1.01	p = .063	1.00	1.00	1.00	p = .193

[a]These findings are based on mulit-level logistic regression analysis

Interpretation of results

When a patient with sore throat symptoms presents him- or herself in a primary care facility, infection is usually the underlying cause [28]. For these symptoms, physicians can send their patient home for a 'wait and see' policy or they can prescribe antibiotics. The results of this study indicate that female physicians are more likely to apply a wait and see policy when seeing a female patient in comparison with the other gender dyads.

Female concordance has been associated with a communication style that is more patient centered [17, 18]. Patient centered communication enhances health outcomes by elevated patients' trust, improved communication and patient satisfaction [17–20, 29]. When communication is patient centered, the physician focuses at hearing and understanding the patients' perspectives. For this, the physician needs to explore the patients ideas and concerns as well as their expectations regarding the physician [30]. It has been shown that addressing patients' ideas, concerns and expectations during a consultation, known as the ICE-model, might lead to fewer medication prescriptions [31]. This is potentially important because a wait and see policy is easier to adopt when patients feel being heard.

In our study, 27.6% of all patients got prescribed antibiotics for their sore throat complaints. This is low in comparison to other countries. In the UK, for example, approximately 56% of all patients with sore throat complaints receive antibiotics from their GP [32]. Traditionally, antibiotic prescription in the Netherlands is lowest of all European countries, with differences up to a threefold [33]. It is unclear how this relates to the outcomes of our study. Therefore, generalizing our findings to countries with much higher antibiotic prescription rate should be done with caution.

Patient age and comorbidity were identified as being predictive for prescribing antibiotics. This was in line with previous research which showed age to be a determinant in the prescription of antibiotics for lower respiratory tract infections and that antibiotics are more often prescribed for patients with comorbidity such as diabetes or chronic obstructive pulmonary disease [34].

Limitations of the study

This study was performed with electronic health records data that were routinely recorded in general practices. This type of data has advantages and disadvantages. Advantages are that the data is cheap, readily available and can be assumed in many respects to represent what actually takes place in clinical practice. However, it also means that circumstances, habits and customs of individual practices in the way data are recorded, can have an impact on the quality of the data [35]. In this study this may have contributed to the fact that we had to exclude 8.5% of all consultations. These consultations had to be excluded because these consultations did not appear to have taken place with the GP but with other practice personnel. The percentage of consultations with the GP is likely to be an underestimate. Some of the consultations may have been taken care of by the GP, but recorded by a practice assistant.

In this study, we would have liked to include age of the GP. It has been shown that the years of experience of the GP correlates with antibiotics prescription [5]. Because, on average, male GPs are older than female GPs [36], age might have been a confounder in this study. Another limitation is that we could not include information on patients' expectations and concerns, which might also influence prescribing behavior [31].

Although the existence of comorbidity was reported by the GP, in this study we regarded comorbidities as present or non-present and did not investigate the role of individual comorbidities. However, COPD and diabetes are examples of diseases which affect susceptibility to disease and therefore possibly influence the prescribing behavior of the GP to a greater extent than most other diseases. In future research it would be important to include these comorbidities separately.

The current study focused solely on sore throat. Therefore, generalizing our findings to other complaints or symptoms should be done with caution. Future research should assess for a broader spectrum of symptoms whether prescription rates are related to gender concordance. Also, sore throat symptoms can be considered relatively gender neutral. This would be different when for example urogenital symptoms were concerned. This could change the effect of gender concordance.

Further research could focus on the effect of gender concordance on antibiotics.

Implications of this study

In recent years the medical community in western societies has experienced a growth in number of female physicians [36]. The results of this study suggest that this feminization could lead to a reduction in the prescription of antibiotics. Female concordance enhances patient centred communication and this might be the underlying explanation for our findings. If so, our results underline the importance of effective communication styles, both by male and female GPs, to contain the prescription of antibiotics.

Conclusion

In this study, we found that gender concordance among females is associated with less prescription of antibiotics for sore throat complaints. In other words, female GPs appear to issue fewer antibiotics prescriptions to female patients than to male patients. Among male GPs, concordance did not appear to have a similar effect. Possibly, our findings can be explained by a different communication style that is handled by female GPs, especially when attending with female patients. Future studies should aim to describe and understand female concordance in more detail, since the findings may suggest that training doctors to adjust their communication style could prevent the prescription of unnecessary antibiotics.

Abbreviations

ATC: Anatomical therapeutical chemical; GP: General Practitioner; ICPC: International classification of primary care; Nivel: Netherlands institute for health services research

Acknowledgments

Not applicable.

Funding

The financial resources required for the publication of this study were made available by UvA-AMC and Nivel.

Authors' contributions

DE, MAMS and GAK wrote the study proposal, analyzed and interpreted the patient data and were the main authors of the manuscript. AK supervised the research project, contributed to the text of the manuscript and was also a major contributor to the study design. RV and KH contributed to the design of the study and the text of the manuscript. AK, RV and KH critically reviewed consecutive draft versions of the manuscript. All authors read and approved the final manuscript.

Authors' information

DE has a master in communications and is currently a medical student in his master phase at the University of Amsterdam – Academic Medical Centre.

MAMS is a medical student in his master phase at the University of Amsterdam – Academic Medical Centre.
GAK is a medical student in his master phase at the University of Amsterdam – Academic Medical Centre.
AK is a professor in social epidemiology and head of the Department of Public Health at the University of Amsterdam – Academic Medical Centre.
RV is programme leader "Big Data & Learning health systems" at the Netherlands Institute for Health Services Research (NIVEL).
KH is postdoctorate researcher at the Netherlands Institute for Health Services Research (NIVEL).

Competing interests

The authors declare that they have no competing interests.

Author details

¹Department of Public Health, Amsterdam UMC, University of Amsterdam, Meibergdreef 9, Amsterdam 1105, AZ, the Netherlands. ²Netherlands Institute for Health Services Research (Nivel), Otterstraat 118-124, Utrecht 3513, CR, the Netherlands.

References

1.   Prestinaci F, Pezzotti P, Pantosti A. Antimicrobial resistance: a global multifaceted phenomenon. Pathogens and global health. 2015;109(7):309–18.
2.   Costelloe C, Metcalfe C, Lovering A, Mant D, Hay AD. Effect of antibiotic prescribing in primary care on antimicrobial resistance in individual patients: systematic review and meta-analysis. BMJ. 2010;340:c2096.
3.   Vazquez-Lago JM, Lopez-Vazquez P, López-Durán A, Taracido-Trunk M, Figueiras A. Attitudes of primary care physicians to the prescribing of antibiotics and antimicrobial resistance: a qualitative study from Spain. Fam Pract. 2012;29(3):352–60.
4.   Teixeira Rodrigues A, Roque F, Falcao A, Figueiras A, Herdeiro MT. Understanding physician antibiotic prescribing behaviour: a systematic review of qualitative studies. Int J Antimicrob Agents. 2013;41(3):203–12.
5.   Akkerman AE, Kuyvenhoven MM, van der Wouden JC, Verheij TJ. Prescribing antibiotics for respiratory tract infections by GPs: management and prescriber characteristics. Br J Gen Pract. 2005;55(511):114–8.
6.   Lado E, Vacariza M, Fernandez-Gonzalez C, Gestal-Otero JJ, Figueiras A. Influence exerted on drug prescribing by patients' attitudes and expectations and by doctors' perception of such expectations: a cohort and nested case-control study. J Eval Clin Pract. 2008;14(3):453–9.
7.   Altiner A, Knauf A, Moebes J, Sielk M, Wilm S. Acute cough: a qualitative analysis of how GPs manage the consultation when patients explicitly or implicitly expect antibiotic prescriptions. Fam Pract. 2004;21(5):500–6.
8.   Coenen S, Francis N, Kelly M, Hood K, Nuttall J, Little P, et al. Are patient views about antibiotics related to clinician perceptions, management and outcome? A multi-country study in outpatients with acute cough. PLoS One. 2013;8(10):e76691.
9.   Bertakis KD. The influence of gender on the doctor–patient interaction. Patient Educ Couns. 2009;76(3):356–60.
10. Adams A, Buckingham CD, Lindenmeyer A, McKinlay JB, Link C, Marceau L, et al. The influence of patient and doctor gender on diagnosing coronary heart disease. Sociology of health & illness. 2008;30(1):1–18.
11. Franks P, Bertakis KD. Physician gender, patient gender, and primary care. J Women's Health. 2003;12(1):73–80.
12. van den Brink-Muinen A. Sekseverschillen en de communicatie tussen huisarts en patiënt. Bijblijven. 2008;24:7–13.
13. Lagro-Janssen AL. Medicine is not gender-neutral: influence of physician sex on medical care. Ned Tijdschr Geneeskd. 2008;152(20):1141–5.
14. STEWART M. Patient characteristics which are related to the doctor-patient interaction. Fam Pract. 1984;1(1):30–6.
15. Grunau GL, Ratner PA, Galdas PM, Hossain S. Ethnic and gender differences in patient education about heart disease risk and prevention. Patient Educ Couns. 2009;76(2):181–8.
16. Van den Brink-Muinen A, van Dulmen S, Messerli-Rohrbach V, Bensing J. Do gender-dyads have different communication patterns? A comparative study in Western-European general practices. Patient Educ Couns. 2002;48(3):253–64.

The influence of gender concordance between general practitioner and patient on antibiotic...

221

17. Sandhu H, Adams A, Singleton L, Clark-Carter D, Kidd J. The impact of gender dyads on doctor-patient communication: a systematic review. Patient Educ Couns. 2009;76(3):348–55.

18. Bertakis KD, Azari R. Patient-centered care: the influence of patient and resident physician gender and gender concordance in primary care. J Womens Health (Larchmt). 2012;21(3):326–33.

19. Schmittdiel JA, Traylor A, Uratsu CS, Mangione CM, Ferrara A, Subramanian U. The association of patient-physician gender concordance with cardiovascular disease risk factor control and treatment in diabetes. J Womens Health (Larchmt). 2009;18(12):2065–70.

20. Pickett-Blakely O, Bleich SN, Cooper LA. Patient-physician gender concordance and weight-related counseling of obese patients. Am J Prev Med. 2011;40(6):616–9.

21. Woolf SH, Grol R, Hutchinson A, Eccles M, Grimshaw J. Clinical guidelines: potential benefits, limitations, and harms of clinical guidelines. BMJ. 1999; 318(7182):527.

22. Dekker AR, Verheij TJ, van der Velden AW. Inappropriate antibiotic prescription for respiratory tract indications: most prominent in adult patients. Fam Pract. 2015;32(4):401–7.

23. Butler CC, Hillier S, Roberts Z, Dunstan F, Howard A, Palmer S. Antibiotic-resistant infections in primary care are symptomatic for longer and increase workload: outcomes for patients with E. coli UTIs. Br J Gen Pract. 2006;56(530):686–92.

24. Wood M, Lamberts H. International classification of primary care: prepared for the world organisation of national colleges, academies and academic associations of general practitioners/family physicians (WONCA) by the ICPC working party. Oxford: Oxford University Press; 1987.

25. NHG-Standaard Acuut hoesten 2011. [cited 2017]. Available from: https://www.nhg.org/standaarden/volledig/nhg-standaard-acuut-hoesten.

26. Tates K, Meeuwesen L, Elbers E, Bensing J. I've come for his throat': roles and identities in doctor-parent-child communication. Child Care Health Dev. 2002;28(1):109–16.

27. Goossens H. Dutch Civil Law. Available from: http://www.dutchcivillaw.com/civilcodebook077.htm.

28. Zwart SDCF. Diagnostiek van alledaagse klachten. 3rd ed: BSL; 2011.

29. Schieber AC, Delpierre C, Lepage B, Afrite A, Pascal J, Cases C, et al. Do gender differences affect the doctor-patient interaction during consultations in general practice? Results from the INTERMEDE study. Fam Pract. 2014;31(6):706–13.

30. Hashim MJ. Patient-Centered Communication: Basic Skills. Am Fam Physician. 2017;95(1):29–34.

31. Matthys J, Elwyn G, Van Nuland M, Van Maele G, De Sutter A, De Meyere M, et al. Patients' ideas, concerns, and expectations (ICE) in general practice: impact on prescribing. Br J Gen Pract. 2009;59(558):29–36.

32. Mehta N, Schilder A, Fragaszy E, H ERE, Dukes O, Manikam L, et al. Antibiotic prescribing in patients with self-reported sore throat. J Antimicrob Chemother. 2017;72(3):914–22.

33. Goossens H, Ferech M, Vander Stichele R, Elseviers M. Outpatient antibiotic use in Europe and association with resistance: a cross-national database study. Lancet (London, England). 2005;365(9459):579–87.

34. Bont J, Hak E, Birkhoff CE, Hoes AW, Verheij TJ. Is co-morbidity taken into account in the antibiotic management of elderly patients with acute bronchitis and COPD exacerbations? Fam Pract. 2007;24(4):317–22.

35. Verheij RA, Curcin V, Brendan BC, McGilchrist MM. Possible sources of Bias in primary care electronic health record data (re) use. J Med Internet Res. 2018; 20(5):e185.

36. van der Velden LF, Hingstman L, Heiligers PJ, Hansen J. Increasing number of women in medicine: past, present and future. Ned Tijdschr Geneeskd. 2008;152(40):2165–71.

Safety work and risk management as burdens of treatment in primary care: insights from a focused ethnographic study of patients with multimorbidity

Gavin Daker-White[1*], Rebecca Hays[2], Thomas Blakeman[3], Sarah Croke[4], Benjamin Brown[5], Aneez Esmail[2] and Peter Bower[2]

Abstract

Background: In primary health care, patient safety failures can arise in service access, doctor-patient relationships, communication between care providers, relational and management continuity, or technical procedures. Through the lens of multimorbidty, and using qualitative ethnographic methods, our study aimed to illuminate safety issues in primary care.

Methods: Data were triangulated from electronic health records (EHRs); observation of primary care consultations; annual interviews with patients, (informal) care providers and GPs. A thematic analysis of observation, interview and field note material sought to describe the patient safety issues encountered and any associated factors or processes. A more detailed longitudinal description of 6 cases was used to contextualise safety issues identified in observation, interviews and EHRs.

Results: Twenty-six patients were recruited. Events which could lead to harm were found in all areas of a framework based on published literature. "Under" and "over" consultation as a precursor of safety failures emerged through thematic analysis of observation and interview material. Other findings concerned workload (for doctors and patients) and the limitations of short consultation times. There were differences in health data collected directly from the patients versus that found in EHRs. Examples included reference to a stroke history and diagnoses for CKD and hypertension. Case study analysis revealed specific issues which appeared contextual to safety concerns, mostly around the management of polypharmacy and patient medication adherence. Clinical imperatives appear around risk management, but the study findings point to a potential conflict with patient expectations around investigation, diagnosis and treatment.

Discussion: Patient safety work involves further burdens on top of existing workload for both clinicians and patients. In this conceptualisation, safety work seemingly forms part of a negative feedback loop with patient safety itself. A line of argument drawn from the triangulation of findings from different sources, points to a tension between the desirability of a minimally disruptive medicine versus safety risks possibly associated with 'under' or 'over' consultation. Multimorbidity acts as a magnifier of tensions in the delivery of health services and quality care in general practice. More attention should be put on system design than patient or professional behaviour.

Keywords: Multimorbidity, Patient safety, Primary care, Qualitative study, Risk, Burden of treatment

* Correspondence: gavin.daker-white@manchester.ac.uk
[1]NIHR Greater Manchester Patient Safety Translational Research Centre (Greater Manchester PSTRC), Division of Population Health, Health Services Research and Primary Care, School of Health Sciences, Faculty of Biology, Medicine and Health, University of Manchester, Manchester Academic Health Science Centre, Manchester, UK
Full list of author information is available at the end of the article

Background

The patient safety literature traditionally draws on incidents [1] such as adverse events [2], which have "root causes" embedded in the safety culture of an organisation [2, 3]. In a synthesis of the literature on patient safety in primary care, a distinction was drawn between "preventable adverse events" (such as "incorrect drug administration") and "process errors" (such as errors in clinical judgement) [4]. However, there are a variety of definitions of medical "error" and the nature of uncertain outcomes in primary care means an error may sometimes only become visible with the benefit of hindsight [5]. Further, "everyday" errors (such as missing test results) may not be conceived of as errors at all [5].

In primary care the elements of safety are as much embedded in communication issues as they are in the technological or administrative aspects of care [6]. However, a qualitative study of US-based family physicians found that most medical errors "arose from healthcare systems dysfunction" [7]. From the patient perspective, "safety" appears as a subjective feeling that is "fluid" and "negotiated" according to ongoing interactions with health services [8]. In this context, patients with clinical multimorbidity [9] are of interest as they are more likely to have a large number of interactions with medical services [10] and prescribed medicines, putting them at increased risk of safety failures [11].

Thus, safety in primary care appears as a potentially nebulous concept [12] although the relevant factors involved can be attributed to patients, doctors and healthcare systems [13]. From our perspective safety incorporates a range of processes or events and can include, variously, serious adverse events, medical errors (e.g. in diagnosis or prescription), technical problems (e.g. failure to access the medical record) and issues in communication and inter-personal relationships involving a patient and the carers around them [13]. Through a lens focused on both doctor and patient, we were interested to see whether we could identify discernible failures and link these to precursor events or the surrounding clinical and social context.

In order to explore patient safety in primary care, we selected to study patients with multimorbidity ("the co-existence of two or more chronic conditions, where one is not necessarily more central than the others"), as they are known to be at increased risk of poor care outcomes [14]. Broadly, the ultimate objective of the wider study was to identify areas in which patients could become more active agents in their own safety management [15]. We have previously reported baseline findings which showed that patients appeared to feel that their safety was threatened "when they felt their needs were ignored, or when they perceived responses as inappropriate or insensitive" [16].

Adverse consequences for patients with multimorbidity may arise in relation to care continuity [17, 18], care transitions [16] and polypharmacy [19]. Complexities of care can create self-management challenges for patients [20] including "treatment burdens" [21], such as dealing with polypharmacy [21] and interpreting sometimes contradictory advice received from different professionals [22]. The consequences of multimorbidity in primary care are influenced by contemporary workloads for general practitioners (GPs), which are seen as "unsustainable" [23]. A report by the UK King's Fund, highlighted the additional workload challenges posed by the rising numbers of people living with multimorbidity [24]. It has been argued that consultation times should be "substantially enhanced" beyond 9.2 min in consequence [24].

Patients with multimorbidity complicate clinical decision-making [25, 26]. A qualitative study of primary care health professionals' views on these issues found a tendency to deal with patients' needs in order of priority "until consultation resources were exhausted, when further management was deferred" [27]. A study of Dutch GPs' views on the clinical management of multimorbidity found that a "personal doctor-patient relationship was considered a major facilitator" whereas "presence of mental health problems was regarded as a complicating factor" [28]. A review and synthesis of related studies pointed to GPs feeling isolated in relation to clinical decision-making and a perceived need for "bidirectional communication" between care providers [29]. Similar issues were evident in a recent Scandinavian study [30]. National Institute for Health and Care Excellence (NICE) guidelines on the clinical management of multimorbidity recommended better co-ordination and tailoring of patient care [31].

"Treatment burden" in multimorbidity has received increasing attention. Gallacher et al. describe the work faced by patients which coalesces around care continuity, communication, access to services, polypharmacy and "fragmented and poorly organized care" [32]. The consequences of treatment burden include poor health outcomes, lack of adherence to prescribed treatments, "avoidable resource use" and a consequential burden for informal carers [33]. Treatment burden varies according to an individual's ability to cope [34] and the personal or social resources available, including "resilience" [35]. May et al. make clear that a patient's "relational networks will often include healthcare and other professionals" [36] although subsequent studies have tended to focus on treatment burden for patients, sometimes with the aim of informing a "minimally disruptive medicine" [37] or in efforts to mobilise patient resources to access health services and enact self-care [38]. A meta-analysis of "active" patient safety incidents (i.e. adverse events) and their precursors (e.g. prescription or diagnostic errors) concluded that "multimorbidity involving mental health may be a key driver of safety incidents" [39].

To date, studies into multimorbidity and safety have focused on polypharmacy [40, 41]. In a thematic analysis of primary care patient safety incident reports in older adults, most unsafe care was related to dispensing and prescription errors, failures in the transfer of information between sites of care and errors in clinical decision-making [42]. Although such errors are important, a meta-synthesis of published studies pointed to patient safety in primary care as a subjective feeling or moral framework as opposed to more tangible or recordable medical errors or adverse events [13]. With notable exceptions [43], previous qualitative studies of patient safety in primary care have tended to adopt a cross-sectional approach and limit data collection methods to individual or group interviews [13]. Although useful, such studies may lack a detailed assessment of the wider context in which problems occur, and cannot explore how problems develop and are managed over time.

The aims of the study were to describe the safety issues identified in a cohort of primary care patients with multimorbidity; and, to explore the clinical and social context in which patient safety concerns arise and play out. These objectives were addressed via a longitudinal, multi-method qualitative study in the form of a focused ethnography [44]. The principle aim of the analysis was to construct a line of argument concerning the circumstances under which patient agency in safety monitoring might be bolstered.

Methods
The study methods are detailed elsewhere [15]. Twenty-six patients were purposefully recruited following identification by participating GPs in Greater Manchester and enrolled for 24 months. Attempts were made to interview patients face-to-face every 12 months and after primary care consultations. On occasion, informal carers were also present at these interviews or were interviewed separately. Patient's GPs and/or practice nurses were interviewed at year 1 and year 2. We aimed to observe at least two primary care consultations each year with each participant. Some participating patients completed a health care diary. Data were extracted from practice electronic health records for each participant at study months 0,12 and 24. Where possible, interviews and observations were audio recorded; with informed consent to use a recorder verbalised at the start of each interview or observation by each participant present. Where one or more participants did not consent to the use of an audio recorder, notes were taken by hand. The fieldworkers (RH, GD-W SC), who were experienced qualitative health researchers, recorded their own impressions and observations as field notes. During the course of the study, one patient dropped out (data excluded) and three died (data retained).

For the purposes of the thematic analysis of interview, observation and diary material, all data were read several times by the first author and selected data which fit our a priori framework [15] was extracted and further organised and analysed by the wider study team with the aid of Quirkos software (www.quirkos.com). The framework was based on the findings of three previous qualitative studies of patient safety in primary care [45–47]. We coded inductively from a subset of interview and observation material (from all participants) that was directly pertinent to patient safety as it fit a taxonomy based on these international studies. We included any surrounding context. We have not shown our working here, as referees pointed out that this data does not add anything to what is already known in the literature. These situations and events could also be used to more easily identify patient and GP participants.

For the case study [48] analysis, we began by comparing information on medical conditions, prescribed medicines and allergies or drug sensitivities as described by patients or found in EHRs. The primary purpose of this exercise was not to discern whether "errors of fact" lay either with the patient or with the system, but rather to identify cases where more detailed analysis could provide context around identified patient safety concerns. A deviant case [49] – where there were no discrepancies between information divulged by patient and practice – was also selected – for comparison, although our analytical approach is primarily descriptive.

For the six cases identified, we analysed all of the data collected for each individual, i.e. EHRs, paper prescriptions (where available), transcripts and field notes from participant interviews and observations of clinical consultations. All data were anonymised at, or immediately following data collection and all participant identifiers are pseudonyms. Ethical approval was obtained. Informed consent was obtained from all participant GPs, patients and carers. Ongoing assent was verbalised in subsequent interviews or observation sessions. Certain unique clinical features of individual cases have been redacted or blurred (e.g. described in less specific terms) and the original datasets are not shown in order to protect participant anonymity.

Results I – Health records analysis
Of 26 patients recruited at baseline (Table 1), 3 died during the course of the study and one withdrew following concerns that the study would saddle them with additional burden. Comparing information on active health conditions, prescribed medicines and allergies or drug sensitivities found discrepancies for all patient

Table 1 Participant characteristics. Demographics of patient participants (from patient reported data at baseline)

		N	%
Gender	Female	14	53.85
	Male	11	42.31
Age group	65–74	10	38.46
	75+	15	57.69
Prescribed medicines	≤6	7	26.92
	7–10	7	26.92
	11+	11	42.31
Long-term conditions	2–3	7	26.92
	4–5	7	26.92
	6+	11	42.31
Requires mobility aid*	Yes	9	34.62
	No	16	61.54
Living status	Alone	7	26.92
	With partner	15	57.69
	With family member	3	11.54
Index of Multiple Deprivation (IMD) Decile**	1–2	9	34.62
	3–4	13	50.00
	5+	3	11.54
Total number of patients		25	100.00

*That is a crutch, stick, walker or wheelchair
**Where 1 is most deprived 10% of Lower Layer Super Output Areas
(data from http://imd-by-postcode.opendatacommunities.org/)

participants, bar one. Thirteen (52% of 25) patients did not mention drug allergies or sensitivities as recorded in their EHR and there were 4 instances where drug allergies mentioned by the patient were not found in the EHR. Sixteen (64% of 25) participating patients did not mention some of the active health conditions recorded in the EHR. However, this was perhaps to be expected in a group of people who had been deliberately selected as having multiple health problems. It was also unsurprising that 4 elderly male participants chose not to disclose to a younger, female researcher that they had erectile dysfunction problems or were in receipt of sildenafil prescriptions.

There were more surprising omissions; principally the participant who appeared not to know that they had previously had a TIA or stroke. In another case, a suspected TIA was mentioned by the patient but not seen in the EHR. Two patients did not mention a diagnosis of hypertension. Three did not mention a CKD diagnosis, although this could have been asymptomatic in the two participants with CKD Stage 3A. In three cases, it appeared as though some of the patient's principal health concerns were not recorded in the EHR as they did not have a definitive diagnostic label or could not be treated effectively, as in a woman with recurrent skin infections, another with "age spots" and a man with a "lazy eye."

On the basis of the above exercise, 6 cases were selected for more detailed consideration as they seemed to highlight potential areas where safety issues would arise or were seen to have arisen. Kathleen was seen at an Urgent Care Centre following a fall in year one and the GP had put a Personalised Care Plan in place which included "admissions avoidance care." Pamela's son was concerned about her medication compliance and the GP suspected cognitive impairment. Deborah was selected primarily because she told the researcher about memory changes which she had withheld from her GP. However, from the GP's perspective, the main safety considerations in her care related to the possible risks of hospital admission resulting from specialised medication that she was taking. Alan was admitted to hospital after collapsing at an event in year 2. This, along with further episodes of "feeling faint," he associated with a statin prescription (although "feeling faint" is not a reported side effect of statins [50]) which was subsequently stopped. Helen was taking more prescribed medicines than any other case considered in detail, and as with Deborah, there were concerns about the possibility of "stomach bleeding or kidney problems" and "ending up in hospital" as a result. Finally, Victoria was selected as she was the only participating patient where no discrepancies were found between medical information collected from herself versus that found in the EHR. She only had three active health conditions, including heart failure and diverticular disease. Further description of each of these cases is considered below.

Comparison of numbers of primary care consultations for the included cases during the 2 year study period mainly underlined the low number of primary care appointments seen in Victoria (the "deviant case") when compared with others. Victoria only had 6 consultations in 24 months (data missing for one month) whereas the remaining participant cases were usually seen in primary care at least once a month. Deborah seemed to have a more overall pattern of regular and consistent use when compared with the others, although she had 3 consultations in month 20. The remaining cases revealed episodes involving periods of large numbers of consultations. Thus, Pamela had 12 consultations in 4 months (months 8–11), Alan had 6 consultations in one month (month 19) and Helen had 23 consultations during months 16–22 inclusive (an average of 3 per month).

Across the study period, participating patients were being prescribed between 7 and 18 items in primary care. Victoria, the "control" was in the lowest position in this regard. Data on secondary care appointments showed that Victoria and Pamela were the only participants not seen in secondary or specialist care for the duration of the study. Alan had only one incident involving secondary care – an emergency admission. Three participants: Kathleen, Deborah and Helen were usually visiting hospitals or specialist clinics every month and each of them had two emergency or urgent care admissions during the course of the study. Combining data on total primary and secondary care appointments over the 24 months of data collection shows that Victoria, the control, had a total of 8 appointments, whereas Kathleen, Pamela and Deborah had between 59 and 67. Helen was also likely in this latter category (with a total of 52 appointments), although data on her secondary care appointments was missing for 5 straight months. On the basis of the included figures, these latter four participants had a mean of 60 total health appointments, or 2.5 per calendar month.

Results II - Case studies

Kathleen

In month 9 of the study Kathleen had a fall and was seen at an urgent care centre. Following this incident, her GP instigated a Personalised Care Plan, including "admission avoidance care." In month 16, Kathleen presented at the surgery feeling "dizzy and wobbly" with "lots" of pain in her back. As part of the examination, the attending GP notes, "I found it very difficult to pinpoint history today" and "I'm not exactly sure how to help."

Katheleen was originally due to go on a list for surgery [details removed] in month 4 but this was put off by the hospital due to the "unpredictability" of surgical loads in the winter months. Whilst Kathleen faced the worry [of whether she would have the operation she needed soon enough], she also reported that a consultant had "said '[details removed] with all its dangers,' so I believe there's some danger in what he's going to do, but there's danger in everything isn't there?" (diary entry, month 15).

Pamela

During month 8, Pamela attended surgery seemingly at the instigation of her son who felt that she was not taking her medicines as prescribed. The attending GP recorded the suspicion that Pamela was "cognitively impaired" and the consultation led the GP to the view that she was "possibly concealing her symptoms." On the son's insistence, Pamela showed the GP [details removed] "which she wasn't going to show or mention." The following month, Pamela presented with memory loss for the first time. An interview with her GP highlighted concerns around whether Pamela was taking her prescribed medicines in light of these memory changes, although a dosette box was being use to facilitate compliance.

Deborah

Deborah's main problems involved rheumatoid and osteo-arthritis, although when describing her symptoms at initial interview she said that "everyday [brings] something different." She lived with her husband who was doing "whatever is needed" domestically. Arthritis had a significant impact on multiple joints. At initial interview she spoke of a bone in her leg which was "wearing away" and "there's not a lot they can do." This view was confirmed during a GP interview, "That's why she comes in all the time … we can't help her properly, we can't cure the problem." This situation had led her to consult a range of alternative practitioners, including a faith healer who "didn't do any good." Deborah further reported that "something had ruptured" in her shoulder but complained that she had not been sent for a scan. In addition to three other health problems, she also reported recent "memory changes" to the interviewer, about which she had "not spoken to anyone" and hoped "it's not Alzheimer's." Deborah was being seen in secondary care for [details removed].

The main safety issue for Deborah concerned the medicines she was taking, which, as her GP put it during an annual interview, could cause "stomach bleeding or kidney problems … that's why she's having these blood tests every month." The root of the safety risks for this participant appeared to be the additional workload created for both patient and primary care physician in relation to the management and monitoring of specialised [details removed] medication which was not licensed for use in primary care. There is an unfortunate irony that these risks were created against a background where none of the specialist medication was perceived to be having much of an effect.

This clinical background led Deborah's GP to conceive of her as a "demanding" patient: "So it seems like the woman is here every week." But the GP added (in annual interview): "even though she's been here only 4 or 5 times in the winter." Data gathered for the 24 month period of the study showed she was actually attending once or twice a month. The EHR also revealed some procedural confusion around a prescription for a specialised medication and associated blood monitoring tests.

Alan

At recruitment, Alan's main contact with health services consisted of 3 monthly blood tests for diabetes with the practise nurse; a condition which he believed he no longer had. The EHR revealed contradictory information around a statin prescription and a few appointment cancellations.

In month 15, Alan was admitted to hospital by ambulance after collapsing at an event. He put this down to commencing statins two weeks previously. Following further episodes of feeling faint, he stopped taking the statin and mentioned this to his GP at a subsequent appointment, who marks the medical record "not for further lipid modifying medication." This decision was confirmed by doctor and patient at a subsequent consultation 4 weeks later. In month 19, another prescription was stopped, which, unlike statins does list dizziness and fainting as potential side-effects.

Of all the cases, Alan appeared least engaged with his health problems, although the work of managing his conditions – whether through eating a healthy diet – or organizing the medications he was taking daily, seemed to fall largely to his wife. However, his symptomology (such as in respect of pain) seemed far less than in the other cases on an everyday basis. When asked what all of his tablets were for during his initial interview, he said, "I don't know you'd have to ask a doctor."

Helen

Helen had a large number of active health conditions and was the biggest user of medications in the case subset. At recruitment she reported, among other conditions, a history of asthma, high blood pressure, diabetes, and heart problems. She described herself as "prone to DVTs," and had previously had a stroke.

In Helen's case, a large number of "main symptoms" and health conditions were identified by both patient and doctor (including hypertension, asthma, and diabetes), although at baseline the patient did not mention CKD, [details of three medical conditions removed] or chest pain. During the course of the study, Helen was also seen in [four hospital departments and one community service – details removed]. She presented at A&E during months 4 (with chest pain) and 14 [details removed]. In month 6, paramedics attend her house concerning [details removed].

By month 12, a more focused trio of symptoms had emerged in the general panoply of ill health, including an ulcer. In the EHR, reference to a lymphoedema first appears at a consultation in month 12. In months 16 and 17 there are face-to-face consultations about her swollen legs. By month 20 (in a long consultation observed by a researcher), the problem has worsened (appearing as "possible DVT" in the EHR) and a referral (with some access problems) is eventually made to an ambulatory care unit. When asked in interview, the GP said, "We don't have an answer," following the investigations on her leg, presenting a "diagnostic dilemma" and "no solution". In remarking that the patient "likes answers, so does [her partner]," however, the GP appears to focus the problematics of this state of affairs onto the patient and partner experiencing the "anxiety that comes with not knowing what's going on."

In safety terms, prescribed medicines were an ever present risk. Helen was previously taken off [a medication which had adverse effects]. She was taking [prescription drug name removed], which can interact with other medications which has to be accounted for in

prescribing. In discussing potential safety concerns around Helen's care, her GP referred to a high chance of her going into chronic kidney failure if she was medicated with diuretics. If she were to use Ace Inhibitors for her CKD, blood tests would need to be undertaken every 2 or 3 days to assess kidney functioning. At the end of the day, there was a danger of her "ending up in hospital."

Victoria

Victoria appeared as a comparatively low user of primary care services with only one episode of hospital care in 24 months (outpatients). At recruitment she reported three health conditions including heart failure. The EHR notes "moderate" diverticular disease which the patient discusses, but not with this precise diagnostic label. Only two potential safety issues were evident. Firstly, the GP mentioned that aspirin had not been requested from the patient for a period of time, although it was suggested that Victoria may have been buying it over the counter. Secondly, the GP referred to an incident involving an infection where it was suggested that "rather than waiting until you need to go to A&E," she could have approached primary care sooner for an antibiotic prescription; thereby avoiding a hospital admission.

Results III – Thematic analysis
Instances of potential contributions to patient safety failures

Characteristics of participating patients at baseline are detailed in Table 1. We found examples of most potential contributors to patient safety failures according to the framework described in the study protocol [15]. For access breakdowns [47], all contributory factors from the taxonomy of events were seen. In the case of communication breakdowns [45], all issues were encountered except for the patient side factors "Inarticulateness" [47] and "lack of confidence" [47] and the staff side factor "failure to respond to adverse drug reactions or painful symptoms" [46]. However, we found additional factors that did not seem to fit the taxonomy: "GP doesn't interact with patient but focuses on computer screen," "health professional approach seen as patronising" and "health professional has 'bad attitude.'" So far as errors of coordination and management continuity [46] were concerned, all factors were found except for the patient contributory factor "comprehension errors" [47] and the staff/system error "wrong chart used for patient" [45]. We found additional factors here, mainly related to the intersection between pressures on GP workload, problems arising from seeing different GPs and the ways in which systematised annual review appointments can lack patient-centredness. In the case of relationship breakdowns [45], there was a very good fit between the taxonomy and the data we gathered, with only the patient contributory factor "selfishness" [47] absent. This descriptive analysis highlights how, in a relatively small sample of patients followed over 2 years, contributors to patient safety failures were both frequent and very varied.

Subsequently, we analysed the data extracted via the framework as a whole and in thematic fashion. As well as those themes that derived from our framework (e.g. access, communication), we encountered additional themes, such as "over or under consultation" and "safety problems inherent in health conditions or treatments." The broad findings coalesced around three main factors, with "work" (for patients) or "workload" (for health workers) as underlying issues: relational tensions in primary care consultations, system constraints in the organisation of care and issues in care continuity.

Relational tensions and 'under' or 'over' consultation

Pressure on GPs' time, and difficulties in securing timely (and lengthy enough) appointments appeared to create anxieties for patients and doctors alike. Some patients avoided seeking help, perhaps believing that their problems were not serious enough ("under consulters"). Other patients, perhaps understood by GPs as being over anxious about their health ("over consulters"), sought repeated appointments, as their complex needs for care and/or emotional support could not be met in a brief appointment slot:

"... if we don't make ... regular appointments then they start ringing in and they'll see perhaps a locum doctor and then another chest x-ray will be done, you know, when one was done three months ago and another...so ...and that's where continuity comes in, you know. ... I think that's where sometimes reviewing patients who are very anxious about their health, on a pre-planned basis, can be helpful because it saves them sort of seeking multiple ... people and getting different opinions, which actually sometimes really worsens her anxiety." (Irene, GP interview, year 2)

When people brought wider concerns from their lives into the consultation room, this could create additional work for GPs, who are "sitting behind a desk rattling through tons and tons and tons of patients in your surgery":"I find it difficult to know what her priorities are ... I think that she verbalises problems with her brother, ... whether it's her brother's health or their relationship. ... So I think she takes on a lot of his problems as well. And then puts a lot of her problems to one side. She's quite a busy person. ... That's her personality and then she becomes busy in the consultation, and it's difficult to control." ([Anonymised], GP interview, year 2)

Prioritisation of conditions is well recognised in multi-morbidity [51] However, the above extract appears to point to a tension, or disconnect, between organisational or system "needs" (10 min appointment slots, prioritisation) and what a patient needs, wants or expects from the consultation.

An elderly woman was understood to be "coping well at home" despite having heart failure. When she died during the course of the study, her death was seen as "unexpected" and her case was referred to the Coroner's Office. But the fact that she did not consult meant that she was not on the practice "radar" and was on reflection seen as an *under consulter*:

"She doesn't consult at all. ... She consulted with [GP], he saw her at home to, sort of; transfer the care of her heart failure to Primary Care. ... [Another GP] arranged with her to see her every three months and to have her blood checked. Then we have not seen her, there was a telephone consultation with [a different GP] because her bloods showed that she was slightly low on folic acid and [a different GP] just talked to her about her diet and gave her some vitamins and then she passed away.

"She was somebody who from our point of view seemed to, despite her heart failure, coping well at home. Although despite her age and her heart failure perhaps an unexpected death, so I think she was referred to the Coroner's Officer, so not on our radar really because she wasn't consulting." (Martha, GP interview, year 2)

In an earlier interview with Martha, it was noteworthy that from the patient's viewpoint one reason why she was consulting infrequently was that she found it difficult to attend the surgery. Furthermore, she had received a letter from the practice regarding a blood pressure reading, which she did not believe had been taken:"I don't go to the surgery, they're supposed to come here, a nurse came to take my blood pressure, two days later got a letter from [my GP] saying, 'Pleased your blood pressure has gone down.' Got another letter two weeks later, saying the same thing, but I hadn't had another test. Then I got another letter from [my GP] saying pleased and she would take your blood pressure next time you come in. I doubt I could get in, would have to take a taxi, don't think I'd manage the stairs." (Martha, health care diary, year 1)

System constraints

Whilst some threats to patient safety follow from the knowledge, behaviour and inter-personal aspects of human actors, others rather follow from protocols, policies and the ways that systems are organised to provide and deliver care [13]. For example, appointments are difficult to organise; especially when arranged at the last minute. Many GPs work part-time and the increasing use of locum GPs can be seen to have an adverse impact on continuity of care [52]. One GP participant pointed to the value in seeing the same practitioner:

GP: It's far easier to judge the progress of a condition and how the patient's coping with a condition if the same person sees them every time. Sometimes a fresh pair of eyes is good. But mostly having the same doctor can help move things along. I suppose, as I mentioned before, having a clear plan of actions, with timescales. And after that timescale, decision points when it's decided what to do next, is what we're doing working, or if it's not, do we need secondary care? (Larry, GP interview, year 2)

Under these circumstances, the onus can fall on the patient to instigate their own clinical monitoring, rather than relying on system generated recall:"We rely on her to come back for the blood tests, so if you're not really careful and there's a bigger practice and many doctors or locums come in, probably sometimes you'll not realise that she hasn't been for two months for the blood tests, prescribe the next month, and then any side effect or danger in protein loss or the kidneys would then go unnoticed till it's probably further advanced." (Deborah, GP interview, year 1)

Another case pointed to a failure to undertake a repeat of an "abnormal" blood test, although it was unclear whether this was a "systems" issue, an oversight by an individual member of staff, confusion over whose role it was to recall the patient, or some combination of all of these factors:GP: ...from the blood tests in February, we have advised that it should be repeated in three months and she has not re-attended.

Interviewer: Would she have been sent a reminder?

GP: She hasn't been sent a reminder, actually, and given that she attended with issues about her memory that is a failing on our part, isn't it. ... [Later] ... And so, perhaps both me and our administrator had not picked up on the fact that her blood tests are due. ... [Later] ... they have not flagged it, we have got a template that flags it up so that they are pulled up by an administrator. ... So, there is a bit of a systems failure going on there. ([Anonymised], GP interview, year 2)

During the observation of one consultation, an interaction concerning the results of a laboratory test appeared to point to a presumption of failure in the transfer of test results, with the GP suggesting that attempting to locate the test result was not worth the work involved:Patient: How did my urine sample go on?

GP: Never got it, so I'm really unsure of what's happened. As you said, you were better, I didn't see any point in chasing this up with the lab, because they're just going to say I can't find it, is that all right? ([Anonymised], observation of consultation, year 2)

This appears as an example of navigating the challenge between maximising the clinical utility of a test whilst minimising the potential for further workload and treatment burden (i.e. redoing a test that may be unnecessary).

Issues in work or workload associated with care continuity

Below, a GP reports about a participating patient's recent referral for expert opinion:

GP: ... they saw her that day, which is great. I had no correspondence for that. She phoned me a week later and they said they will do a scan and I've not heard, we didn't receive any correspondence. So ... so I phoned up [the] unit and said, 'This lady has had a scan, this was an admission avoidance, when is the scan going to be?' They go, 'We don't know, we don't have the records.' So then I had to phone back a week later, they said they'd look into it, then she phoned back saying, 'I've still not heard,' so there's this yoyo that was going around for the best part of two or three weeks, her [removed] were no worse in that time, I did have to see her that once just to reassure myself that nothing had changed. ([Anonymised], GP interview, year 2)

The nature of this scenario creates work and increased workload for the patient, her carers (including health service staff) and suggests "ambiguity and workarounds" [53] between care sectors. Anxiety around clinical decision making in people with multimorbidity or other complexities entails work, and systems constraints exacerbate the work or effort required to resolve the clinical uncertainty.

Another issue related to care transitions was that some specialist medication is not licensed for use in general practice. This was seen to create work for a patient who found it difficult to attend a hospital for screening appointments. This appeared as a potential safety concern:

"... I think the patient probably finds it more difficult to go back to the hospital for the check-ups, which probably in the beginning might be sometimes weekly, so it's a lot of hassle for her but we can't help her there really because it's the licencing and we don't know... And it is a lot of workload involved there, so we sort of... general practice shies away from that a little bit. ... [Later] ... Again, if some of those tablets, let's say, causes stomach bleeding and she's got severe indigestion and thinks, oh, I don't want to go to the doctor again, and then suddenly a vessel bursts in the stomach and then she's got real problems." (Deborah, GP interview, year 1)

Informal carers, typically patients' family members commonly acted as advocates in health service consultations as well as helping out with aspects of home care and management of patient's conditions at home. However, on occasion they were not willing to take on certain tasks expected of them by the formal health service. For example, whilst Michael's's partner had been trained to give a glucose injection should he suffer a diabetic hypo, Helen's partner was not happy to take on what he saw as a strictly medical role. The work required in managing chronic conditions is again highlighted, here with the added consideration of determining who has the capacity to fulfil the required functions related to the management of care.

In the particular context of workload, one GP noted—and seemingly not ironically—that patients who "under consult" are preferable from a workload viewpoint:

Interviewer: And what is it like, having a patient like [removed], whom you don't see very often?

GP: It's great, because you don't see them, so they don't cause you any workload, if I'm being absolutely bloody honest with you. I think it's unsettling when you come to look at their records, and you think, goodness, she has these [removed] conditions and she's not needed to see us. ([Anonymised], GP interview, year 1)

This patient is seen as "great" because they "don't cause you any workload" and attend "appropriately" "for monitoring." Although questions are raised around tensions between managing workload whilst maintaining effective and safe care.

Results IV – Synthesis of research findings

Overall, the findings pointed to various areas of tension impacting on safety. The first of these was around managing underlying anxieties and uncertainties in interactions, both from a patient and a professional perspective. For example, and as expanded in the discussion (see below), there was evidence of a clash between patient expectations to "do something" (as in repeating investigations) and, from the clinical perspective, the risk of that "something" leading to worse outcomes or even harm.

From a patient safety perspective, managing this inherent tension appears as a potentially key element of clinical practice. That requires more work for clinicians, and even more work when dealing with multimorbidity. Handling this tension can lead to real or perceived 'over' consultation – (as exemplified by Irene, cited above). More investigations generate more results which leads to a need for further consultations.

Borderline test results may generate further anxieties, in a kind of negative feedback loop to where we began. This assertion, whilst speculative, brings is to the second area of tension, which involves maximising clinical utility whilst minimising treatment burden. To the ethnographic observer, Helen appeared as someone whose full-time job was organising and attending health appointments. And none of this appeared to address her symptoms or the questions she had about her various conditions. A non-clinician might wonder whether all of this contact with the health service was making her better or worse, with some medications apparently necessary to keep her alive and others which appeared to present the risk of causing her to end up in hospital in their own right.

Systems of care are not necessarily designed to account and effectively reduce the work required to deal with these tensions, and by extension—make things safer. Whether it is possible to effectively deal with the work required to address these tensions in a time bounded routine consultation (and a resource constrained health system) is unclear. Further, our findings show how the current organisation of medical care might exacerbate these constraints. The atypical example in the data of 'under' consultation, illuminated a system run so as to reduce the sense of demand and clinician workload, but this can be at the expense of necessary care. GP participant accounts pointed to a sense of relief in less workload, but with an accompanying realisation that the patient's needs were not necessarily met. Could this be a potential precursor of clinician burn out?

Discussion

Patient safety work involves further burdens on top of existing workload for both clinicians and patients. In this conceptualisation, safety work seemingly forms a negative feedback loop with patient safety itself. A line of argument drawn from the triangulation of findings from different sources, points to a tension between the desirability of a minimally disruptive medicine versus safety risks associated with the way that services are set up, organised and delivered.

What is the potential agency of doctors versus patients in ameliorating clinical iatrogenesis against a background of clinical uncertainty?

By incorporating medical records data and an approach focussed on the detail of purposefully selected cases, we had hoped to reveal discrete safety incidents which we might then link back to precursor events. However, on the rare occasions on which we found an observable and identifiable "safety incident," such as Alan fainting, it is not clear how that might have linked to other safety concerns which had arisen in his case, such as possible antipathy about his state of health, denial of medical diagnosis or cancelling medical appointments. And none of these concerns explain why he linked this incident to a statin prescription; nor why the GP was happy to go along with his view. Although this may have been to appease the patient. Later, another medication was stopped. Perhaps that was the culprit? This example does however underline the reactive nature of the medical system in general terms; and uncertainties around ascribing causes to adverse outcomes, even with the benefit of hindsight. The patient has agency here, and is another factor to be weighed up against clinical guidelines or recommended treatments. Regular diabetes monitoring can prevent serious complications, but Alan believed he did not have the condition; which he felt was temporarily brought on through over consumption of a popular sugary drink when it was on special offer. "Fainting" could be a symptom of diabetes, and if Alan had attended these check-ups more regularly, perhaps he could have avoided blacking out?

For the majority of patients who were more engaged with medicine (even to the point of alleged overuse where anxiety was a compounding clinical feature), there appeared a tension between patient expectations that their GP will "do something," versus GP concerns that "something else" could lead to harm (e.g. kidney injury) or risk hospital admission with the attendant risks. And thus the nub of the matter appears to be a palpable tension for GPs between meeting patient expectations (via patient-centred care) and preventing adverse events. For patients, feeling safe appears to incorporate elements of feeling satisfied with the quality of the clinical relationship and care, which are intrinsically linked to their expectations and previous experience of services [16]. An essential problem here appears to be that patients and GPs are using different conceptualisations of safety (or satisfaction) which might play off against each other. Interesting questions that emerge from this line of argument are firstly whether patients really expect the kinds of "over treatment" that could increase the risk of adverse events that we have implied from our interpretation of the study data? Secondly, how do GPs manage the tightrope walk between meeting patient expectations

to "do something" (which could constitute over treatment and investigation) and "doing no harm," as in offsetting the potential risks of adding more medicines or repeating investigations?

In a time and resource constrained system, could a focus on risk management be compromising patient safety?

Having considered some cases in detail, one gets the sense of an ever present backdrop of risks, appearing largely as tasks for GPs as in "avoid hospital admission," "monitor kidney functioning," or perhaps "be careful about what you prescribe." There are different risks for patients perhaps, e.g. of not getting a diagnosis, of the treatment not working or of the GP overlooking or mis-ascribing something. Plus the risk of not getting a sympathetic hearing, the risk of not being taken seriously or the risk of being blamed for the problem or failure to treat it.

The sense then is that both GP and patient have to be on constant alert to a plethora of risks but that when something does go wrong the reasons for it may be uncertain or difficult to pin down. "Let's stop this drug and see if that helps," perhaps. Within a time constrained and reactive system, however, the context of multimorbidity can mean that all the available time is spent on reacting to the latest crisis, whilst avoiding serious harm through clinical iatrogenesis. In this scenario, there is no time left to address basic patient needs (e.g. "Why isn't this drug working? Where's my test result?") and it could be said that both clinician and patient appear to be in perpetual workaround; or dancing to a system generated script.

One feature or narrative concerning contemporary medical systems is "information chaos": "comprised of various combinations of information overload, information underload, information scatter, information conflict, and erroneous information" [54]. Increased workload, including additional working around "chaotic," complex and inter-twined systems would be expected to increase the likelihood of an error occurring. Data from Primary Care are sparse although a US study of hospital paediatric nurses found that "being rushed" was associated with both medication errors and "burnout." [55]

In circumstances where increasing clinical workload is a driver of safety failures, more work in monitoring or preparing for a possible adverse reaction or serious adverse event (on top of a focus on reacting to the latest medical problem) seemingly forms part of a negative feedback loop whereby the situation becomes less safe. The more people engage with medicine, whether willingly or unwillingly, the more necessarily they are put at risk of potential harm. Given especially the problematics of conditions and syndromes which are either hard to treat or difficult to define clinically and where existing drug lists might prevent the prescription of usual treatments.

The emergence of under or over consultation as a potential driver of patient safety failures highlights a tension between the meta-organisation of health care and the communicative, legalistic or performative aspects of medical consultations in the context of patient centred care

A finding which added to our a priori framework concerning patient safety in primary care highlights the contribution of perceived over or under consulting as having a role in precipitating adverse events. There are highly socialised notions about when it is appropriate to use NHS services [56] and such considerations formed a part of the narrative when participants discussed their own patterns of service use. Avoiding the label of "time-waster" can be a moral imperative for patients [57] and the notion of candidacy is useful in explaining health service utilisation where services are seen as being in short supply [58]. On the other hand, whilst it might suit practitioners if patients don't over consult, this can lead to problems as identified in our findings. Over or under consultation compounds both the discursive aspects of the consultation (where there may be confusion on either side as to the medical reasons for consulting in the first place) and system demands on when patients are seen (as in periodic reviews for patients with, e.g. diabetes or heart disease, which may be viewed as a waste of time by some – results not shown).

Our main findings point to multimorbidity as a magnifier of tensions in the delivery of health services and quality care in general practice. Within this context, older patients with complex and varied healthcare needs encounter almost all potential contributors to patient safety failure, as they negotiate the tensions and limitations of system demands. For GPs, patients and carers, these tensions create additional work which they can struggle to manage and often find frustrating. When the quality of interactions between doctors and their patients begin to fail, or technical problems arise, this can make a bad situation worse in the context of limited consultation times and the perceived scarce or 'rationed' nature of medical resources.

These findings fit with the model of "cumulative complexity" whereby factors "accumulate and interact to complicate patient care" [59]. This model is principally concerned with the balance between the workload created by the demands of care and an individual's capacity to deal with it [59]. The model has previously found to be relevant for people living with multiple chronic conditions [60]. In the introduction, the tendency for a theoretical and empirical focus on patient workload or burdens was noted and a similar preoccupation is evident in the literature concerning patient "capacity" within a framework that is concerned with enabling patients to help themselves more [61]. In this study, whilst we found both patient and staff or system-side threats to safety, "workload" appeared at least as important a patient safety issue when referring to staff as it did to patients. Whilst another strand of health research has illuminated the ways in which health professionals form a part of patients' relational networks [62], the general tendency can rather be to separate out issues for health service staff from those facing patients. The findings of this study point to a need to consider the ways in which care work and clinical responsibilities are allocated, and the consequences for safety when "overworked" health care staff and patients can seemingly attempt to shift care roles or tasks onto one another. Despite repeated calls for patient-centred care, findings point to the possible limits of patient-centredness [63] when safety is at stake.

Implications and future work

A focus on multimorbidity has magnified some of the inherent tensions underpinning everyday interactions in primary health care and the examples of over and under consultation have shone a light on some key system issues that need consideration, particularly when trying to improve the delivery of care for people living with complex health and social care needs. The main learning from the study is very much, how can systems work better for everyone concerned and shift away from a focus on professional (or patient) behaviour. In future work we shall be exploring ways in which patients can take a more active role in reducing harm, such as in knowing how to better communicate with their doctors or having a better knowledge of their own medical records. Such efforts will have to be set against the knowledge that any intervention which is experienced as a burden, or does not fit the patient's self-prioritised needs, is unlikely to succeed.

In relation to potential areas for improving "safety," one route would seem to involve patient education around acceptance of medical risk, which can seemingly cause some considerable anxiety, dissatisfaction and increased service utilisation. From the practitioner perspective, as well as potentially decreasing patient anxieties, such interventions could have the added benefit of reducing GP workload, which appears as a more tangible threat to safety. Particular results concerning doctor-patient communication in memory loss further underline the importance of creating a climate and space in which patients feel free to discuss concerns around their health. A broader research agenda appears concerning the extent to which entrenched systems of top-down medical care can ever fit with contemporary idealised notions of patient-centred care.

Strengths and weaknesses

Traditionally, patient safety research has attempted to explain safety failures by identifying incidents and then historically examining the circumstances that led to failure, as in a study of falls in hospital [64]. We adopted a different tack by following patients over time to discern whether and how adverse events occurred and any precursor, precipitatory or contextual factors. The principal strength of our approach is the longitudinal aspect and the triangulation or comparison of data from different sources. Whilst qualitative research cannot discern frequencies or the probability of events occurring in a given population, it is useful for uncovering context and highlighting areas for further research. The principal weakness of our approach probably concerns observer bias, i.e. the presence of researchers in some consultations may have influenced the behaviour of participating patients or health care workers. Further, people with mental health problems were under represented in the sample and previous research has shown they may be at increased risk of patient safety events [39], e.g. related to polypharmacy or medication adherence.

Conclusion

Multimorbidity creates work for patients, carers and health professionals. The way that the primary care system is currently set up can lead GPs to feel potentially relieved when workload is minimised. However, a focus on managing workload runs the risk of patient safety failures, e.g. when a patient is not seen much by primary care staff. This is potentially relevant for all patients but appears more so for patients living with complex health and social care needs.

Multimorbidity creates burdens for both patients and their doctors which can be seen to create circumstances in which safety can be threatened. The mechanisms by which differential take up of, or access to, primary care consultations may precipitate different types of medical errors or iatrogenic adverse events requires further investigation. Efforts to improve safety in primary care need to tread carefully when intervening in complex clinical management plans, as those which create extra workload for doctors or their patients may cause unintended consequences.

Acknowledgements
Patient advisory input to the study was provided by Wendy Barlow and Brian Minor. We would also like to thank the Multimorbidity Research Advisory Group for their feedback and support. Carly Rolfe and others provided administrative support. We would like to thank the primary care staff and patients who participated.

Funding
This work was funded by the National Institute for Health Research Greater Manchester Primary Care Patient Safety Translational Research Centre (NIHR Greater Manchester PSTRC). The views expressed are those of the authors and not necessarily those of the NHS, the NIHR or the Department of Health.

Authors' contributions
PB conceived of the study. PB, GD-W, RH, and TB and were involved in the design of the study. RH, GD-W and SC collected the data. GD-W, TB, RH, PB, BB, SC, and AE contributed to data analysis and interpretation. The manuscript was drafted by GD-W, TB and RH. All authors read and approved the final manuscript.

Competing interests
The authors declare that they have no competing interests.

Author details
[1]NIHR Greater Manchester Patient Safety Translational Research Centre (Greater Manchester PSTRC), Division of Population Health, Health Services Research and Primary Care, School of Health Sciences, Faculty of Biology, Medicine and Health, University of Manchester, Manchester Academic Health Science Centre, Manchester, UK. [2]NIHR School for Primary Care Research, Division of Population Health, Health Services Research and Primary Care, School of Health Sciences, Faculty of Biology, Medicine and Health, University of Manchester, Manchester Academic Health Science Centre, Manchester, UK. [3]NIHR Collaboration in Applied Health Research and Care Greater Manchester, Division of Population Health, Health Services Research and Primary Care, School of Health Sciences, Faculty of Biology, Medicine and Health, University of Manchester, Manchester Academic Health Science Centre, Manchester, UK. [4]Division of Nursing Midwifery and Social Work, School of Health Sciences, Faculty of Biology, Medicine and Health, University of Manchester, Manchester Academic Health Science Centre, Manchester, UK. [5]Centre for Health Informatics, School of Health Sciences, Faculty of Biology, Medicine and Health, University of Manchester, Manchester Academic Health Science Centre, Manchester, UK.

References
1. Vincent C, Taylor-Adams S, Chapman EJ, Hewett D, Prior S, Strange P, Tizzard A. How to investigate and analyse clinical incidents: clinical risk unit and association of litigation and risk management protocol. BMJ Br Med J. 2000;320(7237):777.
2. Kirk S, Parker D, Claridge T, Esmail A, Marshall M. Patient safety culture in primary care: developing a theoretical framework for practical use. Qual Saf Health Care. 2007;16(4):313–20.
3. Carroll JS, Rudolph JW, Hatakenaka S. Lessons learned from non-medical industries: root cause analysis as culture change at a chemical plant. Qual Saf Health Care. 2002;11(3):266–9.
4. Elder NC, Dovey SM. Classification of medical errors and preventable adverse events in primary care: a synthesis of the literature. J Fam Pract. 2002;51(11):927–32.
5. Elder NC, Pallerla H, Regan S. What do family physicians consider an error? A comparison of definitions and physician perception. BMC Fam Pract. 2006;7(1):73.
6. Rhodes P, Campbell S, Sanders C. Trust, temporality and systems: how do patients understand patient safety in primary care? A qualitative study. Health Expect. 2016;19(2):253–63.
7. Dovey SM, Meyers DS, Phillips RL, Green LA, Fryer GE, Galliher JM, Kappus J, Grob P. A preliminary taxonomy of medical errors in family practice. Qual Saf Health Care. 2002;11(3):233–8.
8. Rhodes P, McDonald R, Campbell S, Daker-White G, Sanders C. Sensemaking and the co-production of safety: a qualitative study of primary medical care patients. Sociol Health Illn. 2016;38(2):270–85.
9. Multimorbidity: clinical assessment and management. NICE guideline [NG56] Published date: 2016. https://www.nice.org.uk/guidance/ng56 accessed 15 Sept 17
10. Fisher K, Griffith L, Gruneir A, Panjwani D, Gandhi S, Sheng LL, Gafni A, Chris P, Markle-Reid M, Ploeg J. Comorbidity and its relationship with health service use and cost in community-living older adults with diabetes: a population-based study in Ontario, Canada. Diabetes Res Clin Pract. 2016;122:113–23.
11. Scott IA, Hilmer SN, Reeve E, Potter K, Le Couteur D, Rigby D, Gnjidic D, Del Mar CB, Roughead EE, Page A, Jansen J. Reducing inappropriate polypharmacy: the process of deprescribing. JAMA Intern Med. 2015;175(5): 827–34.

12. Lamont T, Waring J. Safety lessons: shifting paradigms and new directions for patient safety research. J Health Serv Res Policy. 2015;20:1–8.

13. Daker-White G, Hays R, McSharry J, Giles S, Cheraghi-Sohi S, Rhodes P, Sanders C. Blame the patient, blame the doctor or blame the system? A meta-synthesis of qualitative studies of patient safety in primary care. PLoS One. 2015;10(8):e0128329.

14. Boyd CM, Fortin M. Future of multimorbidity research: how should understanding of multimorbidity inform health system design? Public Health Rev. 2010;32(2):451.

15. Daker-White G, Hays R, Esmail A, Minor B, Barlow W, Brown B, Blakeman T, Bower P. MAXimising involvement in MUltiMorbidity (MAXIMUM) in primary care: protocol for an observation and interview study of patients, GPs and other care providers to identify ways of reducing patient safety failures. BMJ Open. 2014;4(8):e005493.

16. Hays R, Daker-White G, Esmail A, Barlow W, Minor B, Brown B, Blakeman T, Sanders C, Bower P. Threats to patient safety in primary care reported by older people with multimorbidity: baseline findings from a longitudinal qualitative study and implications for intervention. BMC health services research. 2017;17(1):754.

17. Haggerty JL. Ordering the chaos for patients with multimorbidity. BMJ-Br Med J. 2012;345(7876):7.

18. Cowie L, Morgan M, White P, Gulliford M. Experience of continuity of care of patients with multiple long-term conditions in England. J Health Serv Res Policy. 2009;14(2):82–7.

19. Hunt LM, Kreiner M, Brody H. The changing face of chronic illness management in primary care: a qualitative study of underlying influences and unintended outcomes. Ann Fam Med. 2012;10(5):452–60.

20. Bower P, Hann M, Rick J, Rowe K, Burt J, Roland M, Protheroe J, Richardson G, Reeves D. Multimorbidity and delivery of care for long-term conditions in the English National Health Service: baseline data from a cohort study. J Health Serv Res Policy. 2013;18(2_suppl):29–37.

21. Gallacher KI, Batty GD, McLean G, Mercer SW, Guthrie B, May CR, Langhorne P, Mair FS. Stroke, multimorbidity and polypharmacy in a nationally representative sample of 1,424,378 patients in Scotland: implications for treatment burden. BMC Med. 2014;12(1):151.

22. Rosbach M, Andersen JS. Patient-experienced burden of treatment in patients with multimorbidity–a systematic review of qualitative data. PLoS One. 2017;12(6):e0179916.

23. Hawkes N. General practice workload is unsustainable, real time data show. BMJ Br Med J. 2016;353.

24. Baird B, Charles A, Honeyman M, Maguire D, Das P. Understanding pressures in general practice. London: King's Fund; 2016. www.kingsfund.org.uk/publications/pressures-in-general-practice

25. Hobbs FR, Bankhead C, Mukhtar T, Stevens S, Perera-Salazar R, Holt T, Salisbury C. Clinical workload in UK primary care: a retrospective analysis of 100 million consultations in England, 2007–14. Lancet. 2016;387(10035):2323–30.

26. Moffat K, Mercer SW. Challenges of managing people with multimorbidity in today's healthcare systems. BMC Fam Pract. 2015;16(1):129.

27. Bower P, Macdonald W, Harkness E, Gask L, Kendrick T, Valderas JM, Dickens C, Blakeman T, Sibbald B. Multimorbidity, service organization and clinical decision making in primary care: a qualitative study. Fam Pract. 2011;28(5):579–87.

28. Luijks HD, Loeffen MJ, Lagro-Janssen AL, Van Weel C, Lucassen PL, Schermer TR. GPs' considerations in multimorbidity management: a qualitative study. Br J Gen Pract. 2012;62(600):e503–10.

29. Sinnott C, Mc Hugh S, Browne J, Bradley C. GPs' perspectives on the management of patients with multimorbidity: systematic review and synthesis of qualitative research. BMJ Open. 2013;3(9):e003610.

30. Søndergaard E, Willadsen TG, Guassora AD, Vestergaard M, Tomasdottir MO, Borgquist L, Holmberg-Marttila D, Olivarius ND, Reventlow S. Problems and challenges in relation to the treatment of patients with multimorbidity: general practitioners' views and attitudes. Scand J Prim Health Care. 2015;33(2):121–6.

31. National Institute for Health and Care Excellence. Multimorbidity: clinical assessment and management (NICE clinical guideline 56). 2016. www.nice.org.uk/guidance/ng56.

32. Gallacher K, May CR, Montori VM, Mair FS. Understanding patients' experiences of treatment burden in chronic heart failure using normalization process theory. Ann Fam Med. 2011;9(3):235–43.

33. Sav A, King MA, Whitty JA, Kendall E, McMillan SS, Kelly F, Hunter B, Wheeler AJ. Burden of treatment for chronic illness: a concept analysis and review of the literature. Health Expect. 2015;18(3):312–24.

34. Ridgeway JL, Egginton JS, Tiedje K, Linzer M, Boehm D, Poplau S, de Oliveira DR, Odell L, Montori VM, Eton DT. Factors that lessen the burden of treatment in complex patients with chronic conditions: a qualitative study. Patient Prefer Adherence. 2014;8:339.

35. Mair FS, May CR. Thinking about the burden of treatment. Br Med J. 2014;349:g6680.

36. May CR, Eton DT, Boehmer K, Gallacher K, Hunt K, MacDonald S, Mair FS, May CM, Montori VM, Richardson A, Rogers AE. Rethinking the patient: using burden of treatment theory to understand the changing dynamics of illness. BMC Health Serv Res. 2014;14(1):281.

37. Tran VT, Barnes C, Montori VM, Falissard B, Ravaud P. Taxonomy of the burden of treatment: a multi-country web-based qualitative study of patients with chronic conditions. BMC Med. 2015;13(1):115.

38. Boehmer KR, Gionfriddo MR, Rodriguez-Gutierrez R, Dabrh AM, Leppin AL, Hargraves I, May CR, Shippee ND, Castaneda-Guarderas A, Palacios CZ, Bora P. Patient capacity and constraints in the experience of chronic disease: a qualitative systematic review and thematic synthesis. BMC Fam Pract. 2016;17(1):127.

39. Panagioti M, Stokes J, Esmail A, Coventry P, Cheraghi-Sohi S, Alam R, Bower P. Multimorbidity and patient safety incidents in primary care: a systematic review and meta-analysis. PLoS One. 2015;10(8):e0135947.

40. D Kamenski G, Flamm M, Böhmdorfer B, Sönnichsen A. Frequency of medication errors in primary care patients with polypharmacy. Fam Pract. 2012;30(3):313–9.

41. Calderón-Larrañaga A, Poblador-Plou B, González-Rubio F, Gimeno-Feliu LA, Abad-Díez JM, Prados-Torres A. Multimorbidity, polypharmacy, referrals, and adverse drug events: are we doing things well? Br J Gen Pract. 2012;62(605):e821–6.

42. Cooper A, Edwards A, Williams H, Evans HP, Avery A, Hibbert P, Makeham M, Sheikh A, J. Donaldson L, Carson-Stevens A. Sources of unsafe primary care for older adults: a mixed-methods analysis of patient safety incident reports. Age and ageing. 2017;46(5):833–9.

43. Swinglehurst D, Greenhalgh T, Russell J, Myall M. Receptionist input to quality and safety in repeat prescribing in UK general practice: ethnographic case study. BMJ. 2011;343:d6788.

44. Higginbottom G, Pillay JJ, Boadu NY. Guidance on performing focused ethnographies with an emphasis on healthcare research. The Qualitative Report. 2013;18(9):1–6.

45. Kuzel AJ, Woolf SH, Gilchrist VJ, Engel JD, LaVeist TA, Vincent C, Frankel RM. Patient reports of preventable problems and harms in primary health care. Ann Fam Med. 2004;2(4):333–40.

46. Burgess C, Cowie L, Gulliford M. Patients' perceptions of error in long-term illness care: qualitative study. J Health Serv Res Policy. 2012;17(3):181–7.

47. Buetow S, Kiata L, Liew T, Kenealy T, Dovey S, Elwyn G. Approaches to reducing the most important patient errors in primary health-care: patient and professional perspectives. Health Soc Care Community. 2010;18(3):296–303.

48. Baxter P, Jack S. Qualitative case study methodology: study design and implementation for novice researchers. Qual Rep. 2008;13(4):544–59.

49. Patton MQ. Qualitative research. Thousand Oaks: Wiley; 2005.

50. Statins: side effects. https://www.nhs.uk/conditions/statins/side-effects/. Accessed 3 Nov 17.

51. Morris RL, Sanders C, Kennedy AP, Rogers A. Shifting priorities in multimorbidity: a longitudinal qualitative study of patient's prioritization of multiple conditions. Chronic Illn. 2011;7(2):147–61.

52. Croxson CH, Ashdown HF, Hobbs FR. GPs' perceptions of workload in England: a qualitative interview study. Br J Gen Pract. 2017;67(655):e138–47.

53. Spear SJ, Schmidhofer M. Ambiguity and workarounds as contributors to medical error. Ann Intern Med. 2005;142(8):627–30.

54. Beasley JW, Wetterneck TB, Temte J, Lapin JA, Smith P, Rivera-Rodriguez AJ, Karsh BT. Information chaos in primary care: implications for physician performance and patient safety. J Am Board Fam Med. 2011;24(6):745–51.

55. Holden RJ, Scanlon MC, Patel NR, Kaushal R, Escoto KH, Brown RL, Alper SJ, Arnold JM, Shalaby TM, Murkowski K, Karsh BT. A human factors framework and study of the effect of nursing workload on patient safety and employee quality of working life. Qual Saf Health Care. 2011;20(1):15–24.

56. Adamson J, Ben-Shlomo Y, Chaturvedi N, Donovan J. Exploring the impact of patient views on 'appropriate' use of services and help seeking: a mixed method study. Br J Gen Pract. 2009;59(564):e226–33.

Safety work and risk management as burdens of treatment in primary care: insights from a focused...

235

57. Llanwarne N, Newbould J, Burt J, Campbell JL, Roland M. Wasting the doctor's time? A video-elicitation interview study with patients in primary care. Soc Sci Med. 2017;176:113–22.

58. Coyle J. Exploring the meaning of 'dissatisfaction'with health care: the importance of 'personal identity threat. Sociol Health Illn. 1999;21(1):95–123.

59. Shippee ND, Shah ND, May CR, Mair FS, Montori VM. Cumulative complexity: a functional, patient-centered model of patient complexity can improve research and practice. J Clin Epidemiol. 2012;65(10):1041–51.

60. Grembowski D, Schaefer J, Johnson KE, Fischer H, Moore SL, Tai-Seale M, Ricciardi R, Fraser JR, Miller D, LeRoy L. A conceptual model of the role of complexity in the care of patients with multiple chronic conditions. Med Care. 2014;52:S7–14.

61. Coventry PA, Fisher L, Kenning C, Bee P, Bower P. Capacity, responsibility, and motivation: a critical qualitative evaluation of patient and practitioner views about barriers to self-management in people with multimorbidity. BMC Health Serv Res. 2014;14(1):536.

62. Vassilev I, Rogers A, Blickem C, Brooks H, Kapadia D, Kennedy A, Sanders C, Kirk S, Reeves D. Social networks, the 'work'and work force of chronic illness self-management: a survey analysis of personal communities. PLoS One. 2013;8(4):e59723.

63. Rogers A, Kennedy A, Nelson E, Robinson A. Uncovering the limits of patient-centeredness: implementing a self-management trial for chronic illness. Qual Health Res. 2005;15(2):224–39.

64. Healey F, Scobie S, Oliver D, Pryce A, Thomson R, Glampson B. Falls in English and welsh hospitals: a national observational study based on retrospective analysis of 12 months of patient safety incident reports. Qual Saf Health Care. 2008;17(6):424.

Permissions

All chapters in this book were first published in FP, by BioMed Central; hereby published with permission under the Creative Commons Attribution License or equivalent. Every chapter published in this book has been scrutinized by our experts. Their significance has been extensively debated. The topics covered herein carry significant findings which will fuel the growth of the discipline. They may even be implemented as practical applications or may be referred to as a beginning point for another development.

The contributors of this book come from diverse backgrounds, making this book a truly international effort. This book will bring forth new frontiers with its revolutionizing research information and detailed analysis of the nascent developments around the world.

We would like to thank all the contributing authors for lending their expertise to make the book truly unique. They have played a crucial role in the development of this book. Without their invaluable contributions this book wouldn't have been possible. They have made vital efforts to compile up to date information on the varied aspects of this subject to make this book a valuable addition to the collection of many professionals and students.

This book was conceptualized with the vision of imparting up-to-date information and advanced data in this field. To ensure the same, a matchless editorial board was set up. Every individual on the board went through rigorous rounds of assessment to prove their worth. After which they invested a large part of their time researching and compiling the most relevant data for our readers.

The editorial board has been involved in producing this book since its inception. They have spent rigorous hours researching and exploring the diverse topics which have resulted in the successful publishing of this book. They have passed on their knowledge of decades through this book. To expedite this challenging task, the publisher supported the team at every step. A small team of assistant editors was also appointed to further simplify the editing procedure and attain best results for the readers.

Apart from the editorial board, the designing team has also invested a significant amount of their time in understanding the subject and creating the most relevant covers. They scrutinized every image to scout for the most suitable representation of the subject and create an appropriate cover for the book.

The publishing team has been an ardent support to the editorial, designing and production team. Their endless efforts to recruit the best for this project, has resulted in the accomplishment of this book. They are a veteran in the field of academics and their pool of knowledge is as vast as their experience in printing. Their expertise and guidance has proved useful at every step. Their uncompromising quality standards have made this book an exceptional effort. Their encouragement from time to time has been an inspiration for everyone.

The publisher and the editorial board hope that this book will prove to be a valuable piece of knowledge for researchers, students, practitioners and scholars across the globe.

List of Contributors

Tina Mallon, Annette Ernst and Martin Scherer
Department of Primary Medical Care, Center for Psychosocial Medicine, University Medical Center Hamburg-Eppendorf, Hamburg, Germany

Christian Brettschneider and Hans-Helmut König
Department of Health Economics and Health Services Research, Hamburg Center for Health Economics, University Medical Center Hamburg-Eppendorf, Hamburg, Germany

Tobias Luck, Susanne Röhr and Steffi Riedel-Heller
Institute of Social Medicine, Occupational Health and Public Health (ISAP), University of Leipzig, Leipzig, Germany

Siegfried Weyerer and Jochen Werle
Central Institute of Mental Health, Medical Faculty Mannheim, Heidelberg University, Mannheim, Germany

Edelgard Mösch and Dagmar Weeg
Department of Psychiatry, Klinikum rechts der Isar, Technical University of Munich, Munich, Germany

Angela Fuchs and Michael Pentzek
Institute of General Practice, Medical Faculty, Heinrich-Heine-University Düsseldorf, Düsseldorf, Germany

Luca Kleineidam and Kathrin Heser
Department of Psychiatry, University of Bonn, Bonn, Germany

Wolfgang Maier
Department of Psychiatry, University of Bonn, Bonn, Germany
DZNE, German Center for Neurodegenerative Diseases, Bonn, Germany

Birgitt Wiese
Work Group Medical Statistics and IT-Infrastructure, Institute for General Practice, Hannover Medical School, Hannover, Germany

Brenda F. Narice
Clinical Research Fellow in Obstetrics & Gynaecology; Academic Unit of Reproductive and Developmental Unit, University of Sheffield, Sheffield S10 2SF, UK

Brigitte Delaney and Jon M. Dickson
Academic Unit of Primary Medical Care, University of Sheffield, Sheffield S5 7AU, UK

Sabrina T. Wong
School of Nursing, University of British Columbia, T201 2211 Westbrook Mall, Vancouver, BC V6T 2B5, Canada
Centre for Health Services and Policy Research, University of British Columbia, 201-2206 East Mall, Vancouver, BC V6T 1Z3, Canada

William Hogg and Sharon Johnston
Department of Family Medicine, University of Ottawa, 201-600 Peter Morand Cresc, Ottawa, ON K1G 5Z3, Canada
Montfort Hospital Research Institute 713 Montreal Rd, Ottawa, ON K1K 0T2, Canada

Ilisha French
Montfort Hospital Research Institute 713 Montreal Rd, Ottawa, ON K1K 0T2, Canada

Fred Burge and Stephanie Blackman
Department of Family Medicine, Dalhousie University, 5909 Veterans' Memorial Lane, Abbie J. Lane Building, Halifax, NS B3H 2E2, Canada

Stephanie D. Short
Faculty of Health Sciences, Discipline of Behavioral and Social Sciences in Health, The University of Sydney, Science Road, Sydney, NSW 2006, Australia

Muna Habib AL. Lawati
Faculty of Health Sciences, Discipline of Behavioral and Social Sciences in Health, The University of Sydney, Science Road, Sydney, NSW 2006, Australia
Department of Quality Assurance and Patient Safety, Ministry of Health, P.O.Box, 626, Wadi Al Kabir, 117 Muscat, PC, Oman

Sarah Dennis
Ingham Institute for Applied Medical Research, Campbell Street, Liverpool, NSW 2170, Australia Faculty of Health Sciences, Discipline of Physiotherapy, The University of Sydney, 71 East Street, Lidcombe, NSW 2141, Australia

Nadia Noor Abdulhadi
Directorate General of Planning and Studies, Ministry of Health, Muscat, Oman

Karen Busk Nørøxe, Flemming Bro and Peter Vedsted
Research Unit for General Practice, Department of Public Health, Aarhus University, Bartholins Allé 2, 8000 Aarhus C, Denmark

Anette Fischer Pedersen
Research Unit for General Practice & Department of Clinical Medicine, Aarhus University, Aarhus, Denmark

Ariëtte R. J. Sanders and Niek J. de Wit
Julius Centre for Health Sciences and Primary Care, University Medical Centre Utrecht, PO Box 85500 3508, GA, Utrecht, the Netherlands

Tessa Magnée and Peter Verhaak
NIVEL (Netherlands Institute for Health Services Research), PO Box 1568 3500, BN, Utrecht, the Netherlands

Jozien M. Bensing
NIVEL (Netherlands Institute for Health Services Research), PO Box 1568 3500, BN, Utrecht, the Netherlands Faculty of Social and Behavioural Science, Utrecht University, Utrecht, the Netherlands

Elizabeth Halcomb, Elizabeth Smyth and Susan McInnes
School of Nursing, University of Wollongong, Northfields Ave, Wollongong, NSW 2522, Australia

Renaldo Christoffels and Bob Mash
Division of Family Medicine and Primary Care, Stellenbosch University, Box 241, Cape Town 8000, South Africa

Christine M. Everett and Perri Morgan
Duke University School of Medicine, Physician Assistant Program|, 800 South Duke Street, Durham, NC 27701, USA

Valerie A. Smith and George L. Jackson
Center for Health Services Research in Primary Care, Durham Veterans Affairs Medical Center, Durham, NC, USA Department of Population Health Sciences, Duke University School of Medicine, Durham, NC, USA Division of General Internal Medicine, Duke University School of Medicine, Durham, NC, USA

Sandra Woolson, Theodore Berkowitz and Brandolyn White
Center for Health Services Research in Primary Care, Durham Veterans Affairs Medical Center, Durham, NC, USA

David Edelman
Center for Health Services Research in Primary Care, Durham Veterans Affairs Medical Center, Durham, NC, USA Division of General Internal Medicine, Duke University School of Medicine, Durham, NC, USA

Cristina C. Hendrix
Center for Health Services Research in Primary Care, Durham Veterans Affairs Medical Center, Durham, NC, USA Clinical Health Systems & Analytics Division, Duke University School of Nursing, Durham, NC, USA

Henny Sinnema and Daniëlle Volker
Netherlands Institute of Mental Health and Addiction, Trimbos Institute, Postbox 725, 3500, AS, Utrecht, The Netherlands

Berend Terluin
Department of General Practice and Elderly Care Medicine, Amsterdam Public Health Research Institute, VU University Medical Centre, Van der Boechorststraat 7, 1081, BT, Amsterdam, The Netherlands

Michel Wensing
Universitatsklinikum Heidelberg, Im Neuenheimer Feld 130.3, 69120 Heidelberg, Germany

Anton van Balkom
Department of Psychiatry, VU University Medical Centre and GGZinGeest, AJ Ernststraat 887, 1081, HL, Amsterdam, The Netherlands

Johannes Maximilian Just, Linda Bingener, Markus Bleckwenn and Klaus Weckbecker
Institute of General Practice and Family Medicine, Bonn University Clinic, Sigmund-Freud-Street 25, 53127 Bonn, Germany

Rieke Schnakenberg
Institute of General Practice and Family Medicine, Bonn University Clinic, Sigmund-Freud-Street 25, 53127 Bonn, Germany
Department for Health Services Research, Carl von Ossietzky Universität Oldenburg, Post office box 2503, 26111 Oldenburg, Germany

Matthew Cefalu
RAND Corporation, 1776 Main Street, Santa Monica, CA 90407-2138, USA

Lisa S. Meredith
RAND Corporation, 1776 Main Street, Santa Monica, CA 90407-2138, USA
VA HSR&D Center for the Study of Healthcare Innovation, Implementation, and Policy, Los Angeles, CA, USA

Benjamin Batorsky
TriveHive, Boston, MA, USA

Jill E. Darling
USC Center for Economic and Social Research, Los Angeles, CA, USA

Susan E. Stockdale
VA HSR&D Center for the Study of Healthcare Innovation, Implementation, and Policy, Los Angeles, CA, USA
Department of Psychiatry and Biobehavioral Medicine, UCLA School of Medicine, Los Angeles, CA, USA

Elizabeth M. Yano
VA HSR&D Center for the Study of Healthcare Innovation, Implementation, and Policy, Los Angeles, CA, USA
Department of Health Policy and Management, UCLA Fielding School of Public Health, Los Angeles, CA, USA

Lisa V. Rubenstein
VA HSR&D Center for the Study of Healthcare Innovation, Implementation, and Policy, Los Angeles, CA, USA
UCLA Schools of Medicine and Public Health, Los Angeles, CA, USA

Traci D. Yates, Marion E. Davis, Yhenneko J. Taylor, Crystal D. Connor, Katherine Buehler and Melanie D. Spencer
Center for Outcomes Research and Evaluation, Atrium Health, Charlotte, NC, USA

Lisa Davidson
Division of Infectious Disease, Atrium Health, Charlotte, NC, USA

R. Leutgeb, J. Frankenhauser-Mannuß and J. Szecsenyi
Department of General Practice and Health Services Research, University Hospital Heidelberg, Marsilius-Arcades, Western Tower, Im Neuenheimer Feld 130.3, 69120 Heidelberg, Germany

Katja Goetz
Department of General Practice and Health Services Research, University Hospital Heidelberg, Marsilius-Arcades, Western Tower, Im Neuenheimer Feld 130.3, 69120 Heidelberg, Germany
Institute of Family Medicine, University Hospital Schleswig-Holstein, Campus Luebeck, Ratzeburger Alle 160, 23538 Luebeck, Germany

M. Scheuer
Headquarter of Control Centre, District Bergstraße, Gräffstrasse 5, 64646 Heppenheim, Germany

Elisabeth Søndergaard, Ruth K. Ertmann, Susanne Reventlow and Kirsten Lykke
Department of Public Health, University of Copenhagen, Copenhagen, Denmark

Maaike C. M. Ronda, Rimke C. Vos and Guy E. H. M. Rutten
Julius Centre for Health Sciences and Primary Care, University Medical Centre Utrecht, STR 6.131, PO Box 85500, 3508 Utrecht, GA, Netherlands

Lioe-Ting Dijkhorst-Oei
Department of Internal Medicine, Meander Medical Centre, Maatweg 3, 3813 Amersfoort, TZ, Netherlands

Olivia Braillard, Anbreen Slama-Chaudhry and Catherine Joly
Department of Community Medicine, Primary and Emergency Care, Geneva University Hospitals, 1205 Geneva, Switzerland

Nicolas Perone
Department of Community Health and Care, Geneva
University Hospitals, 1205 Geneva, Switzerland

David Beran
Division of Tropical and Humanitarian Medicine,
Geneva University Hospitals and University of
Geneva, 1205 Geneva, Switzerland

**Isabel Gordon, Jonathan Ling, Catherine Hayes
and Ann Crosland**
Faculty of Health Sciences and Wellbeing,
University of Sunderland, City Campus Chester
Road, Sunderland SR1 3SD, UK

Louise Robinson
Newcastle University Institute for Ageing and
Institute for Health & Society, Newcastle University,
Newcastle upon Tyne NE4 5PL, England

Anne K. Santalahti
Turku City Healthcare Center, Turku, Finland

Tero J. Vahlberg
Department of Biostatistics, Faculty of Medicine,
University of Turku, Turku, Finland

Sinikka H. Luutonen
Department of Psychiatry, University of Turku,
Turku, Finland
Department of Psychiatry, Turku University
Hospital, Turku, Finland

Päivi T. Rautava
Department of Public Health, Faculty of Medicine,
University of Turku, Turku, Finland
Turku Clinical Research Centre, Turku University
Hospital, Turku, Finland

Mariko Higuchi
The Department of Internal Medicine, Tsukuba
Central Hospital, 1589-3 Kashiwadachou, Ushiku,
Ibaraki 300-1211, Japan

Keiichiro Narumoto
The Department of Obstetrics and Gynecology,
Kikugawa Municipal General Hospital, 1632
Higashiyokoji, Kikugawa, Shizuoka 439-0022, Japan
Shizuoka Family Medicine Residency Program,
1632 Higashiyokoji, Kikugawa, Shizuoka 439-0022,
Japan

Machiko Inoue
Shizuoka Family Medicine Residency Program,
1632 Higashiyokoji, Kikugawa, Shizuoka 439-0022,
Japan
The Department of Family and Community
Medicine, Hamamatsu University School of
Medicine, 1-20-1 Handayama, Higashi-ku,
Hamamatsu, Shizuoka 431-3192, Japan

Takahiro Goto
Yu Pharmacy, 15-1 Otsudori, Shimada, Shizuoka
427-0056, Japan

**Kasey R Boehmer, Emma Behnken and Victor M
Montori**
Knowledge and Evaluation Research (KER) Unit,
Mayo Clinic, 200 First Street SW, Rochester, MN
55901, USA

Megan Branda
Knowledge and Evaluation Research (KER) Unit,
Mayo Clinic, 200 First Street SW, Rochester, MN
55901, USA
Health Sciences Research, Mayo Clinic, Rochester,
MN, USA

Maria Kyriacou
Phoebe Family Medicine Residency, Albany, GA,
USA

**Daniel Passerman, Denise White-Perkins, Della
A. Rees, Lois Lamerato and Susan Schooley**
Department of Family Medicine, Henry Ford
Hospital, Detroit, MI, USA

Katarzyna Budzynska
Department of Family Medicine, Henry Ford
Hospital, Detroit, MI, USA
Department of Family Medicine, Henry Ford Health
System, 3370 E Jefferson, Detroit, MI 48207, USA

Jinping Xu
Department of Family Medicine and Public Health
Sciences, Wayne State University, Detroit, MI, USA

**D. Eggermont, M. A. M. Smit, G. A. Kwestroo and
A. E. Kunst**
Department of Public Health, Amsterdam UMC,
University of Amsterdam, Meibergdreef 9,
Amsterdam 1105, AZ, the Netherlands

R. A. Verheij and K. Hek
Netherlands Institute for Health Services Research (Nivel), Otterstraat 118-124, Utrecht 3513, CR, the Netherlands

Gavin Daker-White
NIHR Greater Manchester Patient Safety Translational Research Centre (Greater Manchester PSTRC), Division of Population Health, Health Services Research and Primary Care, School of Health Sciences, Faculty of Biology, Medicine and Health, University of Manchester, Manchester Academic Health Science Centre, Manchester, UK

Thomas Blakeman
NIHR Collaboration in Applied Health Research and Care Greater Manchester, Division of Population Health, Health Services Research and Primary Care, School of Health Sciences, Faculty of Biology, Medicine and Health, University of Manchester, Manchester Academic Health Science Centre, Manchester, UK

Sarah Croke
Division of Nursing Midwifery and Social Work, School of Health Sciences, Faculty of Biology, Medicine and Health, University of Manchester, Manchester Academic Health Science Centre, Manchester, UK

Benjamin Brown
Centre for Health Informatics, School of Health Sciences, Faculty of Biology, Medicine and Health, University of Manchester, Manchester Academic Health Science Centre, Manchester, UK

Rebecca Hays, Aneez Esmail and Peter Bower
NIHR School for Primary Care Research, Division of Population Health, Health Services Research and Primary Care, School of Health Sciences, Faculty of Biology, Medicine and Health, University of Manchester, Manchester Academic Health Science Centre, Manchester, UK

Index